neofax®

Sixteenth Edition
2003

by

Thomas E. Young, MD
Clinical Professor
Department of Pediatrics
School of Medicine
University of North Carolina
Chapel Hill, NC

◆

Senior Neonatologist
WakeMed Faculty Physicians
Raleigh, NC

and

Barry Mangum, PharmD
President
Neofax, LLC

Notice

Every effort has been made to ensure that the information herein, particularly that regarding dosage schedules, is accurate and in accord with good medical practice at the time of publication. However, because of ongoing research, changes in government regulations, experience, and the constant flow of information relating to drug therapy and drug reactions, changes in treatment and drug therapy occur.

It is the responsibility of every practitioner to evaluate the appropriateness of a particular opinion in the context of actual clinical situations and with due consideration to new developments and Food and Drug Administration regulations. The authors and publisher cannot be held responsible for any typographic or other errors found in this book.

Please address all comments and suggestions to:

Thomas Young, MD   or   Barry Mangum, PharmD
tyoung@neofax.com   bmangum@neofax.com

Additional copies may be purchased via our website:

www.neofax.com

**Acorn Publishing, Inc.
P.O. Box 17389
Raleigh, NC 27619**

Telephone: (919) 786-1155
Fax: (919) 786-1151

Quotation

Quotation from this edition is permitted if the source is acknowledged. The preferred form is: Young TE, Mangum B: *NeoFax® : A Manual of Drugs Used in Neonatal Care*, ed 16. Raleigh, North Carolina: Acorn Publishing, USA, 2003, p.00.

© Copyright 2003, Acorn Publishing, Inc.

Thomas E. Young and Barry Mangum

Design and layout by Michael P. Sampair, Bleu Aura, Raleigh NC.

ISBN: 1-888703-16-4

Preface

NeoFax continues to grow as we add new outlets for the information. Despite the popularity of handheld computers and other electronic devices, we believe that the book will continue to have a place in NICUs and pharmacies. Sincere thanks to all our colleagues who encourage us to continue this annual journey. We have again made changes based upon feedback from users, and we continue to welcome your comments and suggestions regarding both future content and media formats. And, as always, we couldn't do this every year without the patient support of our wives and children.

Additions to this 16th edition:
- Flecainide
- Lansoprazole
- Piperacillin / tazobactam
- Sucrose

Deletions from previous editions:
- Methicillin
- Mezlocillin
- Tolazoline

Significant updates in this edition:
- Linezolid: new dosing interval with references
- Zidovudine: new dosage with reference
- IVIG: new use (hemolytic jaundice) with references
- Acetaminophen: new dosage with references
- Albuterol: new use (hyperkalemia) with reference
- Aminophylline: new loading dose with reference
- Glucagon: new dose (continuous infusion) with reference
- Enoxaparin, heparin, phentolamine, and protamine were moved from Miscellaneous to the Cardiovascular section

We have continued to use the term "Dex/AA" instead of "TPN" to designate parenteral nutrition solutions that are similar to those routinely used in neonates. Fat emulsions are dealt with separately.

Compatibility information has been updated as usual, based primarily on Trissel's *Handbook of Injectable Drugs,* ed 12, 2003, published by the American Society of Health-System Pharmacists. Drug omissions usually indicate that no information is available in the published literature. The major source of product availability information is the 2003 edition of *Drug Facts and Comparisons,* published by Facts and Comparisons, a Wolters Kluwer Company.

An explanatory note about antibiotic dosing charts:

The antibiotic dosing charts reflect the fact that renal function and drug elimination are most strongly correlated with Postmenstrual Age ("PMA", equivalent to Gestational Age plus Postnatal Age). Postmenstrual Age is therefore used as the primary determinant of dosing interval, with Postnatal Age as the secondary qualifier.

Example: A baby born at 28 weeks gestation is now 21 days old. To determine the dosing interval for cefotaxime, first go to the row on the chart containing his Postmenstrual Age of 31 weeks (30 to 36), and then his Postnatal Age of 21 days (>14) to yield a dosing interval of 8 hours.

Contents

Contents

Contents

Abbreviations

The abbreviations listed below are used in the text.

a/A	arterial-alveolar (gradient)
a/ApO$_2$	arterial-alveolar oxygen tension ratio
ABGs	arterial blood gases
ACTH	adrenocorticotropic hormone
ALT	alanine aminotransferase
AMP	adenosine monophosphate
ANC	absolute neutrophil count
APTT	activated partial thromboplastin time
AST	aspartate aminotransferase
ATP	adenosine triphosphate
ATPase	adenosine triphosphatase
A-V	atrioventricular
BUN	blood urea nitrogen
BPD	bronchopulmonary dysplasia
CBC	complete blood count
CSF	cerebrospinal fluid
CHF	congestive heart failure
CNS	central nervous system
CVP	central venous pressure
DIC	disseminated intravascular coagulation
DNA	deoxyribonucleic acid
D$_5$NS	5% dextrose in normal saline solution
DPPC	dipalmitoyl phosphatidylcholine
D$_5$W	5% dextrose in water solution
D$_{10}$W	10% dextrose in water solution
D$_{15}$W	15% dextrose in water solution
D$_{20}$W	20% dextrose in water solution
DT	diphtheria, tetanus [vaccine]
DTP	diphtheria, tetanus, pertussis [vaccine]
EEG	electroencephalogram
EKG	electrocardiogram
ET	endotracheal
FiO$_2$	fractional inspired oxygen concentration
FRC	functional residual capacity
GABA	gamma-aminobutyric acid
GCSF	granulocyte colony stimulating factor
GE	gastroesophageal
GFR	glomerular filtration rate
GI	gastrointestinal
HBeAg	hepatitis B e antigen
HBIG	hepatitis B immune globulin
HBsAg	hepatitis B surface antigen
Hib	*Haemophilus influenzae* b
HIV	human immunodeficiency virus

continued...

neofax 2003

Abbreviations

IC	intracardiac
IgG	immunoglobulin G
IM	intramuscular
IPV	inactivated polio vaccine (Salk)
IV	intravenous
IVH	intraventricular hemorrhage
IVIG	intravenous immune globulin (human)
Lf	potency of a given weight of an internationally accepted standard preparation of antiserum or antigen
LR	lactated Ringer's solution
NEC	necrotizing enterocolitis
NS	normal saline solution (0.9% sodium chloride)
OPV	oral polio vaccine
PMA	postmenstrual age
PCO_2	partial pressure of carbon dioxide in the blood
PDA	patent ductus arteriosus
PO	by mouth (*per os*)
PO_2	partial pressure of oxygen in the blood
PR	by rectum
PVC	premature ventricular contraction
Q	every (*quaque*)
RDIs	Reference Daily Intakes (replaces US RDAs)
RDS	respiratory distress syndrome
RNA	ribonucleic acid
ROP	retinopathy of prematurity
S-A	sinoatrial node, "pacemaker" of the heart
SC	subcutaneously
SGA	small for gestational age
SVT	supraventricular tachycardia
^{99}Tc-IDA	technetium 99m-image display and analysis
TPN	total parenteral nutrition
TSH	thyroid-stimulating hormone
UAC	umbilical artery catheter
US RDAs	US Recommended Daily Allowances
VLBW	very-low-birth-weight

ANTIBIOTICS

Acyclovir

Dose & Administration

20 mg/kg per dose Q8 hours IV infusion by syringe pump over 1 hour. Increase dosing interval in premature infants <34 weeks PMA, or in patients with significant renal impairment or hepatic failure. Treat localized herpes simplex infections for 14 days, disseminated or CNS infections for 21 days.

Chronic suppression: 75 mg/kg per dose PO Q12 hours.

Uses

Treatment of neonatal herpes simplex infections, varicella zoster infections with CNS and pulmonary involvement, and herpes simplex encephalitis.

Monitoring

Periodic CBC. Serum concentrations two hours after a dose should be approximately 2 mcg/mL. Follow renal and hepatic function. Monitor IV site for phlebitis—if noted, make infusion solution more dilute.

Adverse Effects/Precautions

Neutropenia occurs in approximately 20% of patients - decrease dose or treat with GCSF if ANC remains less than 500/mm^3. Phlebitis may occur at IV site due to alkaline pH of 10. Risk of transient renal dysfunction and crystalluria is minimized by slow infusion rates and adequate patient hydration. Resistant viral strains may emerge during long-term therapy; these patients are at high risk for progressive life-threatening disease.

Pharmacology

Antiviral drug that is preferentially taken up by infected cells; inhibits viral DNA synthesis. Oral absorption is 15 to 30%. Most of administered dose is excreted unchanged in urine, primarily via glomerular filtration. Protein binding and metabolism are minimal. Serum half-life is 3 to 4 hours in patients with normal renal and hepatic function.

Special Considerations/Preparation

Available in 500-mg and 1-g vials. Prepared by dissolving contents of 500-mg vial in 10 mL sterile water for injection. Reconstituted solution is stable at room temperature for 12 hours. **Do not refrigerate.**

Infusion solution concentration should be not greater than 7 mg/mL.

A 5-mg/mL dilution may be made by adding 1 mL of 50 mg/mL concentration to 9 mL of preservative-free normal saline. Dilution is stable for 24 hours at room temperature.

Oral suspension available in 200 mg/5 mL concentration. Store at room temperature.

continued...

Solution Compatibility: D_5W, $D_{10}W$, and NS.

Solution Incompatibility: Dex/AA.

Terminal Injection Site Compatibility: Amikacin, ampicillin, cefazolin, cefotaxime, cefoxitin, ceftazidime, ceftriaxone, chloramphenicol, cimetidine, clindamycin, dexamethasone, erythromycin lactobionate, famotidine, fluconazole, gentamicin, heparin, hydrocortisone succinate, imipenem/cilastatin, linezolid, lorazepam, meropenem, metoclopramide, metronidazole, morphine, nafcillin, oxacillin, penicillin G, pentobarbital, piperacillin, potassium chloride, propofol, ranitidine, remifentanil, sodium bicarbonate, theophylline, ticarcillin/clavulanate, tobramycin, trimethoprim-sulfamethoxazole, vancomycin, and zidovudine.

Incompatibility: Fat emulsion. Aztreonam, cefepime, dobutamine, dopamine, and piperacillin-tazobactam.

Selected References

♦ Kimberlin DW, Lin C-Y, Jacobs RF, et al: Safety and efficacy of high-dose intravenous acyclovir in the management of neonatal herpes simplex infections. *Pediatrics* 2001;108:230-238.

♦ American Academy of Pediatrics. Herpes simplex. In: Pickering LK, ed. *2000 Red Book: Report of the Committee on Infectious Diseases.* 25th ed. Elk Grove Village, IL: American Academy of Pediatrics; 2000: p 313.

♦ Rudd C, Rivadeneira ED, Gutman LT: Dosing considerations for oral acyclovir following neonatal herpes disease. *Acta Paediatr* 1994;83:1237-43.

♦ Whitley R, Arvin A, Prober C, et al: A controlled trial comparing vidarabine with acyclovir in neonatal herpes simplex virus infection. *N Engl J Med* 1991;324:444.

♦ Englund JA, Zimmerman BS, Swierkosz EM, et al: Herpes simplex virus resistant to acyclovir: A study in a tertiary care center. *Ann Intern Med* 1990;112:416.

♦ McDonald L, Tartaglione TA, Mendelman PM, et al: Lack of toxicity in two cases of neonatal acyclovir overdose. *Pediatr Infect Dis J* 1989;8:529.

♦ Sullender WM, Arvin AM, Diaz PS, et al: Pharmacokinetics of acyclovir suspension in infants and children. *Antimicrob Agents Chemother* 1987;31:1722.

♦ Hintz M, Connor JD, Spector SA, et al: Neonatal acyclovir pharmacokinetics in patients with herpes virus infections. *Am J Med* 1982;73(suppl):210.

Text and References updated 3/2002
Compatibilities updated 3/2003

Amikacin

Dose and Administration

During the first week of life:

Gestation (weeks)	Dose (mg/kg/dose)	Interval (hours)
≤27*	18	48
28 to 30	18	36
31 to 33	16	36
≥34	15	24
* or significant asphyxia, PDA, or treatment with indomethacin		

IV infusion by syringe pump over 30 minutes. Administer as a separate infusion from penicillin-containing compounds. IM injection is associated with variable absorption, especially in the very small infant.

First week of life: Serum drug concentrations are usually not necessary except in patients with serious infections or significantly changing fluid or renal status. It is not necessary to wait for 'steady state': Peak levels may be measured after the first dose, and trough levels may be measured before the second dose.

After the first week: Administer an initial dose of 4 mg/kg, then measure a peak serum concentration 30 minutes after end of infusion, and another 12 to 24 hours later to determine dosing interval.

Example: Baby X is born at 28 weeks gestation. At 3 weeks of age, amikacin therapy is begun. A 15 mg/kg dose is administered, with a peak serum concentration of 27 mcg/mL. 24 hours later, the measured serum concentration is 6.7 mcg/mL, yielding a calculated half-life of 12 hours. The predicted serum concentration at 36 hours postdose is 3.4 mcg/mL, and therefore the suggested dosing interval is 36 hours.

Uses

Restricted to treatment of infections caused by gram-negative bacilli that are resistant to other aminoglycosides. Usually used in combination with a β-lactam antibiotic.

Monitoring

Therapeutic serum concentrations:
Peak: 20 to 30 mcg/mL (or C_{max}/MIC ratio greater than 8:1)
(Draw 30 minutes after end of infusion, 1 hour after IM injection.)
Trough: 2 to 5 mcg/mL
Blood samples obtained to monitor drug levels should be spun and refrigerated or frozen as soon as possible. Assess renal function.

Adverse Effects/Precautions

Transient and reversible renal tubular dysfunction may occur, resulting in increased urinary losses of sodium, calcium, and magnesium. Potential vestibular and auditory ototoxicity, especially if treating with other nephrotoxic and/or ototoxic medications (e.g. furosemide, vancomycin). Neuromuscular weakness and respiratory failure may be potentiated when treating concomitantly with pancuronium or other neuromuscular blocking agents, and in patients with hypermagnesemia.

continued...

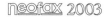

Pharmacology

New dosing recommendations are based on concepts promoted in studies of "once-a-day" dosing in adults: (1) Higher peak concentrations are desirable to increase concentration-dependent bacterial killing; (2) There is a post-antibiotic effect on bacterial killing, especially when treating concurrently with a β-lactam antibiotic; (3) There may be less toxicity with less frequent dosing, due to less renal drug accumulation. Volume of distribution is increased and clearance is decreased in patients with PDA. Serum half-life is also prolonged in premature and asphyxiated newborns. Inactivation of amikacin by penicillin-containing compounds appears to be a time-, temperature-, and concentration-dependent process. This is probably clinically significant only when penicillin-containing compounds are mixed in IV solutions or when blood is allowed to set at room temperature for several hours before serum drug concentration is assayed.

Special Considerations/Preparation

Available in concentrations of 50 and 250 mg/mL. For IV use, dilute with a compatible solution to a concentration of 5 mg/mL.

Solution compatibility: D_5W, $D_{10}W$, $D_{20}W$, and NS.

Terminal Injection Site Compatibility: Dex/AA. Acyclovir, aminophylline, amiodarone, aztreonam, calcium chloride, calcium gluconate, cefazolin, cefepime, cefotaxime, cefoxitin, chloramphenicol, cimetidine, clindamycin, dexamethasone, enalaprilat, epinephrine, esmolol, fluconazole, furosemide, heparin (concentrations ≤1 U/mL), hydrocortisone succinate, hyaluronidase, linezolid, lorazepam, metronidazole, midazolam, morphine, pentobarbital, phenobarbital, potassium chloride, ranitidine, remifentanil, sodium bicarbonate, vancomycin, vitamin K_1, and zidovudine.

Incompatibility: Fat emulsion. Amphotericin B, ampicillin, carbenicillin, heparin (concentrations >1 U/mL), imipenem/cilastatin, methicillin, mezlocillin, nafcillin, oxacillin, penicillin G, phenytoin, propofol, thiopental, and ticarcillin/clavulanate.

Selected References

♦ Kotze A, Bartel PR, Sommers DeK: Once versus twice daily amikacin in neonates: Prospective study on toxicity. *J Paediatr Child Health* 1999;35:283-286.

♦ Langhendries JP, Battisti O, Bertrand JM, et al: Adaptation in neonatology of the once-daily concept of aminoglycoside administration: Evaluation of a dosing chart for amikacin in an intensive care unit. *Biol Neonate* 1998;74:351-362.

♦ Langhendries JP, Battisti O, Bertrand JM, et al: Once-a-day administration of amikacin in neonates: Assessment of nephrotoxicity and ototoxicity. *Dev Pharmacol Ther* 1993;20:220-230.

♦ Hayani KC, Hatzopoulos FK, Frank AL, et al: Pharmacokinetics of once-daily dosing of gentamicin in neonates. *J Pediatr* 1997;131:76-80.

♦ de Hoog M, Schoemaker RC, Mouton JW, van den Anker JN: Tobramycin population pharmacokinetics in neonates. *Clin Pharmacol Ther* 1997;62:392-399.

♦ Giapros VI, Andronikou S, Cholevas VI, Papadopoulou ZL: Renal function in premature infants during aminoglycoside therapy. *Pediatr Nephrol* 1995;9:163.

♦ Daly JS, Dodge RA, Glew RH, et al: Effect of time and temperature on inactivation of aminoglycosides by ampicillin at neonatal dosages. *J Perinatol* 1997;17:42.

♦ Williams BS, Ransom JL, Gal P, et al: Gentamicin pharmacokinetics in neonates with patent ductus arteriosus. *Crit Care Med* 1997;25:273-275.

Text updated 3/2000, Compatibilities updated 3/2002

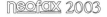

Amphotericin B

Dose & Administration

Initial dose: 0.25 to 0.5 mg/kg IV infusion over 2 to 6 hours.
Maintenance dose: 0.5 to 1 mg/kg IV Q24 to 48 hours.
Dosage modification for renal dysfunction is only necessary if serum creatinine increases >0.4 mg/dL during therapy - hold dose for 2 to 5 days.

Uses

Treatment of systemic fungal infections and severe superficial mycoses.

Monitoring

Monitor CBC, electrolytes, urine output, BUN, and serum creatinine at least every other day. Observe IV site for irritation—phlebitis is common. Serum amphotericin concentrations are not routinely followed.

Adverse Effects/Precautions

Decreases renal blood flow and GFR by 20% to 60%. Injures tubular epithelium with resultant urinary loss of potassium and magnesium, decreased reabsorption of sodium, and renal tubular acidosis. Anemia, thrombocytopenia, hypokalemia, nausea/vomiting, and fever/chills. Consider analgesia before beginning infusion. Cardiac arrest has occurred in patients who received 10 times the recommended dose.

Pharmacology

Amphotericin B binds to ergosterol in the membrane of sensitive fungi and may be fungicidal or fungistatic. The therapeutic concentration range is not well-defined. Highly protein-bound (greater than 90%). Elimination half-life is approximately 15 days. Drug may accumulate in tissues to a significant concentration and be excreted renally for months.

Special Considerations/Preparation

Available as powder for injection in 50-mg vials. Reconstitute using D_5W to a concentration of 5 mg/mL (256 mOsm/kg). Dilute to a concentration no greater than 0.1 mg/mL for infusion. For a 0.1 mg/mL dilution, add 0.2 mL of reconstituted solution to 9.8 mL of D_5W. **Do not mix with saline solution**—the antibiotic will precipitate. **Do not filter this medication when mixed for injection**—the antibiotic will be filtered out. **Protect from light.**

Solution Compatibility: D_5W, $D_{10}W$, $D_{15}W$, and $D_{20}W$.

Solution Incompatibility: Dex/AA and NS.

Terminal Injection Site Compatibility: Heparin, hydrocortisone, sodium bicarbonate, and zidovudine.

Incompatibility: Fat emulsion. Amikacin, aztreonam, calcium chloride, calcium gluconate, cefepime, cimetidine, dopamine, enalaprilat, fluconazole, gentamicin, potassium chloride, linezolid, meropenem, netilmicin, penicillin G, piperacillin-tazobactam, propofol, ranitidine, remifentanil, and tobramycin.

Selected References

♦ Lyman CA, Walsh TJ: Systemically administered antifungal agents: A review of their clinical pharmacology and therapeutic applications. *Drugs* 1992;44:9.

♦ Baley JE, Meyers C, Kliegman RM, et al: Pharmacokinetics, outcome of treatment, and toxic effects of amphotericin B and 5-fluorocytosine in neonates. *J Pediatr* 1990;116:791.

♦ Starke JR, Mason EL, Kramer WG, Kaplan SL: Pharmacokinetics of amphotericin B in infants and children. *J Infect Dis* 1987;155:766.

Compatibilities updated 3/2003

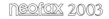

Amphotericin B Lipid Complex

Dose and Administration

1 to 5 mg/kg per dose Q24 hours IV infusion by syringe pump over 2 hours. Begin at 1 mg/kg per dose. Increase daily in 1 mg/kg increments.

Use the higher doses when treating meningitis, osteoarthritis, cryptococcal infections, and Aspergillosis.

Uses

Treatment of systemic fungal infections resistant to conventional amphotericin B therapy or in patients with renal or hepatic dysfunction.

Monitoring

Serum amphotericin B concentrations are not routinely followed. Monitor urine output. Periodic CBC for thrombocytopenia, electrolytes for hypokalemia, BUN, serum creatinine, and hepatic transaminases.

Adverse Effects/Precautions

Anemia, thrombocytopenia, hypokalemia, nausea/vomiting, and fever/chills.

Pharmacology

ABELCET® consists of amphotericin B complexed with two phospholipids in a 1:1 drug-to-lipid ratio. Acts by binding to the sterol component of a cell membrane leading to alterations in the cell wall permeability and death. Penetrates the cell wall of susceptible fungi. Concentrates in the liver and spleen. Less nephrotoxic than conventional amphotericin B. Mean serum half-life in adults 24 to 38 hours. The pharmacokinetics of amphotericin B lipid complex is nonlinear.

Special Considerations/Preparation

Available as a ready-to-use admixture containing 50- and 100-mg ABELCET® in 10- and 20-mL suspension (5 mg/mL) respectively. Shake the vial gently until there is no evidence of any yellow sediment on the bottom. Withdraw the appropriate dose into a syringe using an 18 gauge needle. Remove the needle and replace with the supplied 5 micron filter needle. Inject the drug into a different syringe containing a measured amount of D_5W so that the final infusion concentration is 1 to 2 mg/mL. Shake until thoroughly mixed. Check for complete dispersion. The diluted admixture is stable for 48 hours refrigerated and an additional 6 hours at room temperature.

Do not freeze. Protect from light.

Do not mix ABELCET® with saline solutions.

Solution compatibility: D_5W.

Solution incompatibility: Dex/AA and NS.

Terminal injection site compatibility: No available data.

Selected References

♦ Adler-Shohet F, Waskin H, Lieberman J M: Amphotericin B lipid complex for neonatal invasive candidiasis . *Arch Dis Child Fetal Neonatal Ed* 2001;84:F131-F133.

♦ Walsh TJ, Seibel NL, Arndt C, et al: Amphotericin B lipid complex in pediatric patients with invasive fungal infections. *Pediatr Infect Dis J* 1999;18:702-708.

♦ Wong-Beringer A, Jacobs RA, Guglielmo BJ: Lipid formulations of amphotericin B: Clinical efficacy and toxicities. *Clin Infect Dis* 1998;27:603-618.

Added 3/2000

Dose and Administration

1 to 5 mg/kg per dose Q24 hours IV infusion by syringe pump over 2 hours. Begin at 1 mg/kg per dose. Increase daily in 1 mg/kg increments. Use the higher doses when treating meningitis, osteoarthritis, cryptococcal infections, and Aspergillosis.

Uses

Treatment of systemic fungal infections resistant to conventional amphotericin B therapy or in patients with renal or hepatic dysfunction.

Monitoring

Serum amphotericin B concentrations are not routinely followed. Monitor urine output. Periodic CBC for thrombocytopenia, electrolytes for hypokalemia, BUN, serum creatinine, and hepatic transaminases.

Adverse Effects/Precautions

Anemia, thrombocytopenia, hypokalemia, nausea/vomiting, & fever/chills.

Pharmacology

AmBisome® consists of amphotericin B intercalated within a single bilayer liposomal drug delivery system. Acts by binding to the sterol component of a cell membrane leading to alterations in the cell wall permeability and death. Penetrates the cell wall of susceptible fungi. Concentrates in the liver and spleen but penetrates the CNS less than conventional amphotericin B. Less nephrotoxic than conventional amphotericin B. Mean serum half-life in adults 24 to 38 hours. The pharmacokinetics of amphotericin B liposome is nonlinear.

Special Considerations/Preparation

Available as powder for injection in 50 mg vials. Reconstitute by adding 12 mL of sterile water for injection to a yield a concentration of 4 mg/mL. Immediately shake vial vigorously for 30 seconds. Check for complete dispersion. Reconstituted suspension stable for 24 hours refrigerated. **Do not freeze. Protect from light.**

Before administration, AmBisome® must be diluted with D_5W to a final concentration less than 2 mg/mL. A 1 mg/mL dilution may be made by filtering (using 5 micron filter) 1 mL of reconstituted solution into 3 mL of D_5W. Use one filter per vial of AmBisome®. Use dilution immediately. **Do not mix Ambisome® with saline solutions**–precipitation will occur.

Solution compatibility: D_5W.

Solution incompatibility: Dex/AA and NS.

Terminal injection site compatibility: No available data.

Selected References

♦ Scarcella A, Pasquariello MB, Giugliano B, et al: Liposomal amphotericin B treatment for neonatal fungal infections. *Pediatr Infect Dis J* 1998;17:146-148.

♦ Evdoridou J, Roilides E, Bibashi E, Kremenopoulos G: Multifocal osteoarthritis due to Candida albicans in a neonate: Serum level monitoring of liposomal amphotericin B and literature review. *Infection* 1997;25:112.

♦ Weitkamp JH, Poets CF, Sievers R, et al: Candida infection in very low birthweight infants: Outcome and nephrotoxicity of treatment with liposomal amphotericin B (AmBisome®). *Infection* 1998;26:11-15.

Updated 3/2000

Ampicillin

Dose & Administration

25 to 50 mg/kg per dose by IV slow push, or IM.

Some experts recommend 100 mg/kg/dose when treating meningitis and severe group B streptococcal sepsis.

Dosing Interval Chart

PMA *(weeks)*	PostNatal *(days)*	Interval *(hours)*
≤29	0 to 28 >28	12 8
30 to 36	0 to 14 >14	12 8
37 to 44	0 to 7 >7	12 8
≥45	ALL	6

Uses

Broad-spectrum antibiotic useful against group B *streptococcus, Listeria monocytogenes,* and susceptible *E coli* species.

Monitoring

Serum concentration can be measured but is not usually necessary.

Adverse Effects/Precautions

Very large doses may result in CNS excitation or seizure activity. Hypersensitivity reactions (maculopapular rash, urticarial rash, or fever) are rare in neonates.

Pharmacology

Ampicillin is a semisynthetic penicillin that is bactericidal. Clearance is primarily by the renal route and is inversely related to postnatal age. Serum half-life in term infants younger than 7 days is approximately 4 hours.

Special Considerations/Preparation

Available as powder for injection in 125-, 250-, 500-mg, 1-g, and 2-g vials. Reconstitute using sterile water for injection. Maximum concentration for IV infusion is 100 mg/mL. Mix to a final concentration of 250 mg/mL for IM administration. Reconstituted solution must be used within 1 hour of mixing because of loss of potency.

continued...

Solution Compatibility: D_5W, $D_{10}W$, and NS.

Solution Incompatibility: Dex/AA.

Terminal Injection Site Compatibility: Fat emulsion. Aminophylline, acyclovir, aztreonam, calcium gluconate, cefepime, chloramphenicol, cimetidine, clindamycin, dopamine, enalaprilat, epinephrine, famotidine, furosemide, hydrocortisone succinate, heparin, insulin, lidocaine, linezolid, metronidazole, morphine, phytonadione, potassium chloride, propofol, ranitidine, remifentanil, sodium bicarbonate, tolazoline, and vancomycin.

Incompatibility: Aminoglycoside antibiotics, erythromycin lactobionate, fluconazole, hydralazine, metoclopramide, and midazolam.

Selected References

♦ Shaffer CL, Davey AM, Ransom JL, et al: Ampicillin-induced neurotoxicity in very-low-birth-weight neonates. *Ann Pharmacother* 1998;32:482-484.

♦ Prober CG, Stevenson DK, Benitz WE: The use of antibiotics in neonates weighing less than 1200 grams. *Pediatr Infect Dis J* 1990;9:111.

♦ Kaplan JM, McCracken GH, Horton LJ, et al: Pharmacologic studies in neonates given large dosages of ampicillin. *J Pediatr* 1974;84:571.

♦ Boe RW, Williams CPS, Bennett JV, Oliver TK Jr: Serum levels of methicillin and ampicillin in newborn and premature infants in relation to postnatal age. *Pediatrics* 1967;39:194.

♦ Axline SG, Yaffe SJ, Simon HJ: Clinical pharmacology of antimicrobials in premature infants: II. Ampicillin, methicillin, oxacillin, neomycin, and colistin. *Pediatrics* 1967;39:97.

Updated 3/2001
Compatibilities updated 3/2003

Aztreonam

Dose & Administration

30 mg/kg per dose IV slow push over 5 to 10 minutes, or IM.

To use dosing chart, please refer to explanatory note on page iii

Dosing Interval Chart

PMA *(weeks)*	PostNatal *(days)*	Interval *(hours)*
≤29	0 to 28 >28	12 8
30 to 36	0 to 14 >14	12 8
37 to 44	0 to 7 >7	12 8
≥45	ALL	6

Uses

Treatment of neonatal sepsis caused by susceptible gram-negative organisms (e.g. *E coli*, *H influenzae*, *Klebsiella*, *Pseudomonas*, and *Serratia*). Generally used in combination with ampicillin (empirical treatment of sepsis) or an aminoglycoside (for synergism against *Pseudomonas* and *Enterobacteriaceae*).

Monitoring

Check serum glucose one hour after administration. Measuring serum concentration is not usually necessary. Periodic CBC, AST, ALT.

Adverse Effects/Precautions

Aztreonam contains 780 mg L-arginine per gram of drug (23.4 mg/kg body weight per dose). Adequate amounts of glucose must be provided to prevent hypoglycemia. Side effects are rare but include eosinophilia, elevation of serum transaminases, and phlebitis at the injection site.

Pharmacology

Aztreonam is a synthetically-produced monocyclic β-lactam antibiotic. Although bactericidal against aerobic gram-negative bacteria, it has virtually no activity against aerobic gram-positive and anaerobic bacteria, thereby producing little alteration of bowel flora. Good tissue and fluid penetration has been demonstrated in adults, along with protein-binding of 50 to 65%. Eliminated renally, primarily as unchanged drug. Serum half-life in neonates is 3 to 9 hours. Aztreonam does not interfere with bilirubin-albumin binding.

continued...

Aztreonam

Special Considerations/Preparation

Available as powder for injection in 500-mg, 1-g, and 2-g vials. Reconstitute 500-mg vial with 10 mL of either sterile water for injection or NS (50 mg/mL). **Shake immediately and vigorously.** Reconstituted solution stable for 48 hours at room temperature, 7 days refrigerated.

Solution Compatibility: D_5W, $D_{10}W$, and NS.

Terminal Injection Site Compatibility: Dex/AA and fat emulsion. Amikacin, aminophylline, ampicillin, bumetanide, calcium gluconate, cefazolin, cefepime, cefotaxime, cefoxitin, ceftazidime, ceftriaxone, cimetidine, clindamycin, dexamethasone, dobutamine, dopamine, enalaprilat, famotidine, fluconazole, furosemide, gentamicin, heparin, hydrocortisone succinate, imipenem, insulin, linezolid, metoclopramide, mezlocillin, morphine, netilmicin, piperacillin, piperacillin/tazobactam, potassium chloride, propofol, quinupristin/dalfopristin, ranitidine, remifentanil, sodium bicarbonate, ticarcillin/clavulanate, tobramycin, vancomycin, and zidovudine.

Incompatibility: Acyclovir, amphotericin B, lorazepam, metronidazole, and nafcillin.

Selected References

♦ Uauy R, Mize C, Argyle C, McCracken GH: Metabolic tolerance to arginine: Implications for the safe use of arginine salt-aztreonam combination in the neonatal period. *J Pediatr* 1991;118:965.

♦ Cuzzolin L, Fanos V, Zambreri D, et al: Pharmacokinetics and renal tolerance of aztreonam in premature infants. *Antimicrob Agents Chemother* 1991;35:1726.

♦ Prober CG, Stevenson DK, Benitz WE: The use of antibiotics in neonates weighing less than 1200 grams. *Pediatr Infect Dis J* 1990;9:111.

♦ Likitnukul S, McCracken GH, Threlkeld N, et al: Pharmacokinetics and plasma bactericidal activity of aztreonam in low-birth-weight infants. *Antimicrob Agents Chemother* 1987;31:81.

Added 3/96
Compatibilities updated 3/2003

Cefepime

Dose & Administration

50 mg/kg per dose IV infusion by syringe pump over 30 minutes, or IM. Treatment of pneumonia, urinary tract, or skin infections: Q12 hours. Severe infections and meningitis, especially if due to *P. aeruginosa* or *Enterobacter* spp., administer every 8 hours.

Note: Dose and interval are those recommended for infants older than 2 months of age and children.

To reduce pain at IM injection site, cefepime may be mixed with 1% lidocaine without epinephrine.

Uses

Treatment of serious infections caused by susceptible gram-negative organisms (e.g. *E coli, H influenzae, Enterobacter, Klebsiella, Morganella, Neisseria, Serratia,* and *Proteus* species), especially *Pseudomonas aeruginosa* that are resistant to 3rd generation cephalosporins. Treatment of serious infections caused by susceptible Gram-positive organisms (e.g. *Strep pneumoniae, Strep. pyogenes, Strep. agalactiae, and Staph. aureus*).

Monitoring

Measuring serum concentration is not usually necessary.

Adverse Effects/Precautions

Safety has been documented to be the same as commonly used second- and third-generation cephalosporins. Reported adverse effects are uncommon but include rash, diarrhea, elevated hepatic transaminases, eosinophilia, and positive Coombs' test.

Pharmacology

Cefepime is a new fourth-generation cephalosporin with treatment efficacy equivalent to third-generation cephalosporins. Potential advantages include: more rapid penetration through the cell wall of Gram-negative pathogens; enhanced stability to hydrolysis by β-lactamases; and enhanced affinity for penicillin-binding proteins. The drug distributes widely in body tissues and fluids (i.e. CSF, bile, bronchial secretions, lung tissue, ascitic fluid, middle ear). Protein binding is low (~ 20%), and it is primarily excreted unchanged in the urine. Serum half-life in infants older than 2 months of age is approximately 2 hours. There are no data in preterm or term neonates.

continued...

Special Considerations/Preparation

Available as powder for injection in 500-mg and 1-g, and 2-g vials. Reconstitute 500-mg vial with sterile water for injection to a concentration of 100 mg/mL. Reconstituted solution stable for 24 hours at room temperature, 7 days refrigerated. Protect from light.

Solution Compatibility: D_5W, $D_{10}W$, and NS.

Terminal Injection Site Compatibility: Dex/AA. Amikacin, ampicillin, aztreonam, bumetanide, calcium gluconate, clindamycin, dexamethasone, fluconazole, furosemide, heparin, hydrocortisone succinate, imipenem/cilastatin, lorazepam, methylprednisolone, metronidazole, piperacillin-tazobactam, potassium chloride, ranitidine, sodium bicarbonate, ticarcillin/clavulanate, trimethoprim/sulfamethoxazole, and zidovudine.

Incompatibility: Aminoglycoside antibiotics, aminophylline, acyclovir, amphotericin B, cimetidine, diazepam, dobutamine, dopamine, enalaprilat, famotidine, magnesium sulfate, metoclopramide, morphine, and vancomycin.

Selected References

♦ Blumer JL, Reed MD, Knupp C: Review of the pharmacokinetics of cefepime in children. *Pediatr Infect Dis J* 2001;20:337-342.

♦ Bradley JS, Arrieta A: Empiric use of cefepime in the treatment of lower respiratory tract infections in children. *Pediatr Inf Dis J* 2001;20:343-349.

♦ Saez-Llorens XO, O'Ryan M: Cefepime in the empiric treatment of meningitis in children. *Pediatr Infect Dis J* 2001;20:356-361.

♦ Kessler RE: Cefepime microbiologic profile and update. *Pediatr Inf Dis J* 2001; 20:331-336.

Added 3/2002
Compatibilities updated 3/2003

Cefotaxime

Dose & Administration

50 mg/kg per dose IV infusion by syringe pump over 30 minutes, or IM.

Gonococcal infections: 25 mg/kg per dose IV over 30 minutes, or IM.

To use dosing chart, please refer to explanatory note on page iii

Dosing Interval Chart

PMA (weeks)	PostNatal (days)	Interval (hours)
≤29	0 to 28 >28	12 8
30 to 36	0 to 14 >14	12 8
37 to 44	0 to 7 >7	12 8
≥45	ALL	6

Gonococcal ophthalmia prophylaxis in newborns whose mothers have gonorrhea at the time of delivery: 100 mg/kg IV over 30 minutes or IM, single dose, in addition to topical ophthalmic prophylaxis.

Uses

Treatment of neonatal meningitis and sepsis caused by susceptible gram-negative organisms (e.g. *E coli, H influenzae, Klebsiella,* and *Pseudomonas).* Treatment of disseminated gonococcal infections.

Monitoring

Measuring serum concentration is not usually necessary. Periodic CBC.

Adverse Effects/Precautions

Side effects are rare but include rash, phlebitis, diarrhea, leukopenia, granulocytopenia, and eosinophilia.

Pharmacology

Cefotaxime is one of many third-generation cephalosporin antibiotics. The mechanism of action appears to be by bacterial cell wall disruption. Metabolized in the liver to an active compound, desacetylcefotaxime. The drug distributes widely (i.e. CSF, bile, bronchial secretions, lung tissue, ascitic fluid, middle ear). Excreted renally.

Serum half-life in the premature infant is approximately 3 to 6 hours.

continued...

Special Considerations/Preparation

Available as powder for injection in 500-mg, 1-g, and 2-g vials.
The 500-mg vial is reconstituted with 4.9 mL sterile water for injection to yield a concentration of 100 mg/mL. Reconstituted solution stable for 24 hours at room temperature, 5 days refrigerated.

Solution Compatibility: D_5W, $D_{10}W$, and NS.

Terminal Injection Site Compatibility: Dex/AA and fat emulsion. Acyclovir, amikacin, aztreonam, clindamycin, famotidine, heparin, lorazepam, metronidazole, midazolam, morphine, potassium chloride, remifentanil, propofol, and tolazoline.

Incompatibility: Aminophylline, fluconazole, sodium bicarbonate, and vancomycin.

Selected References

♦ American Academy of Pediatrics: Gonococcal infections. In: Pickering LK, ed. *2000 Red Book: Report of the Committee on Infectious Diseases*, 25th ed. Elk Grove Village, IL: American Academy of Pediatrics, 2000; pp 256-257.

♦ Prober CG, Stevenson DK, Benitz WE: The use of antibiotics in neonates weighing less than 1200 grams. *Pediatr Infect Dis J* 1990;9:111.

♦ Kearns GL, Jacobs RF, Thomas BR, et al: Cefotaxime and desacetylcefotaxime pharmacokinetics in very low birth weight neonates. *J Pediatr* 1989;114:461.

♦ de Louvois J, Mulhall A, Hurley R: The safety and pharmacokinetics of cefotaxime in the treatment of neonates. *Pediatr Pharmacol* 1982;2:275.

♦ Kafetzis DA, Brater DC, Kapiki AN: Treatment of severe neonatal infections with cefotaxime: Efficacy and pharmacokinetics. *J Pediatr* 1982;100:483.

Updated 3/98
Compatibilities updated 3/2003

Cefoxitin

Dose and Administration

25 to 33 mg/kg per dose IV slow push, or IM.

To use dosing chart, please refer to explanatory note on page iii

Dosing Interval Chart

PMA (weeks)	PostNatal (days)	Interval (hours)
≤29	0 to 28 >28	12 8
30 to 36	0 to 14 >14	12 8
37 to 44	0 to 7 >7	12 8
≥45	ALL	6

Uses

Use in neonates is generally limited to treatment of skin, intra-abdominal and urinary tract infections caused by susceptible bacteria – anaerobes (e.g. *Bacteroides fragilis)*, gram positives (e.g. *Staphylococcus aureus, Streptococcus pneumoniae*, and other streptococci except enterococcus) and gram negatives (e.g. *Haemophilus influenzae, Klebsiella* sp., *E. coli, Proteus vulgaris*, and *Neisseria gonorrhoeae)*.

Monitoring

Serum concentrations are not routinely monitored.

Adverse Effects/Precautions

Adverse effects are rare. Transient eosinophilia and elevation of hepatic transaminases have been reported in < 3% of treated patients. Severe overdose can cause tachypnea, pallor, hypotonia, and metabolic acidosis.

Pharmacology

Broad spectrum bactericidal second generation cephalosporin that has enhanced activity against anaerobic bacteria. Inhibits bacterial cell wall synthesis by binding to one or more penicillin-binding proteins. Not inactivated by β-lactamase. Poor CNS penetration. Highly protein bound. Renally excreted as unchanged drug (85 to 90%). Half-life in term neonates is approximately 1.4 hours, and 2.3 hours in preterm neonates —considerably longer than children (0.6 hours) and adults (0.8 hours).

continued...

Special Considerations/Preparation

Available as powder for injection in 1-g, and 2-g vials.

IV administration: Reconstitute 1-g vial with 9.5 mL sterile water for injection to a concentration of 100 mg/mL. A 40 mg/ml dilution may be made by adding 4 mL of reconstituted solution to 6 mL sterile water for injection, or D_5W. Stable for 24 hours at room temperature or 7 days refrigerated.

IM administration: Reconstitute 1-g vial with 4.5 mL of 0.5% Lidocaine solution without epinephrine to a concentration of 200 mg/mL.

Solution Compatibility: D_5W, $D_{10}W$, and NS.

Terminal Injection Site Compatibility: Dex/AA and fat emulsion. Acyclovir, amikacin, aztreonam, cimetidine, clindamycin, famotidine, fluconazole, gentamicin, heparin, insulin, lidocaine, linezolid, magnesium sulfate, morphine, metronidazole, multivitamins, potassium chloride, propofol, ranitidine, remifentanil, sodium bicarbonate, tobramycin and vecuronium.

Incompatibility: Vancomycin

Selected References

♦ Regazzi MB, Chirico G, Cristiani D, et al: Cefoxitin in newborn infants. *Eur J Clin Pharmacol* 1983;25:507-509.

♦ Yogev R, Delaplane D, Wiringa K: Cefoxitin in a neonate. *Ped Infect Dis J* 1983; 2:342-343.

♦ Farmer K: Use of cefoxitin in the newborn. *New Zealand Med J* 1982;95:398.

♦ Marget W: Tenfold overdose of cefoxitin in a newborn. *Infection* 1982;10:243.

♦ Brogden RN, Heel RC, Speight TM, et al: Cefoxitin: A review of its antibacterial activity, pharmacological properties and therapeutic use. *Drugs* 1979;17:1-37.

♦ Feldman WE, Moffitt S, Sprow N: Clinical and pharmacokinetic evaluation of parenteral cefoxitin in infants and children. *Antimicrob Agents Chemother* 1980;17:669-674.

Added 3/2001
Compatibilities updated: 3/2003

Ceftazidime

Dose & Administration

30 mg/kg per dose IV infusion by syringe pump over 30 minutes, or IM. To reduce pain at IM injection site, ceftazidime may be mixed with 1% lidocaine without epinephrine.

To use dosing chart, please refer to explanatory note on page iii

Dosing Interval Chart

PMA (weeks)	PostNatal (days)	Interval (hours)
≤29	0 to 28	12
	>28	8
30 to 36	0 to 14	12
	>14	8
37 to 44	0 to 7	12
	>7	8
≥45	ALL	8

Uses

Treatment of neonatal meningitis and sepsis caused by susceptible gram-negative organisms (e.g. *E coli, H influenzae, Neisseria, Klebsiella,* and *Proteus* species), especially *Pseudomonas aeruginosa*. Resistance among strains of *Serratia* and *Enterobacteriaceae* is increasing.

Monitoring

Measuring serum concentration is not usually necessary.

Adverse Effects/Precautions

Reported adverse effects are uncommon but include rash, diarrhea, elevated hepatic transaminases, eosinophilia, and positive Coombs' test.

Pharmacology

Ceftazidime is one of many third-generation cephalosporins. The drug distributes widely in body tissues and fluids (i.e. CSF, bile, bronchial secretions, lung tissue, ascitic fluid, middle ear). Protein binding is low, and it is excreted unchanged in the urine. Ceftazidime is synergistic with aminoglycosides. Serum half-life in neonates is 3 to 12 hours.

continued...

Special Considerations/Preparation

Available as powder for injection in 500-mg and 1-g, 2-g, and 6-g vials.

Intravenous solution: Reconstitute 500-mg vial with sterile water for injection to a concentration of 50 mg/mL. Reconstituted solution stable for 24 hours at room temperature, 7 days refrigerated.

Intramuscular solution: Prepared by reconstituting 500-mg vial with 2.2 mL of 1% lidocaine without epinephrine to a concentration of 200 mg/mL. Solution is stable for 24 hours at room temperature, 3 days refrigerated.

Ceftazidime mixtures with L-arginine are not approved for pediatric use. All dosage forms approved for pediatric use contain sodium carbonate; when reconstituted, carbon dioxide bubbles will form. Using a vented needle may help reduce spraying and leaking.

Solution Compatibility: D_5W, $D_{10}W$, and NS.

Terminal Injection Site Compatibility: Dex/AA and fat emulsion. Acyclovir, aminophylline, aztreonam, cimetidine, clindamycin, enalaprilat, esmolol, famotidine, heparin, linezolid, metronidazole, morphine, potassium chloride, propofol, ranitidine, remifentanil, sodium bicarbonate, and zidovudine.

Incompatibility: Fluconazole, midazolam, and vancomycin.

Selected References

◆ Prober CG, Stevenson DK, Benitz WE: The use of antibiotics in neonates weighing less than 1200 grams. *Pediatr Infect Dis J* 1990;9:111.

◆ Tessin I, Thiringer K, Trollfors B, Brorson JE: Comparison of serum concentrations of ceftazidime and tobramycin in newborn infants. *Eur J Pediatr* 1988;147:405.

◆ Odio CM, Umana MA, Saenz A, et al: Comparative efficacy of ceftazidime vs. carbenicillin and amikacin for treatment of neonatal septicemia. *Pediatr Infect Dis J* 1987;6:371.

◆ McCracken GH, Threlkeld N, Thomas ML: Pharmacokinetics of ceftazidime in newborn infants. *Antimicrob Agents Chemother* 1984;26:583.

Updated 1/93
Compatibilities updated 3/2003

Ceftriaxone

Dose & Administration

Sepsis and disseminated gonococcal infection: 50 mg/kg Q24 hours.
Meningitis: 100 mg/kg loading dose, then 80 mg/kg Q24 hours .

Uncomplicated gonococcal ophthalmia: 50 mg/kg (maximum 125 mg) single dose.

IV administration: Infusion by syringe pump over 30 minutes.

IM administration: To reduce pain at the injection site, reconstitute with 1% lidocaine without epinephrine.

Uses

Treatment of neonatal sepsis and meningitis caused by susceptible gram-negative organisms (e.g. *E coli, Pseudomonas, Klebsiella, H influenzae*). Treatment of gonococcal infections.

Monitoring

CBC for eosinophilia, thrombocytosis, leukopenia. Serum electrolytes, BUN, creatinine. AST, ALT, bilirubin. Consider abdominal ultrasonography.

Adverse Effects/Precautions

Not recommended for use in neonates with hyperbilirubinemia. Displaces bilirubin from albumin binding sites, resulting in higher free bilirubin serum concentrations. Eosinophilia, thrombocytosis, leukopenia. Increase in bleeding time. Diarrhea. Increase in BUN and serum creatinine. Increase in AST and ALT. Skin rash. Transient gallbladder precipitations occasionally associated with colicky abdominal pain, nausea, and vomiting.

Pharmacology

Ceftriaxone is one of many third-generation cephalosporin antibiotics. The drug distributes widely (i.e. CSF, bile, bronchial secretions, lung tissue, ascitic fluid, middle ear). It is eliminated unchanged by both biliary (40%) and renal mechanisms. Serum half-life in premature infants is 5 to 16 hours. Dosage adjustment is necessary only for patients with combined hepatic and renal failure.

continued...

Special Considerations/Preparation

Intravenous solution: Prepared by reconstituting powder with compatible solution (sterile water for injection, D_5W, or $D_{10}W$) to a concentration of either 40 mg/mL or 100 mg/mL. Reconstituted solution is stable for 3 days at room temperature, 10 days refrigerated. A dark color may appear after reconstitution; however, potency is retained.

To make 100-mg/mL solution: Add 2.4 mL to the 250-mg vial.
To make 40-mg/mL solution: Add 6.2 mL to the 250-mg vial.

Intramuscular solution: Prepared by reconstituting 250-mg vial with 0.9 mL of 1% lidocaine without epinephrine to a concentration of 250 mg/mL. Solution is stable for 24 hours at room temperature, 3 days refrigerated.

Solution Compatibility: D_5W, $D_{10}W$, and NS.

Terminal Injection Site Compatibility: Dex/AA and fat emulsion. Acyclovir, aztreonam, clindamycin, famotidine, heparin, lidocaine, linezolid, metronidazole, morphine, potassium chloride, propofol, remifentanil, sodium bicarbonate, and zidovudine.

Incompatibility: Aminophylline, fluconazole and vancomycin.

Selected References

♦ American Academy of Pediatrics. Gonococcal infections. In: Pickering LK, ed. *2000 Red Book: Report of the Committee on Infectious Diseases. 25th* ed. Elk Grove Village, IL: American Academy of Pediatrics; 2000: pp 256-257.

♦ Centers for Disease Control: 1998 Guidelines for treatment of sexually transmitted diseases. *MMWR* 1998;47:RR-01.

♦ Prober CG, Stevenson DK, Benitz WE: The use of antibiotics in neonates weighing less than 1200 grams. *Pediatr Infect Dis J* 1990;9:111.

♦ Schaad UB, Suter S, Gianella-Borradori A, et al: A comparison of ceftriaxone and cefuroxime for the treatment of bacterial meningitis in children. *N Engl J Med* 1990;332:141.

♦ Fink S, Karp W, Robertson A: Ceftriaxone effect on bilirubin-albumin binding. *Pediatrics* 1987;80:873.

♦ Laga M, Naamara W, Brunham RC, et al: Single-dose therapy of gonococcal ophthalmia neonatorum with ceftriaxone. *N Engl J Med* 1986;315:1382.

♦ Yogev R, Shulman ST, Chadwick E, et al: Once daily ceftriaxone for central nervous system infections and other serious pediatric infections. *Pediatr Inf Dis J* 1986;5:298.

♦ Martin E, Koup JR, Paravicini U, Stoeckel K: Pharmacokinetics of ceftriaxone in neonates and infants with meningitis. *J Pediatr* 1984;105:475.

♦ Schaad UB, Stoeckel K: Single-dose pharmacokinetics of ceftriaxone in infants and young children. *Antimicrob Agents Chemother* 1982;21:248.

References updated 3/2001
Compatibilities updated 3/2003

Cefazolin

Dose & Administration

25 mg/kg per dose IV slow push, or IM.

Dosing Interval Chart

PMA (weeks)	PostNatal (days)	Interval (hours)
≤29	0 to 28 >28	12 8
30 to 36	0 to 14 >14	12 8
37 to 44	0 to 7 >7	12 8
≥45	ALL	6

Uses

Use in neonates is generally limited to perioperative infection prophylaxis and treatment of urinary tract and soft tissue infections caused by susceptible organisms, e.g. penicillin-resistant *Staph. aureus*, *Klebsiella*, and *Proteus*.

Monitoring

Serum concentrations are not routinely monitored.

Adverse Effects/Precautions

Adverse effects are rare, but include phlebitis and eosinophilia.

Pharmacology

First generation cephalosporin that is bactericidal against many gram-positive and a few gram-negative organisms. Inactivated by β-lactamase producing organisms. Poor CNS penetration. Renally excreted as unchanged drug. Half-life in neonates is 3 to 5 hours.

Special Considerations/Preparation

Available as powder for injection in 250-mg, 500-mg, and 1000-mg vials. Reconstitute using NS or sterile water for injection to a concentration of 225 mg/mL. A 20 mg/mL dilution may be made by adding 1-mL of reconstituted solution to 10 mL sterile water for injection, or D_5W.

Solution Compatibility: D_5W, $D_{10}W$, and NS.

Terminal Injection Site Compatibility: Dex/AA and fat emulsion. Acyclovir, amikacin, aztreonam, calcium gluconate, clindamycin, enalaprilat, esmolol, famotidine, fluconazole, heparin, insulin, lidocaine, linezolid, midazolam, morphine, metronidazole, multivitamins, pancuronium bromide, propofol, prostaglandin E_1, ranitidine, remifentanil, and vecuronium.

Incompatibility: Amiodarone, cimetidine, pentobarbital, and vancomycin.

No data are currently available for potassium chloride.

Selected References

♦ Saez-Llorens X, McCracken GH: Clinical pharmacology of antibacterial agents. In: Remington JS, Klein JO (eds): *Infectious Diseases of the Fetus and Newborn Infant*, ed 5. Philadelphia: WB Saunders Co, 2001.

♦ Pickering LK, O'Connor DM, Anderson D, et al: Clinical and pharmacologic evaluation of cefazolin in children. *J Inf Dis* 1973;128:S407.

Added 3/96
Compatibilities updated 3/2003

Dose & Administration

Loading dose: 20 mg/kg IV infusion by syringe pump over 30 minutes.
Maintenance dose: (Begin 12 hours after loading dose.)
Premature infants under 1 month of age: 2.5 mg/kg per dose Q6 hours.
Fullterm infants under 1 week of age and premature infants over 1 month of age: 5 mg/kg per dose Q6 hours.
Fullterm infants over 1 week of age: 12.5 mg/kg per dose Q6 hours.
(Absorption of oral chloramphenicol palmitate is erratic in newborns.)

Uses

A wide-spectrum antimicrobial bacteriostatic agent. May be bactericidal to species such as *H influenzae* and *Neisseria meningitidis*.

Monitoring

Close monitoring of serum concentration is mandatory. Small changes in dose and interval can lead to disproportionately large changes in serum concentration. Therapeutic peak serum concentration: 10 to 25 mcg/mL. Monitor CBC and reticulocyte counts. Assess hepatic and renal function.

Adverse Effects/Precautions

Reversible bone marrow suppression, irreversible aplastic anemia. Serum concentration greater than 50 mcg/mL has been associated with the "gray baby" syndrome (i.e. abdominal distention, pallid cyanosis, vasomotor collapse; may lead to death within hours of onset). Fungal overgrowth.

Pharmacology

Both esters (succinate and palmitate) are biologically inactive prodrugs. Hydrolysis to the active compound is erratic in newborns. Metabolized by hepatic glucuronyl transferase. Hepatically and renally eliminated. Inhibits metabolism of phenobarbital, phenytoin, and other agents.

Special Considerations/Preparation

Chloramphenicol succinate is available as powder for injection in 1-g and 10-g vials. Reconstitute the 1-g vial with 10 mL sterile water for injection, or D_5W to a concentration of 100 mg/mL. Reconstituted solution stable for 4 days refrigerated.

Solution Compatibility: D_5W, $D_{10}W$, and NS.

Terminal Injection Site Compatibility: Dex/AA and fat emulsion. Acyclovir, amikacin, aminophylline, ampicillin, calcium chloride, calcium gluconate, dopamine, enalaprilat, erythromycin lactobionate, esmolol, heparin, hydrocortisone succinate, lidocaine, magnesium sulfate, methicillin, metronidazole, morphine, nafcillin, oxacillin, penicillin G, pentobarbital, potassium chloride, ranitidine, sodium bicarbonate, and vitamin K_1.

Incompatibility: Fluconazole, metoclopramide, phenytoin, and vancomycin.

Selected References

♦ Roberts RJ: *Drug Therapy in Infants*. Philadelphia: WB Saunders Co, 1984, p 70.
♦ Rajchgot P, Prober CG, Soldin S: Initiation of chloramphenicol therapy in the newborn infant. *J Pediatr* 1982;101:1018.
♦ Glazer JP, Danish MA, Plotkin SA, Yaffe SJ: Disposition of chloramphenicol in low birth weight infants. *Pediatrics* 1980;66:573.

Updated 1/91, Compatibilities updated 3/2003

Clindamycin

Dose & Administration

5 to 7.5 mg/kg per dose IV infusion by syringe pump over 30 minutes, or PO.

To use dosing chart, please refer to explanatory note on page iii

Dosing Interval Chart

PMA (weeks)	PostNatal (days)	Interval (hours)
≤29	0 to 28	12
	>28	8
30 to 36	0 to 14	12
	>14	8
37 to 44	0 to 7	12
	>7	8
≥45	ALL	6

Increase dosing interval in patients with significant liver dysfunction.

Uses

Bacteriostatic antibiotic used for the treatment of bacteremia and pulmonary and deep tissue infections caused by anaerobic bacteria and some gram-positive cocci. Clindamycin should not be used in the treatment of meningitis.

Monitoring

Assess liver function. Monitor GI status closely. Therapeutic serum concentration ranges from 2 to 10 mcg/mL (bioassay yields variable results).

Adverse Effects/Precautions

The most serious adverse effect is pseudomembranous colitis, characterized by bloody diarrhea, abdominal pain, and fever. Discontinue clindamycin if any of these signs or symptoms occur, begin bowel rest and TPN, and consider treatment with oral metronidazole.

Pharmacology

Clindamycin inhibits bacterial protein synthesis and is primarily bacteriostatic at therapeutically attainable concentrations. Widely distributed into most tissues, especially the lung. Poor CSF penetration. Oral clindamycin is completely absorbed from the GI tract. Highly protein bound. Almost complete metabolism in the liver, with excretion via bile and feces. Available data in neonates suggest extremely variable clearance, especially in premature infants. No data are available regarding conversion of ester to active drug.

continued...

Special Considerations/Preparation

Oral preparation (clindamycin palmitate) is reconstituted with sterile water for injection, yielding a 75 mg per 5 mL solution.

Do not refrigerate. Stable at room temperature for 2 weeks.

IV preparation (clindamycin phosphate) is available as a 150 mg/mL solution in 2-mL, 4-mL, and 6-mL vials containing 9.45 mg/mL benzyl alcohol. It should be diluted using D_5W, NS, or LR to a concentration of 6 mg/mL, and infused at a rate no greater than 5 mL/min (30 mg/min).

Solution Compatibility: D_5W, $D_{10}W$, and NS.

Terminal Injection Site Compatibility: Dex/AA and fat emulsion. Acyclovir, amikacin, amiodarone, ampicillin, aztreonam, cefazolin, cefepime, cefotaxime, cefoxitin, ceftazidime, ceftriaxone, cimetidine, ciprofloxacin, enalaprilat, esmolol, gentamicin, heparin, hydrocortisone succinate, linezolid, magnesium sulfate, metoclopramide, metronidazole, midazolam, morphine, netilmicin, penicillin G, piperacillin, piperacillin/tazobactam, potassium chloride, propofol, prostaglandin E_1, ranitidine, remifentanil, sodium bicarbonate, tobramycin, and zidovudine.

Incompatibility: Aminophylline, barbiturates, calcium gluconate, fluconazole, and phenytoin.

Selected References

♦ Koren G, Zarfin Y, Maresky D, et al: Pharmacokinetics of intravenous clindamycin in newborn infants. *Pediatr Pharmacol* 1986;5:287.

♦ Bell MJ, Shackelford P, Smith R, Schroeder K: Pharmacokinetics of clindamycin phosphate in the first year of life. *J Pediatr* 1984;105:482.

♦ Feigin RD, Pickering LK, Anderson D, et al: Clindamycin treatment of osteomyelitis and septic arthritis in children. *Pediatrics* 1975;55:213.

♦ Lwin N, Collipp PJ: Absorption and tolerance of clindamycin 2-palmitate in infants below 6 months of age. *Curr Ther Res Clin Exp* 1970;12:648.

Dosing chart revised 3/96
Compatibilities updated 3/2003

Erythromycin

Dose and Administration

Treatment of Pertussis and Chlamydial pneumonitis and conjunctivitis: 12.5 mg/kg per dose PO Q6 hours, E. estolate preferred.

Other infections and prophylaxis: 10 mg/kg per dose PO.

E. estolate (Ilosone®)—Q8 hours.

E. ethylsuccinate (E. E. S.®, EryPed®)—Q6 hours.

Administer with infant formula to enhance absorption of the ethylsuccinate and reduce possible GI side effects.

Severe infections when PO route unavailable: 5 to 10 mg/kg per dose IV infusion by syringe pump over at least 60 minutes Q6 hours.

After reconstitution, dilute to a concentration of 1 to 5 mg/mL for infusion. **Do not administer IM.**

Prophylaxis of ophthalmia neonatorum: Ribbon of 0.5% ointment instilled in each conjunctival sac.

Uses

Treatment of infections caused by *Chlamydia, Mycoplasma,* and *Ureaplasma.* Treatment for and prophylaxis against *Bordetella pertussis.* As a substitute for penicillin in situations of significant allergic intolerance.

Monitoring

Monitor heart rate and blood pressure closely during IV administration. Liver function should be assessed because erythromycin is concentrated in the liver and bile. Observe IV site closely for signs of infiltration. CBC for eosinophilia.

Adverse Effects/Precautions

Hypertrophic pyloric stenosis has been reported in 4% of neonates who received oral erythromycin for pertussis prophylaxis. Two reported cases of severe bradycardia and hypotension occurring during IV administration of erythromycin lactobionate. Intrahepatic cholestasis. Loose stools occur infrequently. Bilateral sensorineural hearing loss has been reported rarely in adults, usually associated with intravenous administration and renal or hepatic dysfunction. The hearing loss occurred after the first few doses and was reversible after discontinuing the drug. Venous irritation is common when using the IV dosage form.

Contraindicated in patients receiving **cisapride** due to precipitation of life-threatening arrhythmias.

Pharmacology

Erythromycin may be bacteriostatic or bactericidal depending on the tissue concentration of drug and the microorganism involved. Serum concentration is higher with the estolate preparation (1 to 2 mcg/mL) and is independent of gestational or postnatal age. IV administration of E. lactobionate to preterm infants, using doses of 6.25 to 10 mg/kg, yielded peak serum concentrations of 1.9 to 3.7 mcg/mL and a half-life of 2 hours. The drug penetrates poorly into the CNS, is concentrated in the liver and bile, and is excreted via the bowel. It is a motilin receptor agonist and induces stomach and small intestine motor activity. Plasma clearance of midazolam is reduced by 50%. Digoxin, midazolam, theophylline and carbamazepine serum concentrations may be significantly increased because of prolongation of their half-life.

continued...

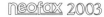

Erythromycin

Special Considerations/Preparation

E. estolate oral suspension is available in concentrations of 125 mg- and 250 mg per 5 mL; E. ethylsuccinate in concentrations of 200 mg- and 400 mg per 5 mL. Refrigeration not required except to preserve taste. Shake suspension well before administering.

Reconstitute IV dosage forms using only sterile water for injection to a concentration of 50 mg/mL (~265-291 mOsm/kg).

A 5-mg/mL dilution may be made by adding 1 mL of reconstituted solution to 9 mL sterile water for injection. Diluted drug should be used within 8 hours. Filter before administration to reduce venous irritation. Use only preservative-free IV erythromycin.

Solution compatibility: NS and sterile water for injection.

Solution incompatibility: D_5W and $D_{10}W$ (unless buffered with 4% sodium bicarbonate to maintain stability).

Terminal injection site compatibility: Dex/AA and fat emulsion. Acyclovir, aminophylline, amiodarone, chloramphenicol, cimetidine, enalaprilat, esmolol, famotidine, heparin, hydrocortisone succinate, lidocaine, lorazepam, magnesium sulfate, methicillin, midazolam, morphine, penicillin G, pentobarbital, potassium chloride, ranitidine, sodium bicarbonate, and zidovudine.

Incompatibility: Ampicillin, fluconazole, furosemide, and metoclopramide.

Selected References

♦ Kaul A: Erythromycin as a prokinetic agent. *J Pediatr Gastroenterol Nutr* 2002; 34:13-15.
♦ Oei J, Lui K: A placebo-controlled trial of low-dose eryhtromycin to promote feed tolerance in preterm infants. *Acta Paediatr* 2001;90:904-908.
♦ American Academy of Pediatrics. Chlamydial Infections, and Pertussis. In: Pickering LK, ed. *2000 Red Book: Report of the Committee on Infectious Diseases.* 25th ed. Elk Grove Village, IL: American Academy of Pediatrics; 2000: p210 and p437.
♦ Pai MP, Graci DM, Amsden GW: Macrolide drug interactions: an update. *Ann Pharmacother* 2000;34:495-513.
♦ Honein MA, Paulozzi LJ, Himelright IM, et al: Infantile hypertrophic pyloric stenosis after pertussis prophylaxis with erythromycin: a case review and cohort study. *Lancet* 1999;354:2101-2105.
♦ Waites KB, Sims PJ, Crouse DT, et al: Serum concentrations of erythromycin after intravenous infusion in preterm neonates treated for *Ureaplasma* urealyticum infection. *Pediatr Infect Dis J* 1994;13:287.
♦ Farrar HC, Walsh-Sukys MC, Kyllonen K, Blumer JL: Cardiac toxicity associated with intravenous erythromycin lactobionate: Two case reports and a review of the literature. *Pediatr Infect Dis J* 1993;12:688.
♦ Ginsburg CM: Pharmacology of erythromycin in infants and children. *Pediatr Infect Dis J* 1986;5:124.
♦ Eichenwald H: Adverse reactions to erythromycin. *Pediatr Infect Dis J* 1986;5:147.
♦ Bass JW: Erythromycin for treatment and prevention of pertussis. *Pediatr Infect Dis J* 1986;5:154.
♦ Patamasucon P, Kaojarern S, Kusmiesz H, Nelson J: Pharmacokinetics of erythromycin ethylsuccinate and estolate in infants under 4 months of age. *Antimicrob Agents Chemother* 1981;19:736.

Referenced Updated 3/2003
Compatibilities updated 3/2003

Fluconazole

Dose & Administration

Systemic infections, including meningitis: 12 mg/kg loading dose, then 6 mg/kg per dose IV infusion by syringe pump over 30 minutes, or PO.

Prophylaxis: 3 mg/kg per dose IV infusion
(Consider only in ELBW infants cared for in NICUs
with high rates of invasive fungal disease)

To use dosing chart, please refer to explanatory note on page iii

Dosing Interval Chart

PMA (weeks)	PostNatal (days)	Interval (hours)
≤29	0 to 14	72
	>14	48
30 to 36	0 to 14	48
	>14	24
37 to 44	0 to 7	48
	>7	24
≥45	ALL	24

Thrush: 6 mg/kg on Day 1, then 3 mg/kg per dose Q24 hours PO.

Uses

Treatment of systemic infections, meningitis, and severe superficial mycoses caused by *Candida* species. Resistance has been reported with *C glabrata* and *C krusei* and in patients receiving long-term suppressive therapy.

Monitoring

Serum fluconazole concentrations are not routinely followed. Assess renal function. Follow AST, ALT, and CBC for eosinophilia.

Adverse Effects/Precautions

Data in neonates are limited. Reversible elevations of transaminases have occurred in 12% of children. Interferes with metabolism of barbiturates and phenytoin. May also interfere with metabolism of caffeine, theophylline, and midazolam.

Contraindicated in patients receiving **cisapride** due to precipitation of life-threatening arrhythmias.

Pharmacology

Water-soluble triazole antifungal agent. Inhibits cytochrome P-450-dependent ergosterol synthesis. Well absorbed after oral administration, with peak serum concentrations reached within 1 to 2 hours. Less than 12% protein binding. Good penetration into CSF after both oral and IV administration. Serum half-life is 30 to 180 hours in severely ill VLBW infants in the first 2 weeks of life and approximately 17 hours in children. Primarily excreted unchanged in the urine.

continued...

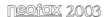

Special Considerations/Preparation

Available as a premixed solution for IV injection in concentrations of 200 mg/100 mL and 400 mg/200 mL in Viaflex® bags (2 mg/mL).

Oral dosage form is available as powder for suspension in concentrations of 10mg/mL and 40 mg/mL. Prepare both concentrations by adding 24 mL distilled water to bottle of powder and shaking vigorously. Suspension is stable at room temperature for 2 weeks. Do not freeze.

Solution Compatibility: D_5W and $D_{10}W$.

Terminal Injection Site Compatibility: Dex/AA and fat emulsion. Acyclovir, amikacin, aminophylline, aztreonam, cefazolin, cefepime, cefoxitin, cimetidine, dexamethasone, dobutamine, dopamine, famotidine, gentamicin, heparin, hydrocortisone succinate, intravenous immune globulin (human), linezolid, lorazepam, meropenem, metoclopramide, metronidazole, midazolam, morphine, nafcillin, nitroglycerin, oxacillin, pancuronium bromide, penicillin G, piperacillin/tazobactam, potassium chloride, phenytoin, propofol, quinupristin/dalfopristin, ranitidine, remifentanil, ticarcillin/clavulanate, tobramycin, vancomycin, vecuronium, and zidovudine.

Incompatibility: Amphotericin B, ampicillin, calcium gluconate, cefotaxime, ceftazidime, ceftriaxone, chloramphenicol, clindamycin, digoxin, erythromycin lactobionate, furosemide, imipenem, piperacillin, ticarcillin, and trimethoprim-sulfamethoxazole.

Selected References

♦ Kaufman D, Boyle R, et al: Fluconazole prophylaxis against fungal colonization and infection in preterm infants. *N Engl J Med* 2001;345:1660-1666.

♦ Huttova M, Hartmanova I, Kralinsky K, et al: Candida fungemia in neonates treated with fluconazole: report of forty cases, including eight with meningitis. *Pediatr Inf Dis J* 1998;17:1012-1015.

♦ Driessen M, Ellis JB, Cooper PA, et al: Fluconazole vs. amphotericin B for the treatment of neonatal fungal septicemia: a prospective randomized trial. *Pediatr Inf Dis J* 1996;15:1107.

♦ Flynn PM, Cunningham CK, Kerkering T, et al: Oropharyngeal candidiasis in immuno-compromised children: a randomized, multicenter study of orally administered fluconazole suspension versus nystatin. The Multicenter Fluconazole Study Group. *J Pediatr* 1995;127:322.

♦ Fasano C, O'Keefe J, Gibbs D: Fluconazole treatment of neonates and infants with severe fungal infections not treatable with conventional agents. *Eur J Clin Microbiol Infect Dis* 1994;13:351.

♦ Saxen H, Hoppu K, Pohjavuori M: Pharmacokinetics of fluconazole in very low birth weight infants during the first two weeks of life. *Clin Pharmacol Ther* 1993;54:269.

♦ Product information, Roerig Division of Pfizer, Inc. *Physicians' Desk Reference*, ed 57. Montvale, NJ: Thomson PDR, 2003, p 2594.

Updated 3/2002
Compatibilities updated 3/2002
References updated 3/2003

Flucytosine

Dose and Administration

12.5 to 37.5 mg/kg per dose Q6 hours PO. Increase dosing interval if renal dysfunction is present.

Uses

Antifungal agent used in combination with amphotericin B or fluconazole for treatment of infections caused by *Candida, Cryptococcus,* and other sensitive fungi.

Monitoring

Desired peak serum concentration ranges from 50 to 80 mcg/mL. Assess renal function. Follow GI status closely. Twice-weekly CBC and platelet counts. Periodic AST, ALT.

Adverse Effects/Precautions

Toxicities are related to serum concentration above 100 mcg/mL, and are usually reversible if the drug is stopped or the dose is reduced. Fatal bone marrow depression (related to fluorouracil production), hepatitis, severe diarrhea, rash. Amphotericin B may increase toxicity by decreasing renal excretion.

Pharmacology

Well absorbed orally. Transformed within cell to fluorouracil, which interferes with RNA synthesis. Excellent penetration into CSF and body tissues. 90% renal elimination of unchanged drug, proportional to GFR. Serum half-life in adults is 3 to 5 hours if renal function is normal, but 30 to 250 hours if renal impairment is present. Limited pharmacokinetic data in premature infants. Resistance develops frequently if used alone. Synergistic with amphotericin even if treating resistant strain.

Special Considerations/Preparation

Flucytosine is available only in 250-mg capsules. A pediatric suspension (10 mg/mL) may be prepared using distilled water; adjust pH from 5 to 7 with dilute sodium hydroxide. The capsule contains talc, which forms large-particle precipitates of inactive compound. The remaining suspension, containing the active drug, may be decanted. Shake well before use. The suspension is stable for 7 days at room temperature.

Selected References

♦ Marr B, Gross S, Cunningham C, et al: Candidal sepsis and meningitis in a very-low-birth-weight infant successfully treated with fluconazole and flucytosine. *Clin Infect Dis* 1994;19:795.

♦ Smego RA, Perfect JR, Durack DT: Combined therapy with amphotericin B and 5-fluorocytosine for *Candida* meningitis. *Rev Infect Dis* 1984;6:791.

♦ Johnson DE, Thompson TR, Green TP, Ferrieri P: Systemic candidiasis in very low-birth-weight infants (<1500 grams). *Pediatrics* 1984;73:138.

♦ Koldin MH, Medoff G: Antifungal chemotherapy. *Pediatr Clin North Am* 1983;30:49.

Updated 3/98

Dose and Administration

Topical: Apply ointment or cream to affected area Q6 hours.
Continue treatment for 3 days after symptoms have subsided.

PO: 1 mL (preterm) to 2 mL (term) of 100,000-U/mL suspension divided and applied with swab to each side of mouth Q6 hours.
Continue treatment for 3 days after symptoms have subsided.

Uses

Treatment of mucocutaneous candidal infections.

Monitoring

Assess response to drug.

Adverse Effects/Precautions

Possible skin rash caused by vehicle in ointment/cream.

Pharmacology

Polyene antifungal similar in structure to amphotericin B. May be fungicidal or fungistatic. Binds to the fungal cell membrane causing disruption of the cell structure. Not absorbed well from the GI tract, skin, or mucous membranes.

Special Considerations/Preparation

Topical ointment/cream: 100,000 U/g in 15- and 30-g tubes. Ointment dissolved in polyethylene and mineral-oil-gel base.

Oral suspension: 100,000 U/mL in 5-, 60-, and 480-mL bottles. Shake well before applying to mouth. Appears to work best when not mixed with formula. Contains <1% alcohol, saccharin, and 50% sucrose.

Selected References

♦ Hoppe JE: Treatment of oropharyngeal candidiasis and candidal diaper dermatitis in neonates and infants: review and reappraisal. *Ped Inf Dis J* 1997;16:885-94.

♦ Faix RG, Kovarik SM, Shaw TR, Johnson RV: Mucocutaneous and invasive candidiasis among very low birth weight (<1500 grams) infants in intensive care nurseries: A prospective study. *Pediatrics* 1989;83:101.

♦ Roberts RJ: *Drug Therapy in Infants.* Philadelphia: WB Saunders Co, 1984, p 81.

♦ Munz D, Powell KR, Pai CH: Treatment of candidal diaper dermatitis: A double-blind placebo-controlled comparison of topical nystatin with topical plus oral nystatin. *J Pediatr* 1982;101:1022.

Updated 3/98

Gentamicin

Dose and Administration

During the first week of life:

Gestation (weeks)	Dose (mg/kg/dose)	Interval (hours)
≤29*	5	48
30 to 33	4.5	48
34 to 37	4	36
≥38	4	24
* or significant asphyxia, PDA, or treatment with indomethacin		

IV infusion by syringe pump over 30 minutes. Administer as a separate infusion from penicillin-containing compounds. IM injection is associated with variable absorption, especially in the very small infant.

First week of life: Serum drug concentrations are usually not necessary except in patients with serious infections or significantly changing fluid or renal status. It is not necessary to wait for 'steady state': Peak levels may be measured after the first dose, and trough levels may be measured before the second dose.

After the first week: Administer an initial dose of 4 mg/kg, then measure a peak serum concentration 30 minutes after end of infusion, and another 12 to 24 hours later to determine dosing interval.

Example: Baby X is born at 28 weeks gestation. At 3 weeks of age, gentamicin therapy is begun. A 4 mg/kg dose is administered, with a peak serum concentration of 8.5 mcg/mL. 24 hours later, the serum concentration is 2.8 mcg/mL, yielding a calculated half-life of 15 hours. The predicted serum concentration at 48 hours postdose is 0.9 mcg/mL, and therefore the suggested dosing interval is 48 hours.

Uses

Treatment of infections caused by aerobic gram-negative bacilli (e.g. *Pseudomonas, Klebsiella, E coli*). Usually used in combination with a β-lactam antibiotic.

Monitoring

Therapeutic serum concentrations:
Peak: 5 to 12 mcg/mL (or C_{max}/MIC ratio greater than 8:1)
(Draw 30 minutes after end of infusion, 1 hour after IM injection.)
Trough: 0.5 to 1 mcg/mL
Blood samples obtained to monitor drug levels should be spun and refrigerated or frozen as soon as possible. Assess renal function.

Adverse Effects/Precautions

Transient and reversible renal tubular dysfunction may occur, resulting in increased urinary losses of sodium, calcium, and magnesium. Potential vestibular and auditory ototoxicity, especially if treating with other nephrotoxic and/or ototoxic medications (e.g. furosemide, vancomycin). Neuromuscular weakness and respiratory failure may be potentiated when treating concomitantly with pancuronium or other neuromuscular blocking agents, and in patients with hypermagnesemia.

continued...

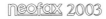

Pharmacology

New dosing recommendations are based on concepts promoted in adult studies of "once-a-day" dosing: (1) Higher peak concentrations are desirable to increase concentration-dependent bacterial killing; (2) There is a post-antibiotic effect on bacterial killing, especially when treating concurrently with a β-lactam antibiotic; (3) There may be less toxicity with less frequent dosing, due to less renal drug accumulation. Volume of distribution is increased and clearance is decreased in patients with PDA. Serum half-life is also prolonged in premature and asphyxiated newborns. Inactivation of gentamicin by penicillin-containing compounds appears to be a time-, temperature-, and concentration-dependent process. This is probably clinically significant only when penicillin-containing compounds are mixed in IV solutions or when blood is allowed to set at room temperature for several hours before serum drug concentration is assayed.

Special Considerations/Preparation

Pediatric injectable solution available in a concentration of 10 mg/mL.

Solution compatibility: D_5W, $D_{10}W$, and NS.

Terminal injection site compatibility: Dex/AA and fat emulsion. Acyclovir, aminophylline, amiodarone, aztreonam, cefoxitin, cimetidine, clindamycin, dopamine, enalaprilat, esmolol, famotidine, fluconazole, insulin, lorazepam, heparin (concentrations ≤1 U/mL), linezolid, magnesium sulfate, meropenem, metronidazole, midazolam, morphine, pancuronium bromide, prostaglandin E_1, ranitidine, remifentanil, tolazoline, vecuronium, and zidovudine.

Incompatibility: Amphotericin B, ampicillin, cefepime, furosemide, imipenem/cilastatin, heparin (concentrations >1 U/mL), indomethacin, methicillin, mezlocillin, nafcillin, oxacillin, penicillin G, propofol, and ticarcillin/clavulanate.

Selected References

♦ Ohler KH, Menke JA, Fuller L: Use of higher dose extended interval aminoglycosides in a neonatal intensive care unit. *Am J Perinatol* 2000;17:285-290.

♦ Lundgren FS, Glasscock GF, Kim EH, Cohen RS: Once-daily gentamicin dosing in newborn infants. *Pediatrics* 1999;103:1228-1234.

♦ Thureen PJ, Reiter PD, Gresores A, et al: Once- versus twice-daily gentamicin dosing in neonates > 34 weeks gestation: Cost-effectiveness analysis. *Pediatrics* 1999;103:594.

♦ Hayani KC, Hatzopoulos FK, Frank AL, et al: Pharmacokinetics of once-daily dosing of gentamicin in neonates. *J Pediatr* 1997;131:76-80.

♦ de Hoog M, Schoemaker RC, Mouton JW, van den Anker JN: Tobramycin population pharmacokinetics in neonates. *Clin Pharmacol Ther* 1997;62:392-99.

♦ Skopnik H, Wallraf R, Nies B, et al: Pharmacokinetics and antibacterial activity of daily gentamicin. *Arch Dis Child* 1992;67:57-61.

♦ Giapros VI, Andronikou S, Cholevas VI, Papadopoulou ZL: Renal function in premature infants during aminoglycoside therapy. *Pediatr Nephrol* 1995;9:163.

♦ Daly JS, Dodge RA, Glew RH, et al: Effect of time and temperature on inactivation of aminoglycosides by ampicillin at neonatal dosages. *J Perinatol* 1997;17:42-45.

♦ Williams BS, Ransom JL, Gal P, et al: Gentamicin pharmacokinetics in neonates with patent ductus arteriosus. *Crit Care Med* 1997;25:273-75.

References updated 3/2001, Compatibilities updated 3/2002

Imipenem-Cilastatin

Dose & Administration

20 to 25 mg/kg per dose Q12 hours IV infusion over 30 minutes.

Uses

Restricted to treatment of non-CNS infections caused by bacteria, primarily Enterobacteriaceae and anaerobes, resistant to other antibiotics.

Monitoring

Periodic CBC and hepatic transaminases. Assess IV site for signs of phlebitis.

Adverse Effects/Precautions

Seizures occur frequently in patients with meningitis, preexisting CNS pathology, and severe renal dysfunction. Local reactions at the injection site and increased platelet counts are the most frequent adverse effects. Others including eosinophilia, elevated hepatic transaminases, and diarrhea also occur in more than 5% of patients.

Pharmacology

Imipenem is a broad-spectrum carbapenem antibiotic combined in a 1:1 ratio with cilastatin, a renal dipeptidase inhibitor with no intrinsic antibacterial activity. Bactericidal activity is due to inhibition of cell wall synthesis. Clearance is directly related to renal function. Serum half-life of imipenem in neonates is 2.5 hours; the half-life of cilastatin is 9 hours.

Special Considerations/Preparation

Available as powder for injection in 250-mg, and 500-mg vials. Reconstitute with 100 mL of compatible diluent. Maximum concentration 5 mg/mL. When reconstituted with NS, solution is stable for 10 hours at room temperature, 48 hours refrigerated. When reconstituted with other compatible diluents, solution is stable for 4 hours at room temperature or 24 hours refrigerated.

Solution Compatibility: D_5W, $D_{10}W$, and NS.

Terminal Injection Site Compatibility: Fat emulsion. Acyclovir, aztreonam, cefepime, famotidine, insulin, linezolid, midazolam, propofol, remifentanil, and zidovudine.

Incompatibility: Amikacin, fluconazole, gentamicin, lorazepam, sodium bicarbonate, and tobramycin.

Selected References

♦ Balfour JA, Bryson HM, Brogden RN: Imipenem/cilastatin: an update of its antibacterial activity, pharmacokinetics and therapeutic efficacy in the treatment of serious infections. *Drugs* 1996;51:99.

♦ Stuart RL, Turnidge J, Grayson mL: Safety of imipenem in neonates. *Pediatr Infect Dis J* 1995;14:804.

♦ Reed MD, Kleigman RM, Yamashita TS, et al: Clinical pharmacology of imipenem and cilastatin in premature infants during the first week of life. *Antimicrob Agents Chemother* 1990;34:1172.

♦ Ahonkhai VI, Cyhan GM, Wilson SE, Brown KR: Imipenem-cilastatin in pediatric patients: and overview of safety and efficacy in studies conducted in the United States. *Pediatr Inf Dis J* 1989;8:740.

♦ Nalin DR, Jacobsen CA: Imipenem/cilastatin therapy for serious infections in neonates and infants. *Scand J Infect Dis* 1987;Suppl.2:46.

Added 3/97
Compatibilities updated 3/2003

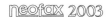

Dose and Administration

PO: 2 mg/kg per dose Q12 hours for one week following birth.

Uses

Used **only** in combination with zidovudine in the treatment of neonates born to HIV-infected women who have had no therapy during pregnancy. (Mother receives oral ZDV and 3TC during labor).

Monitoring

Specific monitoring unnecessary due to short treatment course.

Adverse Effects/Precautions

Limited data on toxicity— none reported in neonates.

Pharmacology

Lamivudine (3TC) is a synthetic nucleoside analog "prodrug" that inhibits HIV replication by interfering with viral reverse transcriptase. It is intracellularly converted in several steps to the active compound, then renally excreted. Poor CNS penetration, CSF:plasma ratio is 1:100. The oral solution is well-absorbed, with 66% bioavailability in children. The serum half-life in preterm infants less than 33 weeks gestation is approximately 14 hours. Viral resistance develops rapidly to monotherapy with lamivudine (3TC).

Special Considerations/Preparation

Available as an oral solution in a concentration of 10 mg/mL. Store at room temperature and protected from light.

Selected References

♦ Perinatal HIV Guidelines Working Group: Public Health Service Task Force recommendations for use of antiretroviral drugs in pregnant HIV-1-infected women with for maternal health and interventions to reduce perinatal HIV-1 transmission in the United States. (update published August 30, 2002 on the HIV/AIDS Treatment Information Service ATIS website: http://www.aidsinfo.nih.gov).

♦ Mueller BU, Lewis LL, Yuen GJ, et al: Serum and cerebrospinal fluid pharmacokinetics of intravenous and oral lamivudine in human immunodeficiency virus-infected children. *Antimicrob Agents Chemother* 1998;42:3187-3192.

♦ Moodley J, Moodley D, Pillay K, et al: Pharmacokinetics and antiretroviral activity of lamivudine alone or when coadministered with zidovudine in human immunodeficiency virus type 1-infected pregnant women and their offspring. *J Inf Dis* 1998;178:1327-1333.

♦ Paediatric European Network for Treatment of AIDS: A randomized double-blind trial of the addition of lamivudine or matching placebo to current nucleoside analogue reverse transcriptase inhibitor therapy in HIV-infected children: the PENTA-4 trial. *AIDS* 1998;12:F151-F160.

♦ Horneff G, Adams O, Wahn V: Pilot study of zidovudine-lamivudine combination therapy in vertically HIV-infected antiretroviral-naïve children. *AIDS* 1998;12:489-494.

References updated 3/2002

Linezolid

Dose & Administration
10 mg/kg/dose Q8 hours by IV infusion over 30 to 120 minutes.

Uses
Limited to treatment of infections caused by gram positive organisms resistant to other antibiotics, e.g. methicillin-resistant *Staph. aureus* and vancomycin-resistant enterococci.

Monitoring
Weekly CBC. Blood pressure if receiving sympathomimetics.

Adverse Effects/Precautions
Thrombocytopenia, anemia, leukopenia, rash, and diarrhea.

Pharmacology
Linezolid is an oxazolidinone agent that has a unique mechanism of inhibition of bacterial protein synthesis. It is usually bacteriostatic, although it may be bactericidal against *S. pneumoniae*, *B. fragilis*, and *C. perfringens*. Completely and rapidly absorbed when administered orally to adults and children. Metabolized by oxidation without cytochrome CYP induction. Excreted in the urine as unchanged drug (30%) and two inactive metabolites. Serum half-life in children is approximately 3 hours.

Special Considerations/Preparation
(Zyvox®) IV injection is supplied as a 2 mg/mL solution in single-use, ready-to-use 100-mL, 200-mL, and 300-mL plastic infusion bags in a foil laminate overwrap. Keep in the overwrap until use. Store at room temperature. Protect from freezing. IV injection may exhibit a yellow color that can intensify over time without affecting potency. An oral suspension is available, 100 mg per 5 mL. Store at room temperature. Use within 21 days after reconstitution. Protect from light.

continued...

Solution Compatibility: D$_5$W, NS, Lactated Ringer's.

Terminal Injection Site Compatibility: Dex/AA. Acyclovir, amikacin, aminophylline, ampicillin, aztreonam, calcium gluconate, cefazolin, cefoxitin, ceftazidime, ceftriaxone, cefuroxime, cimetidine, clindamycin, dexamethasone, digoxin, dobutamine, dopamine, enalaprilat, esmolol, famotidine, fentanyl, fluconazole, furosemide, ganciclovir, gentamicin, heparin, hydrocortisone succinate, imipenem/cilastatin, lidocaine, lorazepam, magnesium, meropenem, methylprednisone, metoclopramide, metronidazole, mezlocillin, midazolam, morphine, naloxone, netilmicin, nicardipine, nitroglycerin, pentobarbital, phenobarbital, piperacillin, piperacillin-tazobactam, potassium chloride, propranolol, ranitidine, remifentanil, sodium bicarbonate, theophylline, ticarcillin, tobramycin, trimethoprim-sulfamethoxazole, vancomycin, vecuronium, and zidovudine.

Incompatibility: Amphotericin B, diazepam, and phenytoin.

Selected References

♦ Jungbluth GL, Welshman IR, Hopkins NK, et al: Impact of gestational and postnatal age on linezolid disposition in neonates and young infants. *Pediatr Res* 2002;51:465A

♦ Kaplan SL: Use of linezolid in children. *Pediatr Inf Dis J* 2002;21:869-872

♦ Kearns GL, Abdel-Rahman SM, Blumer JL, et al: Single dose pharmacokinetics of linezolid in infants and children. *Pediatr Infect Dis J* 2000;19:1178-1184.

♦ Paladino JA: Linezolid: An oxazolidinone antimicrobial agent. *Am J Health-Syst Pharm* 2002;59:2413-2425.

♦ Product information, Pharmacia & UpJohn. *Physicians' Desk Reference*, ed 57. Montvale, NJ: Thomson PDR, 2003, p 2800.

Updated 3/2003

Meropenem

Dose & Administration

Sepsis: 20 mg/kg per dose Q12 hours IV infusion over 30 minutes.
Meningitis and infections caused by Pseudomonas species: 40 mg/kg per dose Q8 hours IV infusion over 30 minutes.

Uses

Treatment of pneumococcal meningitis and other serious infections caused by susceptible gram-negative organisms resistant to other antibiotics.

Monitoring

Periodic CBC (for thrombocytosis and eosinophilia) and hepatic transaminases. Assess IV site for signs of inflammation.

Adverse Effects/Precautions

Diarrhea (4%), nausea/vomiting (1%) and rash (2%). May cause inflammation at the injection site.

Pharmacology

Meropenem is a broad-spectrum carbapenem antibiotic that penetrates well into the CSF and most body tissues. It is relatively stable to inactivation by human renal dehydropeptidase. Plasma protein binding is minimal. Clearance is directly related to renal function, and 70% of a dose is recovered intact in the urine. Hepatic function does not affect pharmacokinetics. Serum half-life of meropenem is 3 hours in preterm and 2 hours in full term neonates.

Special Considerations/Preparation

Available (USA) as powder for injection in 500-mg, and 1000-mg vials. Reconstitute with 100 mL of compatible diluent. Maximum concentration 50 mg/mL. Freshly prepared solutions should be used whenever possible. When reconstituted with NS, solution is stable in the vial for 2 hours at room temperature, 12 hours refrigerated. When reconstituted with D_5W, solution in the vial is stable for 1 hour at room temperature or 8 hours refrigerated.
Solution Compatibility: D_5W, $D_{10}W$, and NS.
Terminal Injection Site Compatibility: Dex/AA and fat emulsion. Acyclovir, aminophylline, atropine, cimetidine, calcium gluconate, dexamethasone, digoxin, dobutamine, dopamine, enalaprilat, fluconazole, furosemide, gentamicin, heparin, insulin, linezolid, metoclopramide, morphine, norepinephrine, phenobarbital, ranitidine, sodium bicarbonate, vancomycin, zidovudine.
Incompatibility: Amphotericin B, and metronidazole.

Selected References

♦ Bradley JS: Meropenem: a new, extremely broad spectrum β-lactam antibiotic for serious infections in pediatrics. *Pediatr Inf Dis J* 1997;16:263-68.

♦ Blumer JL: Pharmacokinetic determinants of carbapenem therapy in neonates and children. *Pediatr Infect Dis J* 1996;15:733-37.

♦ Piyush PR: Compatibility of meropenem with commonly used injectable drugs. *Am J Health-Syst Pharm* 1996;53:2853-55.

♦ Blumer JL, Reed MD, Kearns GL, et al: Sequential, single-dose pharmacokinetic evaluation of meropenem in hospitalized infants and children. *Antimicrob Agents Chemother* 1995;39:1721-25.

♦ Hurst M, Lamb HM: Meropenem: a review of its use in patients in intensive care. *Drugs* 2000;59:653-680.

References updated 3/2001, Compatibilities updated 3/2003

ANTIBIOTICS

(Pseudomonic Acid A)

Dose and Administration

Apply small amounts topically to affected areas 3 times daily.

Uses

Topical use for skin infections caused by *Staphylococcus aureus, S epidermidis, S saprophyticus,* and *Streptococcus pyogenes.*

Monitoring

Assess affected area for continued infection.

Adverse Effects/Precautions

Use only on the skin. No adverse effects reported from topical administration. Routine use may lead to selective bacterial resistance.

Pharmacology

Topical antibacterial produced by fermentation of the organism *Pseudomonas fluorescens.* Inhibits protein synthesis by bonding to bacterial isoleucyl-transfer-RNA synthetase. Highly protein bound. Not absorbed into the systemic circulation after topical administration (older infants and children). Metabolized in the skin to an inactive compound and excreted.

Special Considerations/Preparation

Available in unit-dose packets and 15-g tubes as a 2% ointment (20 mg/g).

Selected References

♦ Zakrzewska-Bode A, Muytjens HL, Liem KD, Hoogkamp-Korstanje JAA: Mupirocin resistance in coagulase-negative staphylococci, after topical prophylaxis for the reduction of colonization of central venous catheters. *J Hosp Infect* 1995;31:189.

♦ Pappa KA: The clinical development of mupirocin. *J Am Acad Dermatol* 1990;22:873.

♦ Leyden JJ: Mupirocin: A new topical antibiotic. *Semin Dermatol* 1987;6:48.

♦ Davies EA, Emmerson AM, Hogg GM, et al: An outbreak of infection with a methicillin-resistant *Staphylococcus aureus* in a special care baby unit: Value of topical mupirocin and of traditional methods of infection control. *J Hosp Infect* 1987;10:120.

Updated 3/98

Metronidazole

Dose & Administration

Loading dose: 15 mg/kg PO or IV infusion by syringe pump over 60 minutes.
Maintenance dose: 7.5 mg/kg PO or IV infusion over 60 minutes. Begin one dosing interval after initial dose.

To use dosing chart, please refer to explanatory note on page iii

Dosing Interval Chart

PMA *(weeks)*	PostNatal *(days)*	Interval *(hours)*
≤29	0 to 28 >28	48 24
30 to 36	0 to 14 >14	24 12
37 to 44	0 to 7 >7	24 12
≥45	ALL	8

Uses

Reserved for treatment of meningitis, ventriculitis, and endocarditis caused by *Bacteroides fragilis* and other anaerobes resistant to penicillin; treatment of serious intra-abdominal infections; and treatment of infections caused by *Trichomonas vaginalis*. Treatment of *C. difficile* colitis.

Monitoring

Measure CSF drug concentrations when treating CNS infections. Trough drug concentration should be greater than minimum inhibitory concentration for organism.

Adverse Effects/Precautions

Metronidazole has been shown to be carcinogenic in mice and rats, and therefore has not been approved for pediatric use. Seizures and sensory polyneuropathy have been reported in a few adult patients receiving high doses over a prolonged period. Drug metabolites may cause brownish discoloration of the urine.

Pharmacology

Metronidazole is bactericidal for many anaerobic organisms. It is well absorbed after oral administration, with peak serum concentrations attained in 1 to 3 hours. Distribution in all tissues throughout the body is excellent. It is less than 20% protein bound. Hydroxylation in the liver occurs in term infants and premature infants exposed to antenatal β-methasone. Unchanged drug and the active metabolite are excreted renally. Elimination half-life is strongly related to gestational age, ranging from 22 to 109 hours.

continued...

Special Considerations/Preparation

Preferred IV preparation is a ready-to-use solution for injection containing 500 mg per 100 mL, in PVC plastic bags or glass vials.

Do not refrigerate (crystals form, but redissolve on warming to room temperature). Osmolarity is 310 mOsm/L, pH is 5 to 7.

Also available as a powder for injection: 500 mg per 5-mL vial.

Supplied as 250 mg and 500 mg for oral administration. Suspension may be prepared by crushing five 250-mg tablets (1250 mg), dissolving powder in 10 mL purified water, then adding cherry syrup to make a total volume of 83 mL. Final concentration is 15 mg/mL.

Protect from light. Suspension is stable for 30 days refrigerated.

Solution Compatibility: D_5W, and NS.

Solution Incompatibility: Manufacturer recommends that if metronidazole is used with a primary IV fluid system, the primary solution should be discontinued during metronidazole infusion.

Terminal Injection Site Compatibility: Dex/AA and fat emulsion. Acyclovir, amikacin, aminophylline, amiodarone, ampicillin, cefazolin, cefepime, cefotaxime, cefoxitin, ceftazidime, ceftriaxone, clindamycin, chloramphenicol, dopamine, enalaprilat, esmolol, fluconazole, gentamicin, heparin, hydrocortisone succinate, linezolid, lorazepam, magnesium sulfate, midazolam, morphine, netilmicin, penicillin G, piperacillin-tazobactam, prostaglandin E_1, remifentanil, and tobramycin.

Incompatibility: Aztreonam, and meropenem.

Selected References

♦ Wenisch C, Parschalk B, Hasenhundl M, et al: Comparison of vancomycin, teicoplanin, metronidazole, and fusidic acid for the treatment of *Clostridium difficile* - associated diarrhea. *Clin Infect Dis* 1996;22:813.

♦ Feder HM Jr: *Bacteroides fragilis* meningitis. *Rev Infect Dis* 1987;9:783.

♦ Roberts RJ: *Drug Therapy in Infants*. Philadelphia: WB Saunders Co, 1984, p 76.

♦ Hall P, Kaye CM, McIntosh N, Steele J: Intravenous metronidazole in the newborn. *Arch Dis Child* 1983;58:529.

♦ Oldenburg B, Speck WT: Metronidazole. *Pediatr Clin North Am* 1983;30:71.

♦ Jager-Roman E, Doyle PE, Baird-Lambert J, et al: Pharmacokinetics and tissue distribution of metronidazole in the newborn infant. *J Pediatr* 1982;100:651.

Updated 3/97
Compatibilities updated 3/2003

Nafcillin

Dose & Administration
25 to 50 mg/kg per dose IV slow push.

Dosing Interval Chart

PMA (weeks)	PostNatal (days)	Interval (hours)
≤29	0 to 28 >28	12 8
30 to 36	0 to 14 >14	12 8
37 to 44	0 to 7 >7	12 8
≥45	ALL	6

Uses
Treatment of infections caused by penicillinase-producing staphylococci, particularly if evidence of renal dysfunction.

Monitoring
Periodic CBC. Observe IV site for signs of extravasation.

Adverse Effects/Precautions
Increase dosing interval in patients with hepatic dysfunction. Irritating to veins—watch for phlebitis. Cases of granulocytopenia have been reported.

Pharmacology
Inhibits synthesis of bacterial cell wall. Better penetration into CSF than methicillin. Excreted via hepatic clearance.

Special Considerations/Preparation
Available as 1-g in 50-mL and 2-g in 100-mL frozen single-dose bags. Thaw bags at room temperature or under refrigeration. Do not force thaw by immersing into water baths or microwaving. pH of resulting solution 6 to 8.5. Reconstituted solution stable for 3 days at room temperature, 21 days refrigerated.

Solution Compatibility: D_5W, $D_{10}W$, and NS.

Terminal Injection Site Compatibility: Dex/AA and fat emulsion. Acyclovir, aminophylline, atropine, chloramphenicol, cimetidine, dexamethasone, enalaprilat, esmolol, famotidine, fentanyl, fluconazole, heparin, lidocaine, morphine, potassium chloride, propofol, sodium bicarbonate, zidovudine.

Incompatibility: Aminoglycoside antibiotics, aztreonam, hydrocortisone succinate, insulin, methylprednisolone, midazolam, and vancomycin.

Selected References
♦ Prober CG, Stevenson DK, Benitz WE: The use of antibiotics in neonates weighing less than 1200 grams. *Pediatr Infect Dis J* 1990;9:111.
♦ Kitzing W, Nelson JD, Mohs E: Comparative toxicities of methicillin and nafcillin. *Am J Dis Child* 1981;135:52.
♦ Banner W, Gooch WM, Burckart G, Korones SB: Pharmacokinetics of nafcillin in infants with low birth weights. *Antimicrob Agents Chemother* 1980;17:691.

Text updated 3/97, Compatibilities updated 3/2000

Dose and Administration

25 to 50 mg/kg per dose IV slow push.

Dosing Interval Chart

PMA (weeks)	PostNatal (days)	Interval (hours)
≤29	0 to 28 >28	12 8
30 to 36	0 to 14 >14	12 8
37 to 44	0 to 7 >7	12 8
≥45	ALL	6

Uses

Treatment of infections caused by penicillinase-producing staphylococci.

Monitoring

Periodic CBC and urinalysis. Irritating to veins—watch for phlebitis. Observe IV site for signs of extravasation.

Pharmacology

Inhibits synthesis of bacterial cell wall. Rapidly excreted renally unchanged. Poor CSF penetration. Good penetration of pleural, pericardial, and synovial fluids.

Adverse Effects/Precautions

Interstitial nephritis associated with hematuria, albuminuria, and casts in urine. Bone marrow depression. Hypersensitivity in the form of a rash. Tolerant strains of staphylococci have been reported.

Special Considerations/Preparation

Available as powder injection in 250-mg, 500-mg, 1-g, 2-g, 4-g, and 10-g vials. Reconstitute 1-g vial with 10 mL of sterile water for injection to make a final concentration of 100 mg/mL. Reconstituted solution is stable for 3 days at room temperature, 7 days refrigerated. A 25-mg/mL dilution may be made by adding 2 mL of reconstituted solution to 6 mL of sterile water for injection. Dilution stable for 4 days refrigerated.

Solution compatibility: D_5W, $D_{10}W$, and NS.

Terminal injection site compatibility: Dex/AA and fat emulsion. Acyclovir, chloramphenicol, dopamine, famotidine, fluconazole, heparin, hydrocortisone succinate, morphine, potassium chloride, sodium bicarbonate, and zidovudine.

Incompatibility: Aminoglycoside antibiotics.

Selected References

♦ Maraqa NF, Gomez MM, Rathore MH, Alvarez AM: Higher occurrence of hepatotoxicity and rash in patients treated with oxacillin, compared with those treated with nafcillin and other commonly used antimicrobials. *Clin Inf Dis* 2002;34:50-54.

♦ Axline SG, Yaffe SJ, Simon HJ: Clinical pharmacology of antimicrobials in premature infants: II. Ampicillin, methicillin, oxacillin, neomycin, and colistin. *Pediatrics* 1967;39:97.

References updated 3/2003

ANTIBIOTICS

Dose and Administration

During the first week of life:

Gestation (weeks)	Dose (mg/kg/dose)	Interval (hours)
≤29*	5	48
30 to 33	4.5	48
34 to 37	4	36
≥38	4	24
* or significant asphyxia, PDA, or treatment with indomethacin		

IV infusion by syringe pump over 30 minutes. Administer as a separate infusion from penicillin-containing compounds. IM injection is associated with variable absorption, especially in the very small infant.

First week of life: Serum drug concentrations are usually not necessary except in patients with serious infections or significantly changing fluid or renal status. It is not necessary to wait for 'steady state': Peak levels may be measured after the first dose, and trough levels may be measured before the second dose.

After the first week: Administer an initial dose of 4 mg/kg, then measure a peak serum concentration 30 minutes after end of infusion, and another 12 to 24 hours later to determine dosing interval.

Example: Baby X is born at 28 weeks gestation. At 3 weeks of age, gentamicin therapy is begun. A 4 mg/kg dose is administered, with a peak serum concentration of 8.5 mcg/mL. 24 hours later, the serum concentration is 2.8 mcg/mL, yielding a calculated half-life of 15 hours. The predicted serum concentration at 48 hours postdose is 0.9 mcg/mL, and therefore the suggested dosing interval is 48 hours.

Uses

Treatment of infections caused by aerobic gram-negative bacilli (e.g. *Pseudomonas, Klebsiella, E coli*). Usually used in combination with a β-lactam antibiotic.

Monitoring

Therapeutic serum concentrations:
Peak: 5 to 12 mcg/mL (or C_{max}/MIC ratio greater than 8:1)
(Draw 30 minutes after end of infusion, 1 hour after IM injection.)
Trough: 0.5 to 1 mcg/mL
Blood samples obtained to monitor drug levels should be spun and refrigerated or frozen as soon as possible. Assess renal function.

Adverse Effects/Precautions

Transient and reversible renal tubular dysfunction may occur, resulting in increased urinary losses of sodium, calcium, and magnesium. Potential vestibular and auditory ototoxicity, especially if treating with other nephrotoxic and/or ototoxic medications (e.g. furosemide, vancomycin). Neuromuscular weakness and respiratory failure may be potentiated when treating concomitantly with pancuronium or other neuromuscular blocking agents, and in patients with hypermagnesemia.

Netilmicin

Pharmacology

New dosing recommendations are based on concepts promoted in adult studies of "once-a-day" dosing: (1) Higher peak concentrations are desirable to increase concentration-dependent bacterial killing; (2) There is a post-antibiotic effect on bacterial killing, especially when treating concurrently with a β-lactam antibiotic; (3) There may be less toxicity with less frequent dosing, due to less renal drug accumulation. Volume of distribution is increased and clearance is decreased in patients with PDA. Serum half-life is also prolonged in premature and asphyxiated newborns. Inactivation of netilmicin by penicillin-containing compounds appears to be a time-, temperature-, and concentration-dependent process. This is probably clinically significant only when penicillin-containing compounds are mixed in IV solutions or when blood is allowed to set at room temperature for several hours before serum drug concentration is assayed.

Special Considerations/Preparation

Available in a concentration of 100 mg/mL in 1.5 mL vials. A 10 mg/mL dilution may be made by adding 1 mL of this solution to 9 mL of sterile water for injection. Dilution is stable for 72 hours refrigerated. Do not freeze.

Solution Compatibility: D_5W, $D_{10}W$, and NS.

Terminal Injection Site Compatibility: Dex/AA and fat emulsion. Aminophylline, atropine, aztreonam, calcium gluconate, cefuroxime, clindamycin, dexamethasone, hydrocortisone succinate, heparin (concentrations ≤1 U/mL), linezolid, iron dextran, isoproterenol, metronidazole, neostigmine, norepinephrine, pancuronium bromide, potassium chloride, remifentanil, sodium bicarbonate, and vitamin K_1.

Incompatibility: Amphotericin B, ampicillin, cefepime, furosemide, heparin (concentrations >1 U/mL), methicillin, mezlocillin, nafcillin, oxacillin, penicillin G, propofol, and ticarcillin/clavulanate.

Selected References

♦ Ohler KH, Menke JA, Fuller L: Use of higher dose extended interval aminoglycosides in a neonatal intensive care unit. *Am J Perinatol* 2000;17:285-290.

♦ Ettlinger JJ, Bedford KA, Lovering AM, et al: Pharmacokinetics of once-a-day netilmicin (6mg/kg) in neonates. *J Antimicrob Chemother* 1996;38:499-505.

♦ Giapros VI, Andronikou S, Cholevas VI, Papadopoulou ZL: Renal function in premature infants during aminoglycoside therapy. *Pediatr Nephrol* 1995;9:163.

♦ Fattinger K, Vozeh S, Olafsson A, et al: Netilmicin in the neonate: Population pharmacokinetic analysis and dosing recommendations. *Clin Pharmacol Ther* 1991;50:55-65.

♦ Kuhn RJ, Nahata MC, Powell DA, et al: Pharmacokinetics of netilmicin in premature infants. *Eur J Clin Pharmacol* 1986;29:635-637.

♦ Noone P: Sisomicin, netilmicin and dibekacin: A review of their antibacterial activity and therapeutic use. *Drugs* 1984;27:548-578.

♦ Daly JS, Dodge RA, Glew RH, et al: Effect of time and temperature on inactivation of aminoglycosides by ampicillin at neonatal dosages. *J Perinatol* 1997;17:42-45.

Added 3/2001
Compatibilities updated 3/2003

Nevirapine

Dose and Administration

PO: 2 mg/kg single dose at 48 to 72 hours of age.

If the mother received nevirapine less than one hour prior to delivery, administer 2 mg/kg as soon as possible after birth, and again at 48 to 72 hours.

Uses

Used **only** in combination with zidovudine in the treatment of neonates born to HIV-infected women who have had no therapy during pregnancy. (Mother receives a single 200-mg oral dose of nevirapine during labor).

Monitoring

Specific monitoring unnecessary due to short treatment course.

Adverse Effects/Precautions

Limited data on toxicity—none reported in neonates.

Pharmacology

Nevirapine is a non-nucleoside antiretroviral agent that inhibits HIV-1 replication by selectively interfering with viral reverse transcriptase without requiring intracellular metabolism. It also inactivates cell-free virions in the genital tract and breast milk. Synergistic antiviral activity occurs when administered with zidovudine. Nevirapine is rapidly absorbed after oral administration to pregnant women and is highly lipophilic, resulting in therapeutic concentrations being readily transferred across the placenta to the fetus. Serum half-life in the neonates is approximately 44 hours. With the maternal/newborn regimen described above, serum concentrations are above 100 mcg/L throughout the first week of life. Nevirapine is extensively metabolized by, and an inducer of, hepatic CYP3A4 and CYP2B6 isoenzymes. Concomitant administration of phenobarbital or phenytoin, CYP3A inducers, may affect plasma concentrations.

Special Considerations/Preparation

Available as an oral suspension in a concentration of 10 mg/mL. Store at room temperature and protect from light.

Selected References

♦ Perinatal HIV Guidelines Working Group: Public Health Service Task Force recommendations for use of antiretroviral drugs in pregnant HIV-1-infected women with for maternal health and interventions to reduce perinatal HIV-1 transmission in the United States. (update published August 30, 2002 on the HIV/AIDS Treatment Information Service ATIS website: http://www.aidsinfo.nih.gov).

♦ Murochnick M, Clarke DF, Dorenbaum A: Nevirapine: pharmacokinetic considerations in children and pregnant women. *Drugs* 2000;39:281-293.

♦ Musoke P, Guay LA, Bagenda D, et al: A phase I/II study of the safety and pharmacokinetics of nevirapine in HIV-1-infected pregnant Ugandan women and their neonates (HIVNET 006). *AIDS* 1999;13:479-486.

Dose and References updated 3/2002

Dose & Administration

7.5 mg/kg/dose Q12 hours by IV infusion over 60 minutes.

Uses

Limited to treatment of infections caused by gram positive organisms resistant to other antibiotics, e.g. methicillin-resistant *Staph. aureus* and vancomycin-resistant *Enterococcus faecium* (not *E faecalis*).

Monitoring

Assess IV site for signs of inflammation.

Adverse Effects/Precautions

Myalgias and arthralgias occur frequently in adults with hepatic or renal failure. Diarrhea, hyperbilirubinemia, and rash were reported infrequently.

Pharmacology

No data are available for infants. Synercid® is a new parenteral antimicrobial agent which consists of two streptogramin antibiotics (quinupristin and dalfopristin in a 30:70 ratio) that inhibit bacterial protein synthesis by binding to separate sites on the bacterial ribosome. Serum half-life of quinupristin in adults ranges from 1 to 3 hours, and of dalfopristin ranges from 5 to 9 hours. 75% is excreted via the biliary route.

Special Considerations/Preparation

Synercid® is supplied as a lyophilized powder in single-dose, 10-mL vials containing 500 mg. Store refrigerated. Reconstitute under aseptic conditions by adding 5 mL of Sterile Water for Injection or D_5W. Before administration, dilute with D_5W to a concentration not exceeding 2 mg/mL. Diluted solution is stable for 5 hours at room temperature, or 54 hours if stored under refrigeration.

Solution Compatibility: D_5W.

Solution Incompatibility: NS.

Terminal Injection Site Compatibility: Aztreonam, fluconazole, and potassium chloride.

Selected References

♦ Gray JW, Darbyshire PJ, Beath SV, et al: Experience with quinupristin/dalfopristin in treating infections with vancomycin-resistant *Enterococcus faecium* in children. *Pediatr Infect Dis J* 2000;19:234-238.

♦ Lamb HM, Figgitt DP, Faulds D: Quinupristin/Dalfopristin: A review of its use in the management of serious gram-positive infections. *Drugs* 1999;58:1061-1097.

♦ Product Information, Aventis Pharmaceuticals: *Physicians' Desk Reference*, ed 57. Montvale, NJ: Medical Economics Data, 2003, p 769.

Added 3/2001

Dose and Administration

» Use only aqueous crystalline penicillin G for IV administration «

Procaine and benzathine penicillin G are for IM administration only.

Meningitis: 75,000 to 100,000 IU/kg per dose IV slow push, or IM.

Bacteremia: 25,000 to 50,000 IU/kg per dose IV slow push, or IM.

Dosing Interval Chart

PMA (weeks)	Postnatal (days)	Interval (hours)
≤29	0 to 28 >28	12 8
30 to 36	0 to 14 >14	12 8
37 to 44	0 to 7 >7	12 8
≥45	All	6

To use dosing chart, please refer to explanatory note on page iii

Group B streptococcal infections: Some experts recommend using 200,000 IU/kg per day for bacteremia and 400,000 IU/kg per day for meningitis, in divided doses at more frequent intervals than those listed above. Consider adding aminoglycoside if tolerance is suspected or confirmed.

Congenital syphilis: Aqueous crystalline penicillin G: 50,000 IU/kg per dose IV slow push given Q12 hours during the first 7 days of life, and Q8 hours thereafter, irrespective of gestational age; or

Procaine penicillin G: 50,000 IU/kg per dose IM, once daily.
Treat for 10 to 14 days.

Gonococcal infection (only with proven penicillin-susceptible isolate):
Use higher doses listed for meningitis and bacteremia.

Uses

Treatment of infections caused by susceptible organisms—congenital syphilis, gonococci, streptococci (non enterococcal).

Monitoring

Follow serum sodium and potassium when using high doses and in patients with renal failure. Observe IV site for signs of extravasation.

Adverse Effects/Precautions

Significant CNS toxicity has been reported in adults with renal failure who developed CSF concentrations >10 mcg/mL. Bone marrow depression, granulocytopenia, and hepatitis are rare. Hypersensitivity has not been seen in neonates.

continued...

Pharmacology

Inhibits synthesis of bacterial cell wall. Excreted unchanged in the urine. CSF penetration is poor, except in inflamed meninges. Concentrates in joint fluid and urine.

Special Considerations/Preparation

Aqueous crystalline penicillin G is available as powder for injection in 1-million, 5-million, 10-million, and 20-million units per vial. Reconstitute 5-million unit vial with 8 mL sterile water for injection to make a final concentration of 500,000 units/mL. Reconstituted solution good for 7 days refrigerated. A 100,000 unit/mL dilution may be made by adding 10 mL of reconstituted solution to 40 mL sterile water for injection. Dilution stable for 4 days refrigerated.

Procaine and benzathine penicillin G for IM injection are available in multiple dosage strengths in vials and Tubex® syringes.

Solution compatibility: D_5W, $D_{10}W$, and NS.

Terminal injection site compatibility: Dex/AA and fat emulsion. Acyclovir, amiodarone, calcium chloride, calcium gluconate, chloramphenicol, cimetidine, clindamycin, dopamine, enalaprilat, erythromycin lactobionate, esmolol, fluconazole, furosemide, heparin, hydrocortisone succinate, lidocaine, methicillin, metronidazole, morphine, pentobarbital, potassium chloride, prostaglandin E_1, ranitidine and sodium bicarbonate.

Incompatibility: Aminoglycoside antibiotics, aminophylline, amphotericin B, and metoclopramide.

Selected References

♦ American Academy of Pediatrics. Syphilis. In: Pickering LK, ed. *2000 Red Book: Report of the Committee on Infectious Diseases. 25th* ed. Elk Grove Village, IL: American Academy of Pediatrics; 2000: pp 553-555.

♦ Centers for Disease Control: 1998 Guidelines for treatment of sexually transmitted diseases. *MMWR* 1998;47:RR-01.

♦ Stoll BJ: Congenital syphilis: evaluation and management of neonates born to mothers with reactive serologic tests for syphilis. *Pediatr Infect Dis J* 1994;13:845.

♦ Prober CG, Stevenson DK, Benitz WE: The use of antibiotics in neonates weighing less than 1200 grams. *Pediatr Infect Dis J* 1990;9:111.

♦ Roberts RJ: *Drug Therapy in Infants.* Philadelphia: WB Saunders Co, 1984, p45.

♦ Pyati SP, Pildes RS, Jacobs NM, et al: Penicillin in infants weighing two kilograms or less with early onset group B streptococcal disease. *N Engl J Med* 1983;308:1383.

♦ McCracken GH Jr, Ginsburg C, Chrane DF, et al: Clinical pharmacology of penicillin in newborn infants. *J Pediatr* 1973;82:692.

References updated 3/2001
Compatibilities updated 3/2001

Piperacillin

ANTIBIOTICS

Dose & Administration

50 to 100 mg/kg per dose IV infusion by syringe pump over 30 minutes, or IM.

To use dosing chart, please refer to explanatory note on page iii

Dosing Interval Chart

PMA (weeks)	PostNatal (days)	Interval (hours)
≤29	0 to 28	12
	>28	8
30 to 36	0 to 14	12
	>14	8
37 to 44	0 to 7	12
	>7	8
≥45	ALL	6

Uses

Semisynthetic penicillin with increased activity against *Pseudomonas aeruginosa* and many strains of *Klebsiella, Serratia, E coli, Enterobacter, Citrobacter,* and *Proteus.* Also effective against group B *Streptococcus.*

Monitoring

Desired peak serum concentration is approximately 150 mcg/mL. Desired trough concentration ranges from 15 to 50 mcg/mL (available as bioassay). Peak serum concentration is lower with IM administration. Observe IV site for signs of extravasation.

Adverse Effects/Precautions

Eosinophilia. Hyperbilirubinemia. Elevations in ALT, AST, BUN, and serum creatinine.

Pharmacology

Piperacillin is a potent, broad-spectrum, semi-synthetic, ureidopenicillin possessing high activity against gram-negative bacteria. Inactivation by β-lactamase-producing bacteria. Synergistic with aminoglycosides. Good penetration into bone; CSF penetration similar to that of other penicillins. Serum half-life depends on gestational age and postnatal age. Primarily excreted renally unchanged.

continued...

Special Considerations/Preparation

Available as powder for injection in 2-g, 3-g, and 4-g vials. Reconstitute 2-g vial with 4 mL of sterile water for injection to make a final concentration of 400 mg/mL. Reconstituted solution stable for 24 hours at room temperature, 2 days refrigerated. A 100 mg/mL dilution may be made by adding 2.5 mL of reconstituted solution to 7.5 mL sterile water for injection. Dilution stable for 7 days refrigerated.

IM Administration: Use 400 mg/mL concentration.

Solution Compatibility: D_5W, $D_{10}W$, and NS.

Terminal Injection Site Compatibility: Dex/AA and fat emulsion. Acyclovir, aminophylline, aztreonam, clindamycin, enalaprilat, esmolol, famotidine, heparin, hydrocortisone succinate, linezolid, lorazepam, midazolam, morphine, potassium chloride, propofol, ranitidine, remifentanil, and zidovudine.

Incompatibility: Aminoglycoside antibiotics, fluconazole, and vancomycin.

Selected References

♦ Kacet N, Roussel-Delvallez M, Gremillet C, et al: Pharmacokinetic study of piperacillin in newborns relating to gestational and postnatal age. *Pediatr Inf Dis J* 1992;11:365.

♦ Prober CG, Stevenson DK, Benitz WE: The use of antibiotics in neonates weighing less than 1200 grams. *Pediatr Infect Dis J* 1990;9:111.

♦ Reed MD, Myers CM, Yamashita TS, Blumer JL: Developmental pharmacology and therapeutics of piperacillin in gram-negative infections. *Dev Pharmacol Ther* 1986;9:102.

♦ Plazek M, Whitelaw A, Want S, et al: Piperacillin in early neonatal infection. *Arch Dis Child* 1983;58:1006.

Updated 3/97
Compatibilities updated 3/2003

Piperacillin-Tazobactam

Dose & Administration

50 to 100 mg/kg per dose IV infusion by syringe pump over 30 minutes.

To use dosing chart, please refer to explanatory note on page iii

Dosing Interval Chart

PMA (weeks)	PostNatal (days)	Interval (hours)
≤29	0 to 28	12
	>28	8
30 to 36	0 to 14	12
	>14	8
37 to 44	0 to 7	12
	>7	8
≥45	ALL	8

Uses

Treatment of non-CNS infections, caused by susceptible β-lactamase producing bacteria, including many strains of *E. coli, Enterobacter, Klebsiella, Haemophilus influenzae, Proteus mirabilis, Pseudomonas spp.,* and *Staph. aureus.* Also effective against group *B Streptococcus.*

Monitoring

Observe IV site for signs of extravasation.

Adverse Effects/Precautions

Eosinophilia. Hyperbilirubinemia. Elevations in ALT, AST, BUN, and serum creatinine.

Pharmacology

Zosyn® combines the extended-spectrum antibiotic piperacillin with the β-lactamase inhibitor tazobactam in a 8:1 ratio. Piperacillin is primarily eliminated unchanged by renal mechanisms, whereas tazobactam undergoes significant hepatic metabolism. The mean half-life of piperacillin and tazobactam in neonates is approximately 1.5 hours. CNS penetration is modest (limited data). Sodium content is 2.35 mEq per gram of piperacillin.

continued...

Special Considerations/Preparation

Available as powder for injection in 2-g, 3-g, 4-g, and 36-g preservative free vials. Reconstitute 2-g vial with 10 mL of sterile water for injection to make a final concentration of 200 mg/mL. Reconstituted solution stable for 24 hours at room temperature, 2 days refrigerated.

Solution Compatibility: D_5W, $D_{10}W$, and NS.

Terminal Injection Site Compatibility: Dex/AA and fat emulsion. Aminophylline, aztreonam, bumetanide, calcium gluconate, cefepime, cimetidine, clindamycin, dexamethasone, dopamine, enalaprilat, esmolol, fluconazole, furosemide, heparin, hydrocortisone succinate, linezolid, lorazepam, metoclopramide, metronidazole, morphine, potassium chloride, ranitidine, remifentanil, sodium bicarbonate, trimethoprim-sulfamethoxazole, and zidovudine.

Incompatibility: Acyclovir, aminoglycoside antibiotics, amphotericin B, dobutamine, famotidine, and vancomycin.

Selected References

♦ Pilley T, Pillay D, Adhikari M, Sturn A: Piperacillin/tazobactam in the treatment of Klebsiella pneumoniae infections in neonates. *Am J Perinatol* 1998;15:47-51.

♦ Reed MD, Goldfarb J, Yamashita TS, Blumer JL: Piperacillin and tazobactam in infants and children. *Antimicrob Agents Chemother* 1994;38:2817-26.

♦ Schoonover L, Occhipinti D, Rodvold K, et al: Piperacillin/tazobactam: A new β-lactam/β-lactamase inhibitor combination. *Ann Pharmacother* 1995;29:501-14.

♦ Prober CG, Stevenson DK, Benitz WE: The use of antibiotics in neonates weighing less than 1200 grams. *Pediatr Infect Dis J* 1990;9:111.

Added 3/2003

Rifampin

Dose and Administration

PO: 10 to 20 mg/kg per dose Q24 hours. May administer with feedings.

IV: 5 to 10 mg/kg per dose Q24 hours, given via syringe pump over 30 minutes.

Do not administer IM or SC.

Prophylaxis for high-risk contacts of invasive meningococcal disease: 5 mg/kg per dose PO Q12 hours, for 2 days.

Prophylaxis for high-risk contacts of invasive H influenzae type b disease: 10 mg/kg per dose PO Q24 hours, for 4 days.

Uses

Used in combination with vancomycin or aminoglycosides for treatment of persistent staphylococcal infections. Prophylaxis against infections caused by *N meningitidis* and *H influenzae* type b .

Monitoring

Monitor hepatic transaminases and bilirubin. Periodic CBC for thrombocytopenia. Observe IV site for signs of extravasation.

Adverse Effects/Precautions

Causes orange/red discoloration of body secretions (e.g. sweat, urine, tears, sputum). Induces hepatic microsomal enzymes, enhancing metabolism of some drugs (e.g. cimetidine, dexamethasone, digoxin, enalapril, fluconazole, propranolol, and zidovudine). Extravasation may cause local irritation and inflammation.

Pharmacology

Rifampin is a semisynthetic antibiotic with a wide spectrum of antibacterial activity against staphylococci, most streptococci, *H influenzae, Neisseria sp., Legionella, Listeria,* some *Bacteroides* species, Mycobacterium tuberculosis, and certain atypical mycobacterium. Enterococci and aerobic gram-negative bacilli are generally resistant. Not used as monotherapy because resistance may develop during therapy. Inhibits transcription of DNA to RNA by binding to the beta subunit of bacterial RNA-polymerase. Well absorbed orally. Rapidly deacetylated to desacetylrifampin (active metabolite) and undergoes enterohepatic circulation. Nearly all of the rifampin excreted into the bile is deacetylated within 6 hours. Serum half-life ranges from 1 to 3 hours.

continued...

Special Considerations/Preparation

Available as a lyophilized powder for injection in 600-mg vials. Reconstitute with sterile water for injection to make a final concentration of 60 mg/mL. Reconstituted solution is stable for 24 hours at room temperature. Further dilution is required - maximum concentration for infusion is 6 mg/mL. A 3-mg/mL dilution may be made by adding 0.5 mL of reconstituted solution to 9.5 mL of D_5W or NS. Dilution made with D_5W is stable for 4 hours at room temperature. Dilution made with NS is stable for 2 hours. Do not use if solution precipitates.

A neonatal suspension may be prepared by mixing 5 mL (300 mg) of the reconstituted IV solution with 25 mL of simple syrup to make a final concentration of 10 mg/mL. Shake well before use. Suspension is stable for 4 weeks at room temperature or refrigerated. Also available in 150- and 300-mg capsules. Preparation of oral suspension using capsules yields variable dosage bioavailability.

Solution compatibility: D_5W and NS. No data available on Dex/AA or fat emulsion.

Terminal injection site compatibility: No data available.

Selected References

♦ Tan TQ, Mason EO, Ou C-N, et al: Use of intravenous rifampin in neonates with persistent staphylococcal bacteremia. *Antimicrob Agents Chemother* 1993;37:2401.

♦ Koup JR, William-Warren J, Viswanathan CT, et al: Pharmacokinetics of rifampin in children. II. Oral bioavailability. *Ther Drug Monit* 1986;8:17.

♦ Koup JR, William-Warren J, Weber A, et al: Pharmacokinetics of rifampin in children. I. Multiple dose intravenous infusion. *Ther Drug Monit* 1986;8:11.

♦ McCracken GH, Ginsburg CM, Zweighaft TC, et al: Pharmacokinetics of rifampin in infants and children: relevance to prophylaxis against Haemophilus influenzae type B disease. *Pediatrics* 1980;66:17

♦ Nahata MC, Morosco RS, Hipple TF: Effect of preparation method and storage on rifampin concentration in suspensions. *Ann Pharmacother* 1994;28:182.

Added 3/98

Ticarcillin-Clavulanate

Dose and Administration
75 to 100 mg/kg per dose IV infusion by syringe pump over 30 minutes.

To use dosing chart, please refer to explanatory note on page iii

Dosing Interval Chart

PMA (weeks)	Postnatal (days)	Interval (hours)
≤29	0 to 28 >28	12 8
30 to 36	0 to 14 >14	12 8
37 to 44	0 to 7 >7	12 8
≥45	All	6

Uses
Treatment of non-CNS infections, caused by susceptible ß-lactamase producing bacteria, including many strains of *E. coli, Enterobacter, Klebsiella, Haemophilus influenzae, Proteus mirabilis, Pseudomonas spp.,* and *Staph. aureus.*

Monitoring
Serum concentrations are not routinely monitored. Assess renal function prior to therapy. Measure serum sodium concentrations and hepatic transaminases periodically. Observe IV site for signs of extravasation.

Adverse Effects/Precautions
Eosinophilia. Hyperbilirubinemia. Elevations in ALT, AST, BUN, and serum creatinine. Hypernatremia may be exacerbated in ELBW patients.

Pharmacology
Timentin® combines the extended-spectrum antibiotic ticarcillin with the ß-lactamase inhibitor clavulanic acid in a 30:1 ratio. Ticarcillin is primarily eliminated unchanged by renal mechanisms, whereas clavulanate undergoes significant hepatic metabolism. As a result the mean half-life of ticarcillin in neonates is 4.2 hours compared to a mean half-life of 2 hours for clavulanate. CNS penetration is modest (limited data). Sodium content is 4.75 mEq per gram, therefore each dose will contain 0.35 to 0.48 mEq per kg body weight.

continued...

Special Considerations/Preparation

Available as powder for injection in 3.1-g vials. Reconstitute vial by adding 13.1 mL of sterile water for injection to make a final concentration of 200 mg/mL of ticarcillin. Reconstituted solution stable for 6 hours at room temperature, 72 hours refrigerated. May be further diluted prior to administration in a compatible solution. Dilutions stable for 24 hours at room temperature, 3 days refrigerated, and 7 days frozen.

Solution compatibility: D_5W, LR, and NS.

Terminal injection site compatibility: Dex/AA and fat emulsion. Acyclovir, aztreonam, cefepime, famotidine, fluconazole, heparin, insulin, morphine, propofol, remifentanil, and theophylline.

Incompatibility: Aminoglycoside antibiotics, sodium bicarbonate and vancomycin.

Selected References

♦ Rubino CM, Gal P, Ransom JL: A review of the pharmacokinetic and pharmacodynamic characteristics of ß-lactam/ß-lactamase inhibitor combination antibiotics in premature infants. *Pediatr Inf Dis J* 1998;17:1200-1210.

♦ Reed MD: A reassessment of ticarcillin/clavulanic acid dose recommendations for infants, children, and adults. *Pediatr Infect Dis J* 1998;17:1195-1199.

Added 3/2002

Tobramycin

Dose and Administration

During the first week of life:

Gestation (weeks)	Dose (mg/kg/dose)	Interval (hours)
≤29*	5	48
30 to 33	4.5	48
34 to 37	4	36
≥38	4	24
* or significant asphyxia, PDA, or treatment with indomethacin		

IV infusion by syringe pump over 30 minutes. Administer as a separate infusion from penicillin-containing compounds. IM injection is associated with variable absorption, especially in the very small infant.

First week of life: Serum drug concentrations are usually not necessary except in patients with serious infections or significantly changing fluid or renal status. It is not necessary to wait for 'steady state': Peak levels may be measured after the first dose, and trough levels may be measured before the second dose.

After the first week: Administer an initial dose of 4 mg/kg, then measure a peak serum concentration 30 minutes after end of infusion, and another 12 to 24 hours later to determine dosing interval.

Example: Baby X is born at 28 weeks gestation. At 3 weeks of age, gentamicin therapy is begun. A 4 mg/kg dose is administered, with a peak serum concentration of 8.5 mcg/mL. 24 hours later, the serum concentration is 2.8 mcg/mL, yielding a calculated half-life of 15 hours. The predicted serum concentration at 48 hours postdose is 0.9 mcg/mL, and therefore the suggested dosing interval is 48 hours.

Uses

Treatment of infections caused by aerobic gram-negative bacilli (e.g. *Pseudomonas, Klebsiella, E coli*). Usually used in combination with a β-lactam antibiotic.

Monitoring

Therapeutic serum concentrations:
    Peak: 5 to 12 mcg/mL (or C_{max}/MIC ratio greater than 8:1)
(Draw 30 minutes after end of infusion, 1 hour after IM injection.)
    Trough: 0.5 to 1 mcg/mL
Blood samples obtained to monitor drug levels should be spun and refrigerated or frozen as soon as possible. Assess renal function.

Adverse Effects/Precautions

Transient and reversible renal tubular dysfunction may occur, resulting in increased urinary losses of sodium, calcium, and magnesium. Potential vestibular and auditory ototoxicity, especially if treating with other nephrotoxic and/or ototoxic medications (e.g. furosemide, vancomycin). Neuromuscular weakness and respiratory failure may be potentiated when treating concomitantly with pancuronium or other neuromuscular blocking agents, and in patients with hypermagnesemia.

continued...

Pharmacology

New dosing recommendations are based on concepts promoted in adult studies of "once-a-day" dosing: (1) Higher peak concentrations are desirable to increase concentration-dependent bacterial killing; (2) There is a post-antibiotic effect on bacterial killing, especially when treating concurrently with a β-lactam antibiotic; (3) There may be less toxicity with less frequent dosing, due to less renal drug accumulation. Volume of distribution is increased and clearance is decreased in patients with PDA. Serum half-life is also prolonged in premature and asphyxiated newborns. Inactivation of tobramycin by penicillin-containing compounds appears to be a time-, temperature-, and concentration-dependent process. This is probably clinically significant only when penicillin-containing compounds are mixed in IV solutions or when blood is allowed to set at room temperature for several hours before serum drug concentration is assayed.

Special Considerations/Preparation

Pediatric injectable solution available in a concentration of 10 mg/mL.

Solution Compatibility: D_5W, $D_{10}W$, and NS.

Terminal Injection Site Compatibility: Dex/AA and fat emulsion. Acyclovir, amiodarone, aztreonam, calcium gluconate, cefoxitin, clindamycin, dopamine, enalaprilat, esmolol, fluconazole, furosemide, insulin, heparin (concentrations ≤1 U/mL), linezolid, metronidazole, midazolam, morphine, ranitidine, remifentanil, theophylline, tolazoline, and zidovudine.

Incompatibility: Amphotericin B, ampicillin, cefepime, imipenem/cilastatin, indomethacin, heparin (concentrations >1 U/mL), methicillin, mezlocillin, nafcillin, oxacillin, penicillin G, propofol, and ticarcillin/clavulanate.

Selected References

♦ Ohler KH, Menke JA, Fuller L: Use of higher dose extended interval aminoglycosides in a neonatal intensive care unit. *Am J Perinatol* 2000;17:285-290.

♦ Lundgren FS, Glasscock GF, Kim EH, Cohen RS: Once-daily gentamicin dosing in newborn infants. *Pediatrics* 1999;103:1228-1234.

♦ Thureen PJ, Reiter PD, Gresores A, et al: Once- versus twice-daily gentamicin dosing in neonates > 34 weeks gestation: Cost-effectiveness analysis. *Pediatrics* 1999;103:594.

♦ Hayani KC, Hatzopoulos FK, Frank AL, et al: Pharmacokinetics of once-daily dosing of gentamicin in neonates. *J Pediatr* 1997;131:76-80.

♦ de Hoog M, Schoemaker RC, Mouton JW, van den Anker JN: Tobramycin population pharmacokinetics in neonates. *Clin Pharmacol Ther* 1997;62:392-399.

♦ Skopnik H, Wallraf R, Nies B, et al: Pharmacokinetics and antibacterial activity of daily gentamicin. *Arch Dis Child* 1992;67:57-61.

♦ Giapros VI, Andronikou S, Cholevas VI, Papadopoulou ZL: Renal function in premature infants during aminoglycoside therapy. *Pediatr Nephrol* 1995;9:163.

♦ Daly JS, Dodge RA, Glew RH, et al: Effect of time and temperature on inactivation of aminoglycosides by ampicillin at neonatal dosages. *J Perinatol* 1997;17:42-45.

♦ Williams BS, Ransom JL, Gal P, et al: Gentamicin pharmacokinetics in neonates with patent ductus arteriosus. *Crit Care Med* 1997;25:273-275.

Updated 3/2000
Compatibilities updated 3/2003

Vancomycin

Dose & Administration

IV infusion by syringe pump over 60 minutes.

Meningitis: 15 mg/kg per dose

Bacteremia: 10 mg/kg per dose

To use dosing chart, please refer to explanatory note on page iii

Dosing Interval Chart

PMA (weeks)	PostNatal (days)	Interval (hours)
≤29	0 to 14 >14	18 12
30 to 36	0 to 14 >14	12 8
37 to 44	0 to 7 >7	12 8
≥45	ALL	6

Uses

Drug of choice for serious infections caused by methicillin-resistant staphylococci (e.g. *S aureus* and *S epidermidis*) and penicillin-resistant pneumococci.

Monitoring

Serum trough concentrations should be followed in neonates because of changes in renal function related to maturation and severity of illness. Peak concentrations have not been clearly demonstrated to correlate with efficacy, but monitoring these has been recommended when treating meningitis.

    Trough: 5 to 10 mcg/mL

    Peak: 30 to 40 mcg/mL (when treating meningitis)

        (Draw 30 minutes after end of infusion.)

Assess renal function. Observe IV site for signs of extravasation and phlebitis.

Adverse Effects/Precautions

Nephrotoxicity and ototoxicity: Enhanced by aminoglycoside therapy.

Rash and hypotension (red man syndrome): Appears rapidly and resolves within minutes to hours. Lengthening infusion time usually eliminates risk for subsequent doses.

Neutropenia: Reported after prolonged administration (more than 3 weeks).

Phlebitis: May be minimized by slow infusion and dilution of the drug.

Pharmacology

Bactericidal—interferes with cell wall synthesis, inhibits RNA synthesis, and alters plasma membrane function. Diffuses readily and is widely distributed in most body fluids. CSF concentrations in premature infants ranged from 26 to 68% of serum concentrations. Small amount of hepatic metabolism.

continued...

Special Considerations/Preparation

Available as powder for injection in 500-mg and 1-g vials. Reconstitute 500-mg vial with 10 mL sterile water for injection to make a final concentration of 50 mg/mL. Reconstituted solution stable for 14 days refrigerated. A 5 mg/mL dilution may be made by adding 10 mL of this reconstituted solution to a 90-mL normal saline minibag. Dilution stable for 4 days refrigerated.

Solution Compatibility: D_5W, $D_{10}W$, and NS.

Terminal Injection Site Compatibility: Dex/AA and fat emulsion. Acyclovir, amikacin, ampicillin, aminophylline, amiodarone, aztreonam, calcium gluconate, cimetidine, enalaprilat, esmolol, famotidine, fluconazole, heparin (concentrations ≤1 U/mL), hydrocortisone succinate, insulin, linezolid, lorazepam, meropenem, midazolam, morphine, pancuronium bromide, potassium chloride, propofol, ranitidine, remifentanil, sodium bicarbonate, tolazoline, vecuronium, and zidovudine.

Incompatibility: Cefazolin, cefepime, cefotaxime, cefoxitin, ceftazidime, ceftriaxone, chloramphenicol, dexamethasone, heparin (concentrations >1 U/mL), methicillin, mezlocillin, nafcillin, pentobarbital, phenobarbital, piperacillin, piperacillin-tazobactam, ticarcillin, and ticarcillin/clavulanate.

Selected References

♦ de Hoog M, Schoemaker RC, Mouton JW, van den Anker JN: Vancomycin population pharmacokinetics in neonates. *Clin Pharmacol Ther* 2000;67:360-367.

♦ Ahmed A: A critical evaluation of vancomycin for treatment of bacterial meningitis. *Pediatr Inf Dis J* 1997;16:895-903.

♦ Trissel LA, Gilbert DL, Martinez JF: Concentration dependency of vancomycin hydrochloride compatibility with β-lactam antibiotics during simulated y-site administration. *Hosp Pharm* 1998;33:1515-1520.

♦ Reiter PD, Doron MW: Vancomycin cerebrospinal fluid concentrations after intravenous administration in premature infants. *J Perinatol* 1996;16:331-335.

♦ Schilling CG, Watson DM, McCoy HG, Uden DL: Stability and delivery of vancomycin hydrochloride when admixed in a total parenteral nutrition solution. *JPEN* 1989;13:63.

♦ Lacouture PG, Epstein MF, Mitchell AA: Vancomycin-associated shock and rash in newborn infants. *J Pediatr* 1987;111:615.

♦ Schaible DH, Rocci mL, Alpert GA, et al: Vancomycin pharmacokinetics in infants: Relationships to indices of maturation. *Pediatr Infect Dis J* 1986;5:304.

Updated 3/2002
Compatibilities updated 3/2003

Zidovudine (ZDV, AZT)

Dose & Administration

IV: 1.5 mg/kg per dose, given via infusion pump over 1 hour.
PO: 2 mg/kg per dose.

Dosing Interval Chart

Gestational Age (weeks)	Postnatal Age (days)	Interval (hours)
≤29	0 to 28	12
	>28	8
30 to 34	0 to 14	12
	>14	8
≥35	ALL	6

Do not administer IM.

Begin treatment within 6 to 12 hours of birth, and continue for 6 weeks. Initiation of post-exposure prophylaxis after the age of 2 days is not likely to be effective. Subsequent treatment is based on HIV culture results and clinical status.

Uses

Treatment of neonates born to HIV-infected women.

Monitoring

CBC at the beginning of therapy, then every other week to assess for anemia, thrombocytopenia, and neutropenia.

Adverse Effects/Precautions

Anemia and neutropenia occur frequently, and are associated with serum concentrations greater than 3 µmol/L. Mild cases usually respond to a reduction in dose. Severe cases may require cessation of treatment and/or transfusion. Concomitant treatment with fluconazole significantly reduces zidovudine metabolism - dosing interval should be prolonged.

Pharmacology

Zidovudine is a nucleoside analog that inhibits HIV replication by interfering with viral reverse transcriptase. It is converted intracellularly in several steps to a triphosphate derivative, metabolized via hepatic glucuronidation, then renally excreted. Protein binding is approximately 25%. Zidovudine distributes into cells by passive diffusion and is relatively lipophilic. The CSF: plasma ratio is 0.24. The relationship between serum concentration and clinical efficacy is unclear. The oral syrup is well-absorbed, but only 65% bioavailable due to significant first-pass metabolism. The serum half-life in term newborns is 3 hours, declining to 2 hours after 2 weeks of age. In preterm infants less than 33 weeks gestation, half-life during the first two weeks of life ranges from 5 to 10 hours, decreasing to 2 to 6 hours afterward.

continued...

Zidovudine (ZDV, AZT)

Special Considerations/Preparation

Available as a syrup for oral use in a concentration of 10 mg/mL.
The IV form is supplied in a concentration of 10 mg/mL in a 20 mL single-use vial. **Dilute before IV administration to a concentration not exceeding 4 mg/mL.** A dilution of 4 mg/mL may be prepared by adding 4 mL of the 10-mg/mL concentration to 6 mL D_5W. After dilution the drug is stable at room temperature for 24 hours. Both forms should be stored at room temperature and protected from light.

Solution Compatibility: D_5W and NS.

Terminal Injection Site Compatibility: Dex/AA and fat emulsion. Acyclovir, amikacin, amphotericin B, aztreonam, cefepime, ceftazidime, ceftriaxone, cimetidine, clindamycin, dexamethasone, dobutamine, dopamine, erythromycin lactobionate, fluconazole, gentamicin, heparin, imipenem, linezolid, lorazepam, meropenem, metoclopramide, morphine, nafcillin, oxacillin, piperacillin, piperacillin-tazobactam, potassium chloride, ranitidine, remifentanil, tobramycin, trimethoprim-sulfamethoxazole, and vancomycin.

Incompatibility: Blood products and protein solutions.

Selected References

♦ Capparelli EV, Mirochnick MH, Danker WM: Pharmacokinetics and tolerance of zidovudine in preterm infants. *J Pediatr* 2003;142:47-52.

♦ Perinatal HIV Guidelines Working Group: Public Health Service Task Force recommendations for use of antiretroviral drugs in pregnant HIV-1-infected women with for maternal health and interventions to reduce perinatal HIV-1 transmission in the United States. (update published August 30, 2002 on the HIV/AIDS Treatment Information Service ATIS website: http://www.aidsinfo.nih.gov).

♦ American Academy of Pediatrics. Antiretroviral therapy. In: Pickering LK, ed. *2000 Red Book: Report of the Committee on Infectious Diseases.* 25th ed. Elk Grove Village, IL: American Academy of Pediatrics; 2000: pp 681-682.

♦ Mirochnick MH, Capparelli EV, Conner J: Pharmacokinetics of zidovudine in infants: A population analysis across studies. *Clin Pharmacol Ther* 1999;66:16-24.

♦ Acosta EP, Page LM, Fletcher CV: Clinical pharmacokinetics of zidovudine. *Drugs* 1996;30:251.

♦ Conner EM, Sperling RS, Gelber R, et al: Reduction of maternal-infant transmission of human immunodeficiency virus type 1 with zidovudine treatment. *N Engl J Med* 1994;331:1173.

♦ Boucher FD, Modlin JF, Weller S: Phase I evaluation of zidovudine administered to infants exposed at birth to the human immunodeficiency virus. *J Pediatr* 1993;122:137.

♦ Product Information, GlaxoSmithKline: *Physicians' Desk Reference,* ed 57. Montvale, NJ: Thomson PDR, 2003, p 1629.

Dosing and References updated 3/2003
Compatibilities updated 3/2003

BIOLOGICALS

BIOLOGICALS

Recommended Childhood Immunization Schedule United States, 2003

range of recommended ages
catch-up vaccination
preadolescent assessment

Vaccine ► / Age ►	Birth	1 mo	2 mos	4 mos	6 mos	12 mos	15 mos	18 mos	24 mos	4-6 yrs	11-12 yrs	13-18 yrs
Hepatitis B[1]	Hep B #1 only if mother HBsAg (-)	Hep B #2			Hep B #3						Hep B series	
Diphtheria, Tetanus, Pertussis[2]			DTaP	DTaP	DTaP		DTaP	DTaP		DTaP	Td	
Haemophilus influenzae Type b[3]			Hib	Hib	Hib	Hib	Hib					
Inactivated Polio			IPV	IPV		IPV		IPV		IPV		
Measles, Mumps, Rubella[4]						MMR #1				MMR #2	MMR #2	MMR #2
Varicella[5]						Varicella	Varicella		Varicella		Varicella	
Pneumococcal[6]			PCV	PCV	PCV	PCV			PCV	PCV	PPV	
Hepatitis A[7]									Hepatitis A series			
Influenza[8]					Influenza (yearly)							

------- Vaccines below this line are for selected populations

Approved by the Advisory Committee on Immunization Practices (www.cdc.gov/nip/acip) the American Academy of Pediatrics (www.aap.org), and the American Academy of Family Physicians (www.aafp.org).

1. **Hepatitis B vaccine (HepB)**. All infants should receive the first dose of hepatitis B vaccine soon after birth and before hospital discharge; the first dose may also be given by age 2 months if the infant's mother is HBsAg-negative. Only monovalent HepB can be used for the birth dose. Monovalent or combination vaccine containing HepB may be used to complete the series. Four doses of vaccine may be administered when a birth dose is given. The second dose should be given at least 4 weeks after the first dose, except for combination vaccines which cannot be administered before age 6 weeks. The third dose should be given at least 16 weeks after the first dose and at least 8 weeks after the second dose. The last dose in the vaccination series (third or fourth dose) should not be administered before age 6 months.

Infants born to HBsAg-positive mothers should receive HepB and 0.5 mL Hepatitis B Immune Globulin (HBIG) within 12 hours of birth at separate sites. The second dose is recommended at age 1-2 months. The last dose in the vaccination series should not be administered before age 6 months. These infants should be tested for HBsAg and anti-HBs at 9-15 months of age.

Infants born to mothers whose HBsAg status is unknown should receive the first dose of the HepB series within 12 hours of birth. Maternal blood should be drawn as soon as possible to determine the mother's HBsAg status; if the HBsAg test is positive, the infant should receive HBIG as soon as possible (no later than age 1 week). The second dose is recommended at age 1-2 months. The last dose in the vaccination series should not be administered before age 6 months.

2. **Diphtheria and tetanus toxoids and acellular pertussis vaccine (DTaP)**. The fourth dose of DTaP may be administered as early as age 12 months, provided 6 months have elapsed since the third dose and the child is unlikely to return at age 15-18 months. **Tetanus and diphtheria toxoids (Td)** is recommended at age 11-12 years if at least 5 years have elapsed since the last dose of tetanus and diphtheria toxoid-containing vaccine. Subsequent routine Td boosters are recommended every 10 years.

3. *Haemophilus influenzae* **type b (Hib) conjugate vaccine**. Three Hib conjugate vaccines are licensed for infant use. If PRP-OMP (PedvaxHIB® or ComVax® [Merck]) is administered at ages 2 and 4 months, a dose at age 6 months is not required. DTaP/Hib combination products should not be used for primary immunization in infants at ages 2, 4 or 6 months, but can be used as boosters following any Hib vaccine.

4. **Measles, mumps, and rubella vaccine (MMR)**. The second dose of MMR is recommended routinely at age 4-6 years but may be administered during any visit, provided at least 4 weeks have elapsed since the first dose and that both doses are administered beginning at or after age 12 months. Those who have not previously received the second dose should complete the schedule by the 11-12 year old visit.

5. **Varicella vaccine**. Varicella vaccine is recommended at any visit at or after age 12 months for susceptible children, i.e. those who lack a reliable history of chickenpox. Susceptible persons aged ≥13 years should receive two doses, given at least 4 weeks apart.

6. **Pneumococcal vaccine**. The heptavalent pneumococcal conjugate vaccine (PCV) is recommended for all children age 2-23 months. It is also recommended for certain children age 24-59 months. Pneumococcal polysaccharide vaccine (PPV) is recommended in addition to PCV for certain high-risk groups. See *MMWR* 2000;49(RR-9):1-38.

7. **Hepatitis A vaccine**. Hepatitis A vaccine is recommended for children and adolescents in selected states and regions, and for certain high-risk groups; consult your local public health authority. Children and adolescents in these states, regions, and high risk groups who have not been immunized against hepatitis A can begin the hepatitis A vaccination series during any visit. The two doses in the series should be administered at least 6 months apart. See *MMWR* 1999;48(RR-12);1-37.

8. **Influenza vaccine**. Influenza vaccine is recommended annually for children age ≥6 months with certain risk factors (including but not limited to asthma, cardiac disease, sickle cell disease, HIV, diabetes, and household members of persons in groups at high risk; see *MMWR* 2002;51(RR-3);1-31), and can be administered to all others wishing to obtain immunity. In addition, healthy children age 6-23 months are encouraged to receive influenza vaccine if feasible because children in this age group are at substantially increased risk for influenza-related hospitalizations. Children aged ≤12 years should receive vaccine in a dosage appropriate for their age (0.25 mL if age 6-35 months or 0.5 mL if aged ≥3 years). Children aged <8 years who are receiving influenza vaccine for the first time should receive two doses separated by at least 4 weeks.

For additional information about vaccines, including precautions and contraindications for immunization and vaccine shortages, please visit the National Immunization Program Web site at www.cdc.gov/nip or call the National Immunization Information Hotline at 800-232-2522 (English) or 800-232-0233 (Spanish).

Thimerosal in Vaccines

Vaccine	Brand Name	Manufacturer	% Thimerosal Concentration[1]	Mercury µg/0.5 mL
DTaP	Infanrix®	GlaxoSmithKline	0	0
	Daptacel™	Aventis Pasteur	0	0
	Tripedia®	Aventis Pasteur	0	0
DT	All Products		.01	25
DTwP-Hib	Tetramune	Wyeth Lederle	.01	25
Hib	ActHIB®	Aventis Pasteur	0	0
	TriHIBit	Aventis Pasteur	0	0
	HibTITER® - Multidose	Wyeth Lederle	.01	25
	- Single dose		0	0
	PedvaxHIB® liquid	Merck	0	0
	COMVAX™[2]	Merck	0	0
Hepatitis B virus	Engerix-B®	GlaxoSmithKline	Trace	<0.5
	Recombivax HB	Merck	0	0
IPV	IPOL™	Aventis Pasteur	0	0
Pneumococcal	Prevnar®	Wyeth Lederle	0	0

[1] A concentration of 1:10,000 is equivalent to a 0.01 concentration. Thimerosal is approximately 50% Hg by weight. A 1:10,000 concentration contains 25 µg of Hg per 0.5 mL.

[2] COMVAX™ is not approved for use under 6 weeks of age because of decreased response to the Hib component.

American Academy of Pediatrics Committee on Infectious Diseases and Committee on Environmental Health, *Pediatrics* 1999;104:570-573. Table revised March 2001 using manufacturers' updated product prescribing information.

DT Vaccine

(Diphtheria and tetanus toxoids for pediatric use)

Dose and Administration

0.5 mL IM in the anterolateral thigh. Immunize premature infants according to their postnatal age. Please refer to most recent AAP/ACIP immunization schedule.

When giving multiple vaccines, use a separate syringe for each and give at different sites. Care should be taken to draw back on the plunger of the syringe before injection to be certain the needle is not in a blood vessel.

Uses

Immunoprophylaxis against diphtheria and tetanus for infants who have a contraindication for pertussis vaccine.

Monitoring/Adverse Effects

Observe injection site for erythema, induration (common), palpable nodule (uncommon), or sterile abscess (rare). Fever (common) may be treated with acetaminophen, 15 mg/kg per dose Q4 hours. Other common, self-limited, systemic effects are drowsiness, fretfulness, and anorexia. Rare anaphylactic reactions (i.e. hives, swelling of the mouth, hypotension, breathing difficulty, and shock) have been reported.

Precautions/Contraindications

Infants with stable neurologic conditions, including well-controlled seizures, may be vaccinated. Infants who have had prior seizures are at increased risk for seizures following DT vaccination; acetaminophen should be used to prevent postvaccination fever.

Pharmacology

Diphtheria and tetanus toxoids are prepared by formaldehyde treatment of the respective toxins. DT vaccine is an aluminum-salt-adsorbed preparation.

Special Considerations/Preparation

DT vaccine (for pediatric use) is available from several manufacturers in 0.5-mL Tubex® and 5-mL vials. Store refrigerated. Do not freeze. Shake vial well before withdrawing each dose. Do not use if product contains clumps that cannot be resuspended with vigorous shaking. Normal appearance is a turbid whitish suspension.

Selected References

♦ American Academy of Pediatrics. Tetanus. In: Pickering LK, ed. *2000 Red Book: Report of the Committee on Infectious Diseases*. 25th ed. Elk Grove Village, IL: American Academy of Pediatrics; 2000: pp 6-13 and 566.

♦ Advisory Committee on Immunization Practices: Diphtheria, tetanus, and pertussis: Recommendations for vaccine use and other preventive measures. *MMWR* 1991;40(RR-10):1.

References updated 3/2001

BIOLOGICALS

DTaP Vaccine

(Diphtheria and tetanus toxoids and acellular pertussis vaccine adsorbed)

Dose and Administration

0.5 mL IM in the anterolateral thigh. Shake vial vigorously before withdrawing each dose. Immunize premature infants according to their postnatal age. Please refer to the most recent AAP/ACIP immunization schedule.

When giving multiple vaccines, use a separate syringe for each and give at different sites. Care should be taken to draw back on the plunger of the syringe before injection to be certain the needle is not in a blood vessel.

Uses

Preferred immunoprophylaxis against diphtheria, tetanus, and pertussis.

Monitoring/Adverse Effects

Minor reactions, such as drowsiness, irritability, fever, anorexia, and pain/erythema/induration at the injection site are similar to those observed with DTwP vaccine, but are significantly less frequent. Moderate to severe reactions are also less frequent. See Precautions/Contraindications below.

Precautions/Contraindications

It is prudent to delay the initial dose of DTaP vaccine in infants with neurologic disorders until further observation and study have clarified their neurologic status and the effect of treatment. Those infants with stable neurologic conditions, including well-controlled seizures, may be vaccinated. Infants who have had prior seizures are at increased risk for seizures following DTP vaccination; acetaminophen should be used to prevent postvaccination fever.

Precautions to further DTaP vaccination (the benefits of administering DTaP may exceed risks in areas with a high incidence of pertussis; otherwise administer DT vaccine):

1) Temperature of $\geq 40.5\,°C$ (105 °F) within 48 hours with no other cause. (Frequency approximately 1 per 3000 doses)
2) Hypotonic-hyporesponsive collapse or shock-like state within 48 hours. (Frequency approximately 1 per 10,000 doses)
3) Inconsolable crying (≥ 3 hours) occurring within 48 hours. (Frequency approximately 1 per 2000 doses)
4) Convulsions with or without fever occurring within 3 days. (Frequency approximately 1 per 14,000 doses)

continued...

Contraindications to further DTaP vaccination: In children who develop encephalopathy within 7 days following any DTP vaccination, DT vaccine should be substituted for the remaining doses. In children who develop an immediate anaphylactic reaction, further immunization with any of the three antigens should be deferred.

Pharmacology

DTaP vaccines are aluminum-salt-adsorbed preparations. All acellular pertussis vaccines contain inactivated pertussis toxoid, but vary in the inclusion and concentration of four other pertussis antigens. Diphtheria and tetanus toxoids are prepared by formaldehyde treatment of the respective toxins. Daptacel™, Infanrix® and Tripedia® are thimerosal-free. Each dose of Daptacel™ contains 15 Lf diphtheria toxoid, 5 Lf tetanus toxoid, 5 mcg fimbriae types 2 and 3, 5 mcg FHA, and 3 mcg pertactin, with 3.3 mg 2-phenoxyethanol as a preservative. Each dose of Infanrix® contains 25 Lf diphtheria toxoid, 10 Lf tetanus toxoid, 25 mcg inactivated toxin, 25 mcg FHA, and 8 mcg pertactin, with 2.5 mg 2-phenoxyethanol as a preservative. Each dose of Tripedia® contains 6.7 Lf diphtheria toxoid, 5 Lf tetanus toxoid, 23.4 mcg inactivated toxin, and 23.4 mcg FHA.

Special Considerations/Preparation

FDA-licensed DTaP vaccines as of March 2003: Infanrix® (SmithKline Beecham), available in single dose vials, Daptacel™ (Aventis Pasteur), available in single dose vials, and Tripedia® (Aventis Pasteur), available in single dose vials and in a 15-dose (7.5 mL) vial. Store refrigerated at 2 °C to 8 °C (36 °F to 46 °F). **Do not freeze.** SHAKE VIAL WELL before withdrawing dose. Do not use if product contains clumps that cannot be resuspended with vigorous shaking. Normal appearance is a turbid whitish suspension.

Selected References

♦ American Academy of Pediatrics. Tetanus. In: Pickering LK, ed. *2000 Red Book: Report of the Committee on Infectious Diseases. 25th* ed. Elk Grove Village, IL: American Academy of Pediatrics; 2000: pp 6-13 and 566.

♦ American Academy of Pediatrics, Committee on Infectious Diseases : Acellular pertussis vaccine: recommendations for use as the initial series in infants and children. *Pediatrics* 1997;99:282.

♦ Centers for Disease Control and Prevention: Update: vaccine side effects, adverse reactions, contraindications, and precautions. Recommendations of the Advisory Committee on Immunization Practices (ACIP). *MMWR* 1996;45(RR-12):1-35.

♦ Product information, GlaxoSmithKline: *Physicians' Desk Reference,* ed 56. Montvale, NJ: Medical Economics Data, 2002, p 1562.

♦ Product information, Aventis Pasteur: *Physicians' Desk Reference,* ed 57. Montvale, NJ: Thomson PDR, 2003, pp 790 and 811.

References updated 3/2003

Epoetin alfa

Dose & Administration
200 to 400 Units/kg/dose, 3 to 5 times per week, for 2 to 6 weeks.
Total dose **per week** is 600 to 1400 Units per kg.
Administer SC, or IV over at least 4 hours (even continuously in TPN).
Supplemental iron therapy should be initiated concurrently.

Uses
To stimulate erythropoiesis and decrease the need for erythrocyte transfusions in high-risk preterm infants. Those most likely to benefit are infants with birth weights < 800 g and phlebotomy losses > 30 mL/kg.

Monitoring
Weekly CBC to check for neutropenia and monitor RBC response.

Adverse Effects/Precautions
The only adverse effect in premature neonates is neutropenia, which occurs rarely and resolves with discontinuation of the drug.

Pharmacology
Epoetin alfa is a 165-amino acid glycoprotein manufactured by recombinant DNA technology that has the same biological effects as endogenous erythropoietin. It acts on mature erythroid progenitors, CFU-E, by binding to cell surface receptors and stimulating differentiation and cell division. Noticeable effects on hematocrit and reticulocyte counts occur within 2 weeks. Adequate iron and protein intake is necessary for epoetin to be effective (additional Vitamin E intake may be necessary as well). Subcutaneously administered drug appears to be pharmacodynamically as effective as IV, despite only 40% bioavailability. Half- life of r-HuEPO in preterm infants is approximately 12 hours. Doses reported in the literature are all stated as Units/kg **per week**. Efficacy may be dose dependent in the range of 500 to 1500 Units/kg per week (see meta-analysis by Garcia et al), but no differences were observed in the randomized trial by Maier et al.

Special Considerations/Preparation
Available in preservative-free, single-use, 1-mL vials containing 2000, 3000, 4000, or 10,000 Units formulated in an isotonic, sodium chloride/sodium citrate buffered solution with 2.5 mg human albumin. **Do not shake.** Undiluted epoetin is stable in plastic syringes for 2 weeks. For IV infusions, dilute epoetin in 2 mL of solutions containing at least 0.05% protein and infuse over 4 hours- these dilutions are stable for 24 hours. Product support for use in neonates is handled by Ortho Biotech, Inc. (Procrit®). A multidose 2-mL vial is also available from Amgen (Epogen®) containing 20,000 Units in a 1% (10 mg/mL) benzyl alcohol solution.

continued...

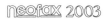

Selected References

♦ Ohls R: Human recombinant erythropoietin in the prevention and treatment of anemia of prematurity. *Paediatr Drugs* 2002;4:111-121.

♦ Garcia MG, Hutson AD, Christensen RD: Effect of recombinant erythropoietin on "late" transfusions in the neonatal intensive care unit: A meta-analysis. *J Perinatol* 2002;22:108-111.

♦ Donato H, Vain N, Rendo P, et al: Effect of early versus late administration of human recombinant human erythropoietin on transfusion requirements in premature infants: Results of a randomized, placebo-controlled, multicenter trial. *Pediatrics* 2000;105:1066.

♦ Maier RF, Obladen M, Kattner E, et al: High- versus low-dose erythropoietin in extremely low birth weight infants. *J Pediatr* 1998;132:866-870.

♦ Ohls RK, Christensen RD: Stability of recombinant human epoetin alfa in commonly used neonatal intravenous solutions. *Ann Pharmacother* 1996;30:466.

♦ Shannon KM, Keith JF, Mentzer WC, et al: Recombinant human erythropoietin stimulates erythropoiesis and reduces erythrocyte transfusions in very low birth weight preterm infants. *Pediatrics* 1995;95:1.

♦ Ohls RK, Osborne KA, Christensen RD: Efficacy and cost analysis of treating very low birth weight infants with erythropoietin during their first two weeks of life: A randomized placebo controlled trial. *J Pediatr* 1995;126:421.

♦ Meyer MP, Meyer JH, Commerford A, et al: Recombinant erythropoietin in the treatment of the anemia of prematurity: Results of a double-blind, placebo-controlled study. *Pediatrics* 1994;93:918.

References updated 3/2003

Haemophilus b (Hib)
Conjugate Vaccine

Dose & Administration

0.5 mL IM in the anterolateral thigh. Please refer to the most recent AAP/ACIP immunization schedule. It is recommended that premature infants should be immunized according to their postnatal age; however, inadequate seroconversion may occur in chronically ill premature infants.

For HbOC and PRP-T, second and third doses are given at 2-month intervals, followed by a fourth dose given at age 15 months.

For PRP-OMP, only the second dose is given after a 2-month interval; the third dose is given at age 15 months.

When giving multiple vaccines, use a separate syringe for each and give at different sites. Care should be taken to draw back on the plunger of the syringe before injection to be certain the needle is not in a blood vessel.

Uses

Immunoprophylaxis against invasive disease caused by *Haemophilus influenzae* type b.

Monitoring

Observe injection site for local reactions.

Adverse Effects/Precautions

Soreness at the injection site with local erythema, swelling, tenderness, and fever.

Pharmacology

Three conjugate vaccines are currently approved for use in infants older than 2 months of age. These vaccines are derived from *H influenzae* type b capsular polysaccharide, polyribosylribitol phosphate (PRP), which is linked to a T-cell-dependent protein antigen to enhance immunogenicity.

continued...

Haemophilus b (Hib) Conjugate Vaccine

Special Considerations/Preparation

Manufacturer	Abbreviation	Trade Name	Carrier Protein
Wyeth Lederle	HbOC	HibTITER®	CRM_{197} (a nontoxic mutant diphtheria toxin)
Aventis Pasteur	PRP-T	ActHIB®	Tetanus toxoid
Merck & Co, Inc	PRP-OMP Liquid	PedvaxHIB®	OMP (an outer membrane protein complex of *N meningitidis*)

BIOLOGICALS

HibTITER® is a clear, colorless solution supplied in single dose (preservative-free) and multidose (thimerosal-containing) vials. Discard if discolored or turbid. Store refrigerated at 2 °C to 8 °C (36 °F to 46 °F). **Do not freeze.**

ActHIB® is supplied as lyophilized powder. Store the lyophilized vaccine and diluent refrigerated at 2 °C to 8 °C (36 °F to 46 °F). **Do not freeze.** Reconstitute using only the 0.4% saline diluent provided in prefilled single-use 0.6-mL syringe and use immediately. Reconstituted vaccine is a clear, colorless solution.

Liquid PedvaxHIB® is supplied in single dose vials. It is a slightly opaque white suspension. Shake well before withdrawal and use. Store refrigerated at 2 °C to 8 °C (36 °F to 46 °F). **Do not freeze**.

Selected References

♦ American Academy of Pediatrics. *Haemophilus influenzae* Infections. In: Pickering LK, ed. *2000 Red Book: Report of the Committee on Infectious Diseases. 25th* ed. Elk Grove Village, IL: American Academy of Pediatrics; 2000: pp 266-8.

♦ Washburn LK, O'Shea TM, Gillis DC, et al: Response to *Haemophilus influenzae* type b conjugate vaccine in chronically ill premature infants. *J Pediatr* 1993;123:791.

♦ Recommendations for use of *Haemophilus* b conjugate vaccines and a combined diphtheria, tetanus, pertussis, and *Haemophilus* b vaccine: Recommendations of the Advisory Committee on Immunization Practices (ACIP). *MMWR* 1993;42 (RR-13):1.

♦ Product information, Wyeth-Lederle Pharmaceuticals: *Physicians' Desk Reference,* ed 57. Montvale, NJ: Medical Economics Data, 2003, p 3402.

♦ Product information, Aventis Pasteur: *Physicians' Desk Reference,* ed 57. Montvale, NJ: Medical Economics Data, 2003, p 786.

♦ Product information, Merck & Co: *Physicians' Desk Reference,* ed 57. Montvale, NJ: Medical Economics Data, 2003, p 2052.

References Updated 3/200

Hib Conjugate-Hepatitis B Combination Vaccine

Dose and Administration

0.5 mL IM in the anterolateral thigh. Please refer to the most recent AAP/ACIP immunization schedule. It is recommended that premature infants should be immunized according to their postnatal age; some data, however, suggest delaying the first dose in chronically ill premature infants due to inadequate seroconversion against *H influenzae*.

When giving multiple vaccines, use a separate syringe for each and give at different sites. Care should be taken to draw back on the plunger of the syringe before injection to be certain the needle is not in a blood vessel.

Uses

COMVAX™ is indicated for vaccination against invasive disease caused by Haemophilus influenzae type b and against infection caused by all known subtypes of hepatitis B virus in infants 6 weeks to 15 months of age born to HBsAg-negative mothers. COMVAX™ should not be used in infants younger than 6 weeks of age.

Monitoring

Observe injection site for local reactions.

Adverse Effects/Precautions

Local pain and tenderness may occur at the injection site.

Pharmacology

COMVAX™ (preservative-free) combines the antigenic components of Recombivax HB® and PedvaxHIB®. Each 0.5 mL dose contains 5 mcg HBsAg and 7.5 mcg *Haemophilus b* -PRP.

Special Considerations/Preparation

Supplied in 0.5-mL unit-dose syringes and multiple-use vials. Store refrigerated. Do not freeze.

Selected References

♦ American Academy of Pediatrics. *Haemophilus influenzae* Infections. In: Pickering LK, ed. *2000 Red Book: Report of the Committee on Infectious Diseases. 25th* ed. Elk Grove Village, IL: American Academy of Pediatrics; 2000: p 267 and 294.

♦ Product information, Merck & Co: *Physicians' Desk Reference,* ed 56. Montvale, NJ: Medical Economics Data, 2002, p 2056.

References updated 3/2002

Hepatitis B Immune Globulin (Human)

Dose and Administration

0.5 mL IM in the anterolateral thigh. Give as soon as it is determined that the mother is HBsAg-positive, within 7 days of birth.

When given at the same time as the first dose of hepatitis B vaccine, use a separate syringe and a different site. Care should be taken to draw back on the plunger of the syringe before injection to be certain the needle is not in a blood vessel.

Uses

Passive immunization of newborns whose mothers have acute hepatitis B infection at the time of delivery, or who are HBsAg-positive. Infants born to mothers who are HBeAg-positive have the highest risk.

Monitoring

No specific monitoring required.

Adverse Effects/Precautions

Local pain and tenderness may occur at the injection site.

Do not administer IV because of the risk of serious systemic reactions. Serious complications of IM injections are rare. Universal precautions should be used with neonates born to HBsAg-positive mothers until they have been bathed carefully to remove maternal blood and secretions.

Pharmacology

Hepatitis B Immune Globulin (human) is a hyperimmune globulin solution prepared from pooled plasma of individuals with high titers of antibody to hepatitis B surface antigen (anti-HBsAg). All donors are HBsAg-negative and HIV-antibody negative. Nabi-HB™ (Nabi) and BayHep B™ (Bayer) are solvent detergent treated and thimerosal free hepatitis B immune globulin preparations.

Special Considerations/Preparation

Refrigerate. Supplied in 0.5-mL unit-dose syringes and multiple-use vials.

Selected References

♦ American Academy of Pediatrics. Hepatitis. In: Pickering LK, ed. *2000 Red Book: Report of the Committee on Infectious Diseases. 25th* ed. Elk Grove Village, IL: American Academy of Pediatrics; 2000: pp 298-300.

♦ Zeldis JB, Crumpacker CS: Hepatitis, in Remington JS, Klein JO (eds): *Infectious Diseases of the Fetus and Newborn Infant,* ed 4. Philadelphia: WB Saunders Co, 1995, p 828.

References updated 3/2001

Hepatitis B Vaccine
(Recombinant)

Dose and Administration

Engerix-B® 10 mcg (0.5 mL) or Recombivax HB® 5 mcg (0.5 mL) IM.

Maternal HBsAg-Positive: Administer first dose before 12 hours of age regardless of gestational age (administer HBIG also).

An infant whose mother's HBsAg status is unknown at delivery should be immunized at birth (within 12 hours). Additional administration of HBIG should depend on results of serologic screening of the mother, which should be done as soon as possible, but not later than 7 days after birth.

Preterm infants with birth weights less than 2 kg have lower seroconversion rates. For infants born to mothers who are HBsAg-positive or HBsAg-unknown, the initial dose given within 12 hours of birth should not be counted in the required 3-dose series. For infants born to HBsAg-negative mothers, delay the first dose until either term PMA or 2 months postnatal age.

Please refer to the most recent AAP/ACIP immunization schedule for subsequent doses. Engerix-B® also has an alternative four-dose schedule: Birth, 1, 2, and 12 to 18 months of age.

Uses

Immunoprophylaxis against hepatitis B. Safe for use in infants born to HIV-positive mothers, although it may be less effective.

Monitoring

Testing for immunity 3 months after completion of the vaccination series is recommended for infants born to HBsAg-positive mothers and, perhaps, for premature infants who received an early first dose.

Adverse Effects/Precautions

The only common side effect is soreness at the injection site. Fever greater than 37.7 °C occurs in 1 to 6%.

continued...

Hepatitis B Vaccine (Recombinant)

Pharmacology

Recombinant hepatitis B vaccines are produced by *Saccharomyces cerevisiae* (common baker's yeast) that has been genetically modified to synthesize HBsAg. Both vaccines are inactivated (noninfective) products that contain HBsAg protein adsorbed to aluminum hydroxide, and may be interchanged with comparable efficacy.

Special Considerations/Preparation

Recombivax HB® for infant use is supplied in 0.5 mL single-dose vials containing 5 mcg. Engerix-B® is supplied in 0.5 mL single-dose vials and 0.5 mL single-dose prefilled disposable syringes containing 10 mcg. The vaccine should be used as supplied; do not dilute. **Shake well before withdrawal and use.** Store refrigerated at **2 °C to 8 °C (36 °F to 46 °F). Do not freeze**–destroys potency.

Selected References

♦ American Academy of Pediatrics. Hepatitis B. In: Pickering LK, ed. *2000 Red Book: Report of the Committee on Infectious Diseases. 25th* ed. Elk Grove Village, IL: American Academy of Pediatrics; 2000: pp 292-295.

♦ Centers for Disease Control and Prevention: Update: vaccine side effects, adverse reactions, contraindications, and precautions. Recommendations of the Advisory Committee on Immunization Practices (ACIP). *MMWR* 1996;45(RR-12):1.

♦ Losonsky GA, Wasserman SS, Stephens I: Hepatitis B vaccination of premature infants: a reassessment of current recommendations for delayed immunization. *Pediatrics* 1999;103(2). URL: http://www.pediatrics.org/cgi/content/full/103/2/e14.

♦ West DJ, Margolis HS: Prevention of hepatitis B virus infection in the United States: A pediatric perspective. *Pediatr Infect Dis J* 1992;11:866.

♦ Centers for Disease Control: Hepatitis B virus: A comprehensive strategy for eliminating transmission in the United States through universal childhood vaccination: Recommendations of the Advisory Committee on Immunization Practices (ACIP). *MMWR* 1991;40 (RR-13):1.

Updated 3/2001

Intravenous Immune Globulin (Human)

BIOLOGICALS

Dose & Administration
Usual dosage of IVIG: 500 to 750 mg/kg per dose over 2 to 6 hours.

See next page for product-specific information.

Uses
Adjuvant treatment of fulminant neonatal sepsis and hemolytic jaundice. Most studies used a single dose, although additional doses have been given at 24 hour intervals.Other reported uses include treatment of immune thrombocytopenia and oral administration for treatment of diarrhea caused by rotavirus.

Monitoring
Frequent monitoring of heart rate and blood pressure. Check IV site for signs of phlebitis.

Adverse Effects/Precautions
Rare cases of hypoglycemia, transient tachycardia, and hypotension that resolved after stopping the infusion have been reported. No short-term or long-term adverse effects have been reported in neonates. Animal studies have demonstrated reticuloendothelial system blockade when higher doses (>1 g/kg) have been used. All donor units are nonreactive to HBsAg and HIV. Note: Hepatitis C has been reported in at least 137 patients who received Gammagard® (Hyland/Baxter) and Polygam® (Baxter/distributed by the American Red Cross) prior to the worldwide recall on February 23, 1994. The manufacturing process of these products now includes a solvent/detergent treatment to inactivate hepatitis C and other membrane-enveloped viruses.

Pharmacology
IVIG is a plasma-derived, concentrated form of IgG antibodies present in the donor population. Significant lot-to-lot variation of specific antibodies may occur with all products. No significant differences in clinical outcomes using the different products have been seen. All preparations are reported to contain more than 92% IgG monomers and a normal distribution of IgG subclasses. Total IgG titers in treated, septic neonates remain elevated for approximately 10 days.

continued...

Intravenous Immune Globulin (Human)

Special Considerations/Preparation

Reconstitute lyophilized products with supplied diluent. All products are preservative-free. Shelf life varies, but is at least 2 years when stored properly.

Solution Compatibility: D_5W, $D_{15}W$, and Dex/AA.

Terminal Injection Site Compatibility: Fluconazole.

Brand	Form	Storage	Preparation*
Gamimune® N (Bayer Pharm.)	5% solution, 10% maltose, pH 4.25	Refrigerate Do not freeze	Allow to come to room temperature.
Gammagard® S/D (Baxter)	0.5 g, 2% glucose, pH 6.8	Room temperature	Rotate gently. Do not shake.
Sandoglobulin® (Novartis)	1, 3, 6, and 12 g 5% or 10% sucrose, pH 6.6	Room temperature	3% and 6% solution. Do not shake.
Gammar®-P (Aventis)	1, 2.5, 5, and 10 g, 5% sucrose, pH 6.8	Room temperature Do not freeze	5% solution
Panglobulin® (American Red Cross)	6 g and 12 g, sucrose, pH 6.8	Room temperature	5% solution
Venoglobulin®, -S (Alpha Therapeutics)	5, 10, & 20 g, 5% & 10% D-sorbitol, pH 5.8	Refrigerate	5% and 10% solution
Polygam®, S/D (American Red Cross)	2.5, 5, and 10 g 5% glucose pH 6.8	Room temperature	5% and 10% solution
IVEEGAM® -EN (Baxter)	0.5, 1, 2.5, and 5 g 5% glucose, pH 7.0	Refrigerate	5% solution

* Reconstitute lyophilized products with supplied diluent. All products are preservative free. Shelf life varies, but is at least 2 years, when stored properly.

Selected References

♦ Jensen HB, Pollock BH: Meta-analyses of the effectiveness of intravenous immune globulin for prevention and treatment of neonatal sepsis. *Pediatrics* 1997;99(2):e2.

♦ Weisman LE, Stoll BJ, Kueser TJ: Intravenous immunoglobulin therapy for early-onset sepsis in premature neonates. *J Pediatr* 1992;121:434.

♦ Christensen RD, Brown MS, Hall DC, et al: Effect on neutrophil kinetics and serum opsonic capacity of intravenous administration of immune globulin to neonates with clinical signs of early-onset sepsis. *J Pediatr* 1991;118:606.

♦ Sandberg K, Fasth A, Berger A, et al: Preterm infants with low immunoglobulin G levels have increased risk for neonatal sepsis byt do not benefit from prophylactic immunoglobulin G. *J Pediatr* 2000;137:623-628.

♦ Gottstein R, Cooke RWI: Systematic review of intravenous immunoglobulin in haemolytic disease of the newborn. *Arch Dis Child Fetal Neonatal Ed* 2003; 88:F6-F10.

♦ Tanyer G, Suklar Z, Dallar Y, et al: Multiple dose IVIG treatment of neonatal immune hemolytic jaundice. *J Trop Pediatr* 2001:47:50-53.

Text updated 3/2003, Preparation Chart updated 3/2002

Pneumococcal 7-Valent Conjugate Vaccine

Dose & Administration

0.5 mL IM in the anterolateral thigh. Please refer to the most recent AAP/ACIP immunization schedule. Immune responses in premature infants have not been studied.

Shake vial vigorously before withdrawing dose.

Do not mix with other vaccines.

When giving multiple vaccines, use a separate syringe for each and give at different sites. Care should be taken to draw back on the plunger of the syringe before injection to be certain the needle is not in a blood vessel.

Uses

Immunoprophylaxis against invasive disease caused by *S. pneumoniae*.

Monitoring

Observe injection site for erythema, induration (common), palpable nodule (uncommon), or sterile abscess (rare). Fever (common) may be treated with acetaminophen, 15 mg/kg per dose Q4 hours. Other common, self-limiting, systemic effects are drowsiness, fretfulness, and anorexia.

Adverse Effects/Precautions

Hypersensitivity to any component of the vaccine, including diphtheria toxoid, is a contraindication to the vaccine.

Pharmacology

Prevnar® is a sterile solution of saccharides of the capsular antigens of *Streptococcus pneumoniae* serotypes 4, 6B, 9V, 14, 18C, 19F, and 23F individually conjugated to diphtheria CRM_{197} protein. The seven serotypes account for approximately 80% of invasive pneumococcal disease in children in the United States. Each dose contains 0.125 mg aluminum as aluminum phosphate adjuvant.

Special Considerations/Preparation

Prevnar® is supplied in 0.5-mL single-dose vials. After being shaken vigorously, it should appear as a homogeneous white suspension. The vaccine should not be used if it cannot be resuspended. Store refrigerated at 2 °C to 8 °C (36 °F to 46 °F). **Do not freeze.**

Incompatibility: Selected References

♦ American Academy of Pediatrics, Committee on Infectious Diseases: Recommendations for the prevention of pneumococcal infections, including the use of pneumococcal conjugate vaccine (Prevnar®), pneumococcal polysaccharide vaccine, and antibiotic prophylaxis. *Pediatrics* 2000;106:362-366.

♦ Shinefield H, Black S, Ray P, et al: Efficacy, immunogenicity and safety of heptavalent pneumococcal conjugate vaccine in low birth weight and preterm infants. *Pediatr Infect Dis J* 2002;21:182-186.

♦ Product information, Wyeth Pharmaceuticals: *Physicians' Desk Reference*, ed 57, Montvale, NJ: Thomson PDR, 2003, p 3455.

References update 3/2003.

Poliovirus Vaccine
Enhanced-Inactivated

Dose & Administration
0.5 mL injected **subcutaneously** in the midlateral thigh. Immunize premature infants according to their postnatal age. Please refer to the most recent immunization schedule.

When giving multiple vaccines, use a separate syringe for each and give at different sites. Care should be taken to draw back on the plunger of the syringe before injection to be certain the needle is not in a blood vessel.

Uses
Preferred initial immunoprophylaxis against poliomyelitis in the United States. Specific indications also include hospitalized infants, and infants with contraindications for OPV (e.g. immunodeficiency, HIV-positive, those with immunodeficient contacts).

Monitoring
No specific monitoring required.

Adverse Effects/Precautions
Occasional reactions include erythema and tenderness at the injection site. Trace components may infrequently cause allergic reactions.

Pharmacology
Sterile suspension of types 1, 2, and 3 poliovirus inactivated with formaldehyde. The vaccine produced using a microcarrier culture technique of monkey kidney cells has enhanced potency. Contains traces of streptomycin, neomycin, and polymyxin B.

Special Considerations/Preparation
IPOL™ (Aventis Pasteur) is a clear, colorless solution, available in 0.5 mL single-dose syringes. Do not use if the vaccine is turbid or discolored. Refrigerate at 2 °C to 8 °C (36 °F to 46 °F). **Do not freeze.**

Selected References
♦ American Academy of Pediatrics. Poliovirus Infections. In: Pickering LK, ed. *2000 Red Book: Report of the Committee on Infectious Diseases. 25th* ed. Elk Grove Village, IL: American Academy of Pediatrics; 2000: pp 467-468.

♦ Product information, Aventis Pasteur: *Physicians' Desk Reference,* ed 57. Montvale, NJ: Medical Economics Data, 2003, p 802.

♦ American Academy of Pediatrics, Committee on Infectious Diseases: Poliomyelitis prevention: recommendations for use of inactivated poliovirus vaccine and live oral poliovirus vaccine. *Pediatrics* 1997;99:300.

References updated 3/2003

BIOLOGICALS

Palivizumab

Dose and Administration

15 mg/kg per dose IM, preferably in the anterolateral aspect of the thigh. The first dose should be administered prior to commencement of the RSV season.

Repeat monthly throughout RSV season.

Uses

Immunoprophylaxis against severe RSV lower respiratory tract infections in high risk infants: those younger than 24 months of age with chronic lung disease or congenital heart disease, those younger than 12 months of age who were born at less than 28 weeks gestation, those younger than 6 months of age who were born at less than 32 weeks gestation, and those infants born at 32 to 35 weeks gestation with an additional risk factor. There are no data regarding treatment of established RSV disease.

Monitoring

Observe injection site for induration and swelling.

Adverse Effects/Precautions

Pain and swelling at the injection site in 2% of recipients. Other adverse events, such as fever (3%) and rash (1%), occur at similar frequencies in patients who received either palivizumab or placebo.

Pharmacology

Humanized monoclonal antibody produced by recombinant DNA technology. This composite of human (95%) and murine (5%) antibody sequences inhibits RSV replication. The mean half-life is 20 days with significant interpatient variability. Adequate antibody titers are maintained for one month following a 15-mg/kg dose. Palivizumab does not interfere with administration of other vaccines.

Special Considerations/Preparation

Synagis® is supplied in single use vials containing 50 mg and 100 mg lyophilized product without preservative. Store refrigerated at 2 to 8 °C (36 to 46 °F). **Do not freeze.**

Reconstitute by slowly adding 0.6 mL sterile water for injection to a 50 mg vial, or 1 mL sterile water for injection to a 100 mg vial. The vial should be gently swirled for 30 seconds to avoid foaming. **Do not shake.** Let stand at room temperature for a minimum of 20 minutes until the solution clarifies. Use within 6 hours of reconstitution.

Selected References

♦ The Impact-RSV Study Group: Palivizumab, a humanized respiratory syncytial virus monoclonal antibody, reduces hospitalization from respiratory syncytial virus infection in high-risk infants. *Pediatrics* 1998;102:531-537.

♦ American Academy of Pediatrics Committee on Infectious Diseases and Committee on Fetus and Newborn: Prevention of respiratory syncytial virus infections: indications for the use of palivizumab and update on the use of RSV-IGIV. *Pediatrics* 1998;102:1211-1216.

♦ Subramanian KNS, Weisman LE, Rhodes T, et al: Safety, tolerance and pharmacokinetics of a humanized monoclonal antibody to respiratory syncytial virus in premature infants and infants with bronchopulmonary dysplasia. *Pediatr Infect Dis J* 1998;17:110-115.

♦ Groothuis JR: Safety and tolerance of palivizumab administration in a large northern hemisphere trial. *Pediatr Inf Dis J* 2001;20:628-629.

Updated 3/2003

RSV Immune Globulin

Respiratory Syncytial Virus Immune Globulin Intravenous

Dose and Administration

750 mg/kg per dose over approximately 3 hours.
Begin infusion rate at 1.5 mL/kg/hr for first 15 minutes. If no change in clinical condition, increase to 3 mL/kg/hr for the next 15 minutes, then to a maximum of 6 mL/kg/hr for the remainder of the infusion.
Repeat monthly during RSV season.

Uses

Immunoprophylaxis against severe RSV lower respiratory tract infections in high risk infants: primarily those younger than 24 months of age with chronic lung disease, those younger than 12 months of age who were born at less than 28 weeks gestation, and those younger than 6 months of age who were born at less than 32 weeks gestation. RSV-IGIV is not efficacious in the treatment of RSV respiratory infections.

Monitoring

Monitor vital signs and oxygen saturation frequently during infusion.

Adverse Effects/Precautions

Do not use in patients with cyanotic congenital heart disease. Do not use in patients with a history of a prior reaction to human immune globulin preparations, or those with selective IgA deficiency. Volume infused is 15 mL/kg: some patients will develop respiratory distress due to fluid overload; furosemide or bumetanide should be available for management. Fever occurs in 3%. Measles / mumps / rubella and varicella vaccines should be delayed until 9 months after the last dose.

Pharmacology

RespiGam® is purified from pooled adult human plasma selected for high titers of neutralizing antibody (IgG) against RSV. A solvent-detergent viral inactivation process is used to decrease the possibility of transmission of blood borne pathogens.

Special Considerations/Preparation

Available in 50 mL (2500 mg) and 20 mL (1000 mg) single-use vials. Refrigerate at 2 °C to 8 °C (36 °F to 46 °F). **Do not freeze. Do not shake.**

Selected References

♦ American Academy of Pediatrics, Committee on Infectious Diseases, Committee on Fetus and Newborn: Respiratory syncytial virus immune globulin intravenous: indications for use. *Pediatrics* 1997;99:645-50.

♦ The PREVENT study group: Reduction of respiratory syncytial virus hospitalization among premature infants and infants with bronchopulmonary dysplasia lsyncytial virus immune globulin prophylaxis. *Pediatrics* 1997;99:93.

♦ Rodriguez WJ, Gruber WC, Groothuis JR, et al: Respiratory syncytial virus immune globulin treatment of RSV lower respiratory tract infections in previously healthy children. *Pediatrics* 1997;100:937-42.

♦ Product information, MedImmune, 1996.

Updated 3/98

CARDIOVASCULAR DRUGS

Adenosine

Dose and Administration
Starting dose: 50 mcg/kg rapid IV push (1 to 2 seconds).
Increase dose in 50 mcg/kg increments Q2 minutes until return of sinus rhythm. Usual maximum dose: 250 mcg/kg.
Infuse as close to IV site as possible. Flush IV with saline immediately.
Intraosseous administration has also been reported to be successful.

Uses
Acute treatment of sustained paroxysmal supraventricular tachycardia. It may also be useful in establishing the cause of the SVT.

Monitoring
Continuous EKG and blood pressure monitoring.

Adverse Effects/Precautions
Flushing, dyspnea, and irritability occur frequently, but usually resolve within 1 minute. Transient (duration <1 minute) arrhythmias may occur between termination of SVT and onset of normal sinus rhythm. Apnea has been reported in one preterm infant. Recurrence of SVT occurs in approximately 30% of treated patients. Theophylline and caffeine diminish adenosine's effect by competitive antagonism.

Pharmacology
Adenosine is the pharmacologically active metabolite of ATP. It acts by depressing sinus node automaticity and A-V node conduction. It does **not** have negative inotropic effects. Response should occur within 2 minutes of the dose. Estimated serum half-life is 10 seconds.

Special Considerations/Preparation
Supplied in 2 mL vials containing 6 mg adenosine dissolved in NS. Contains no preservative. Store at room temperature. **Do not refrigerate;** crystallization will occur. Solution must be clear at the time of use.
Dilutions can be made with NS for doses <0.2 mL (600 mcg). Use 1 mL (3000 mcg) with 9 mL NS to make a solution with a final concentration of 300 mcg/mL.

Selected References
♦ Paret G, Steinmetz D, Kuint J et al: Adenosine for the treatment of paroxysmal supraventricular tachycardia in fullterm and preterm newborn infants. *Am J Perinatol* 1996;13:343-46.

♦ Friedman FD: Intraosseous adenosine for the termination of supraventricular tachycardia in an infant. *Ann Emerg Med* 1996;28:356-58.

♦ Crosson JE, Etheridge SP, Milstein S et al: Therapeutic and diagnostic utility of adenosine during tachycardia evaluation in children. *Am J Cardiol* 1994;74:155-60.

♦ Till J, Shinebourne EA, Rigby ML, et al: Efficacy and safety of adenosine in the treatment of supraventricular tachycardia in infants and children. *Br Heart J* 1989;62:204.

♦ Overholt ED, Rhuban KS, Gutgesell HP, et al: Usefulness of adenosine for arrhythmias in infants and children. *Am J Cardiol* 1988;61:336.

Updated 3/98

Captopril

Dose and Administration
Initial dose: 0.01 to 0.05 mg/kg per dose PO Q8 to 12 hours.
Adjust dose and interval based on response. Administer 1 hour before feeding.

Uses
Treatment of moderate to severe hypertension. Afterload reduction in patients with congestive heart failure.

Monitoring
Frequent assessment of blood pressure, particularly after the first dose. Periodic assessment of renal function and serum potassium.

Adverse Effects/Precautions
Neonates are more sensitive to the effects of captopril than are older infants and children. Significant decreases in cerebral and renal blood flow have occurred in premature infants with chronic hypertension who received higher doses (0.15 to 0.30 mg/kg per dose) than those recommended above. These episodes occurred unpredictably during chronic therapy, and some were associated with neurologic (seizures, apnea, lethargy) and renal (oliguria) complications. **The use of captopril is contraindicated in** patients with bilateral renovascular disease or with unilateral renal artery stenosis in a solitary kidney, as the loss of adequate renal perfusion could precipitate acute renal failure. Hyperkalemia occurs primarily in patients receiving potassium-sparing diuretics or potassium supplements.

Pharmacology
Captopril is an angiotensin-converting enzyme (ACE) inhibitor that blocks the conversion of angiotensin I to angiotensin II, a potent vasoconstrictor. It thereby decreases plasma and tissue concentrations of angiotensin II and aldosterone, and increases plasma and tissue renin activity. Captopril also prevents the breakdown of bradykinin, a potent vasodilator. Vascular resistance is reduced without reflex tachycardia. Beneficial effects are thought to be caused by a combination of afterload reduction and long-term inhibition of salt and water retention. Bioavailability is good in neonates, although food will decrease absorption. Onset of action is 15 minutes after a dose, with peak effects seen in 30 to 90 minutes. Duration of action is usually 2 to 6 hours, but may be significantly longer (>24 hours).

Special Considerations/Preparation
Captopril oral suspension can be made by dissolving 6.25 mg (one half of a scored 12.5 mg tablet) in 10 mL of sterile water, adding 1000 mg of sodium ascorbate for injection (4 mL of 250 mg/mL solution) to decrease oxidation, then adding sufficient water to make a final volume of 200 mL. The final concentration is 0.03 mg/mL captopril and 5 mg/mL sodium ascorbate. Solution is stable for 14 days at room temperature, 56 days refrigerated. Some undissolved excipients will remain visible.

Selected References
♦ Nahata MC, Morosco RS, Hipple TF: Stability of captopril in three liquid dosage forms. *Am J Hosp Pharm* 1994;51:95.
♦ Perlman JM, Volpe JJ: Neurologic complications of captopril treatment of neonatal hypertension. *Pediatrics* 1989;83:47.
♦ O'Dea RF, Mirkin BL, Alward CT: Treatment of neonatal hypertension with captopril. *J Pediatr* 1988;113:403.

Added 1/94

Alteplase

Tissue Plasminogen Activator (t-PA)

Dose & Administration

200 mcg/kg per hour (0.2 mg/kg per hour). Duration of therapy is 6 to 48 hours. If administering directly into the thrombus, dose may be increased after 6 hours to a maximum of 500 mcg/kg per hour. If localized bleeding occurs, stop infusion for 1 hour and restart using 100 mc/kg per hour. Discontinue heparin several hours prior to initiation of therapy.

Note: Reports in the literature are a collection of cases gathered over several years. Some authors used loading doses, others did not. Infused doses ranged from 20 to 500 mcg/kg per hour. Complications were most often linked with higher doses and longer duration of therapy.
Call 1-800-NOCLOTS for case reporting and treatment guidance.

Uses

Dissolution of intravascular thrombi of recent onset that are either intraarterial or life-threatening. Adjuvant treatment of infective endocarditis vegetations.

Monitoring

Follow coagulation studies (PT, aPTT, fibrinogen, fibrin split products) prior to therapy and at least daily during treatment. Maintain fibrinogen levels greater than 100 mg/dL and platelets > 50,000/mm^3. Echocardiography to assess clot lysis at least every 12 hours (Q6 h optimal). Cranial ultrasound to assess for hemorrhage prior to therapy.

Adverse Effects/Precautions

Intracranial hemorrhage may occur, especially in premature infants treated for prolonged periods. Bleeding from venipuncture sites occurs in approximately half of treated patients. The risk of complications increases at doses above 450 mcg/kg per hour.

Pharmacology

Alteplase binds strongly and specifically to fibrin in a thrombus and converts the entrapped plasminogen to plasmin. This initiates local fibrinolysis with limited systemic proteolysis. Alteplase has a shorter half-life than streptokinase and does not cause anaphylactic reactions. It is cleared rapidly from the plasma, primarily via the liver.

continued...

CARDIOVASCULAR

Special Considerations/Preparation

Available as a lyophilized powder for injection in a 50-mg and 100-mg vials. Reconstitute only with sterile water for injection supplied. Gently swirl, **do not shake**, after reconstitution. Reconstituted solutions and dilutions are stable for 8 hours at room temperature.

Solution Compatibility: NS, and D_5W

Terminal Injection Site Compatibility: Lidocaine, morphine, and propranolol.

Incompatibility: Dobutamine, dopamine, and heparin.

Selected References

♦ Manco-Johnson M, Nuss R: Neonatal thrombotic disorders. *NeoReviews* 2000;1:e201.

♦ Hartmann J, Hussein A, Trowitzsch E, et al: Treatment of neonatal thrombus formation with recombinant tissue plasminogen activator: six years experience and review of the literature. *Arch Dis Child Fetal Neonatal Ed* 2001;85:F18-F22.

♦ Marks KA, Zucker N, Kapelushnik J, et al: Infective endocarditis successfully treated in extremely low birth weight infants with recombinant tissue plasminogen activator. *Pediatrics* 2002,109:153-158.

♦ Weiner GM, Castle VP, DiPietro MA, Faix RG: Successful treatment of neonatal arterial thromboses with recombinant tissue plasminogen activator. *J Pediatr* 1998;133:133-136.

Uses and references updated 3/2003
Compatibilities updated 3/2003

CARDIOVASCULAR

Amiodarone

Dose & Administration

IV Loading dose: 5 mg/kg IV infusion given over 30 to 60 minutes, preferably in a central vein.

Maintenance infusion: 7 to 15 mcg/kg per minute (10 to 20 mg/kg per 24 hours). Begin at 7 mcg/kg per minute and titrate by monitoring effects. **Prepare fresh drug Q24 hours due to degradation of amiodarone in solution. Consider switching to oral therapy within 24 to 48 hours.**

PO: 5 to 10 mg/kg per dose Q12 hours.

Uses

Treatment of life-threatening or drug-resistant refractory supraventricular (SVT), ventricular tachyarrhythmias (VT), and postoperative junctional ectopic tachycardia (JET) - see Adverse Effects.

Monitoring

Continuous EKG and blood pressure (for IV). Follow AST and ALT. Monitor T_3, T_4, and TSH. Observe IV site for extravasation.

Adverse Effects/Precautions

Short term toxicity: Bradycardia and hypotension (possibly associated with rapid rates of infusion). Polymorphic ventricular tachycardia. Irritating to the peripheral vessels (concentrations > 2 mg/mL). Administer through central vein if possible.

Long term toxicity: Hyperthyroidism (due to inhibition of T_4 to T_3) and hypothyroidism (due to high concentration of inorganic iodine). Contains 2% benzyl alcohol (20mg/mL). Hepatitis and cholestatic hepatitis (rare). Photosensitivity (10%), nausea and vomiting (10%), optic neuritis (4 to 9%), and pulmonary fibrosis (4 to 9%) have been reported with prolonged oral use in adults.

Pharmacology

Class III antiarrhythmic agent that is an iodinated benzofuran compound. Electrophysiologic activity is accomplished by prolonging the duration of the action potential and increasing the effective refractory period. Increases cardiac blood flow and decreases cardiac work and myocardial oxygen consumption. Highly protein bound (95%) in adults. Extensively metabolized to an active metabolite by the cytochrome CYP3A4 isoenzyme system (limited in preterm infants). Drug-drug interaction potentially occur when given in combination with drugs that inhibit cytochrome CYP3A4: phenytoin, fosphenytoin, clarithromycin, erythromycin, azole antifungals (e.g. fluconazole, ketoconazole, itraconazole), protease inhibitors (e.g. indinavir, ritonavir), class IA and class III antiarrhythmics (e.g. quinidine, procainamide, sotalol) and cimetidine (amiodarone levels increase). Amiodarone prevents the elimination of digoxin resulting in high digoxin levels. Half-life reported to be 26 to 107 days in adults. No data in preterm infants. Accumulates in tissues; serum levels can be detected for months. Contains 37.3% iodine by weight. Adheres to PVC tubing: low infusion rates in neonates may lead to reduced drug delivery during continuous infusions. Oral absorption is variable with approximately 50% bioavailability.

continued...

Amiodarone

Special Considerations/Preparation

IV: Available as 50 mg/mL concentration in 3 mL ampules. Contains 2% (20 mg/mL) of benzyl alcohol and 10% (100 mg/mL) polysorbate (Tween) 80 as a preservative. Store at room temperature and protect from light. **Infusions greater than 1 hour, amiodarone IV concentrations should not exceed 2 mg/mL unless using a central line.**

PO: Supplied in 200 mg tablets. An oral suspension with a final concentration of 5 mg/mL may be made as follows: crush a 200 mg tablet, slowly mix in 20 mL of 1% methylcellulose, then add in 20 mL of simple syrup to make a total volume of 40 mL. Stable for six weeks at room temperature and three months refrigerated when stored in glass or plastic.

Solution Compatibility: D_5W, and NS.

Solution Incompatibility: No data available for Dex/AA solutions.

Terminal Injection Site Compatibility: Amikacin, clindamycin, dobutamine, dopamine, erythromycin, esmolol, furosemide, gentamicin, insulin, isoproterenol, lidocaine, metronidazole, midazolam, morphine, nitroglycerin, penicillin G, potassium chloride, tobramycin, and vancomycin.

Incompatibility: Aminophylline, cefazolin, heparin, mezlocillin, sodium bicarbonate and sodium nitroprusside.

No data available for Dex/AA solutions.

Selected References

♦ Etheridge SP, Craig JE, Compton SJ. Amiodarone is safe and highly effective therapy for supraventricular tachycardia in infants. *Am Heart J* 2001;141:105-110.

♦ Yap SC, Hoomtje T, Sreeram N: Polymorphic ventricular tachycardia after use of intravenous amiodarone for postoperative junctional ectopic tachycardia. *Internat J Cardiol* 2000;76:245-247.

♦ Drago F, Mazza A, Guccione P, et al: Amiodarone used alone or in combination with propranolol: A very effective therapy for tachycarrhythmias in infants and children. *Pediatr Cardiol* 1998;19:445-449.

♦ Grandy J, Wonko N, Kantoch MJ, et al: Risks of intravenous amiodarone in neonates. *Can J Cardiol* 1998;14:855-858.

♦ Bowers PN, Fields J, Schwartz D, et al: Amiodarone induced pulmonary fibrosis in infancy. *PACE* 1998;21:1665-1667.

♦ Nahata MC: Stability of amiodarone in an oral suspension stored under refrigeration and at room temperature. *Ann Pharmcother* 1997;31:851-852.

♦ Pramar YV: Chemical stability of amiodarone hydrocortisone in intravenous fluids. *Int J Pharm Comp* 1997;1:347-348.

♦ Perry JC, Fenrich AL, Hulse JE, et al: Pediatric use of intravenous amiodarone: Efficacy and safety in critically ill patients from a multicenter protocol. *J Am Coll Cardiol* 1996;27:1246-1250.

♦ Soult JA, Munoz M, Lopez JD, et al: Efficacy and safety of intravenous amiodarone for short-term treatment of paroxysmal supraventricular tachycardia in children. *Pediatr Cardiol* 1995;16:16-19.

♦ Figa FH, Gow RW, Hamilton RM, et al: Clinical efficacy and safety of intravenous amiodarone in infants and children. *Am J Cardiol* 1994;74:573-577.

Added 3/2001
Compatibilities updated: 3/2003
References updated: 3/2003

CARDIOVASCULAR

Atropine

Dose & Administration

IV: 0.01 to 0.03 mg/kg per dose IV over 1 minute, or IM. Dose can be repeated Q10 to 15 minutes to achieve desired effect, with a maximum total dose of 0.04 mg/kg.

ET: 0.01 to 0.03 mg/kg per dose immediately followed by 1 mL NS.

PO: Begin with 0.02 mg/kg per dose given Q4 to 6 hours. May increase gradually to 0.09 mg/kg per dose.

Uses

Reversal of severe sinus bradycardia, particularly when parasympathetic influences on the heart (digoxin, beta-blocker drugs, hyperactive carotid sinus reflex) predominate. Also used to reduce the muscarinic effects of neostigmine when reversing neuromuscular blockade.

Monitoring

Heart rate.

Adverse Effects/Precautions

Cardiac arrhythmias can occur, particularly during the first 2 minutes following IV administration; usually a simple A-V dissociation, more often caused by smaller rather than larger doses. Fever, especially in brain-damaged infants. Abdominal distention with decreased bowel activity. Esophageal reflux. Mydriasis and cycloplegia.

Pharmacology

Anticholinergic. Increases heart rate by decreasing the effects of the parasympathetic system while increasing the effects of the sympathetic system. Peak tachycardia is 12 to 16 minutes after dose is given. Relaxes bronchial smooth muscle, thus reducing airway resistance and increasing dead space by 30%. Motor activity in the stomach and small and large intestines is reduced. Esophageal sphincter tone is reduced. Salivary secretion is inhibited. Duration of action is 6 hours. Primarily excreted renally unchanged.

continued...

Special Considerations/Preparation

IV, ET, or IM: Supplied as 0.4 mg/mL, 0.8 mg/mL, and 1 mg/mL for injection.

PO: Give IV dosage form PO.

Prepare IV or PO dilution by mixing 1 mL of injectable atropine (0.4 mg/mL) in 4 mL of sterile water for injection to yield final concentration of 0.08 mg/mL.

Stable for 28 days refrigerated.

Solution Compatibility: D_5W, $D_{10}W$, and NS.

Terminal Injection Site Compatibility: Dex/AA. Cimetidine, dobutamine, famotidine, fentanyl, furosemide, glycopyrolate, heparin, hydrocortisone succinate, meropenem, metoclopramide, midazolam, morphine, nafcillin, netilmicin, pentobarbital, potassium chloride, propofol, prostaglandin E_1, ranitidine, and sodium bicarbonate.

Incompatibility: No data are currently available.

Selected References

♦ Miller BR, Friesen RH: Oral atropine premedication in infants attenuates cardiovascular depression during Halothane anesthesia. *Anesth Analg* 1988;67:180.

♦ Roberts RJ: *Drug Therapy in Infants.* Philadelphia: WB Saunders Co, 1984, p 284.

♦ Adams RG, Verma P, Jackson AJ, Miller RL: Plasma pharmacokinetics of intravenously administered atropine in normal human subjects. *J Clin Pharmacol* 1982;22:477.

♦ Kattwinkel J, Fanaroff AA, Klaus M: Bradycardia in preterm infants: Indications and hazards of atropine therapy. *Pediatrics* 1976;58:494.

♦ Unna KR, Glaser K, Lipton E, Patterson PR: Dosage of drugs in infants and children: I. Atropine. *Pediatrics* 1950;6:197.

Text updated 1/91
Compatibilities updated 3/2001

CARDIOVASCULAR

Digoxin

Dose & Administration

Loading doses: ("Digitalization") are generally used only when treating arrhythmias and acute congestive heart failure. Give over 24 hours as 3 divided doses. Administer IV slow push over 5 to 10 minutes.

Oral doses should be 25% greater than IV doses. Do not administer IM.

Total Loading Dose			Maintenance Dose			
PMA (weeks)	IV (mcg/kg)	PO (mcg/kg)	PMA (weeks)	IV (mcg/kg)	PO (mcg/kg)	Interval (hours)
≤29	15	20	≤29	4	5	24
30 to 36	20	25	30 to 36	5	6	24
37 to 48	30	40	37 to 48	4	5	12
≥49	40	50	≥49	5	6	12

Note: These beginning doses are based primarily on studies that measured echocardiographic changes and EKG signs of toxicity and take into account renal maturation. We recommend titrating dosage based on clinical response. Decrease dose proportional to the reduction in creatinine clearance.

Uses

Treatment of heart failure caused by diminished myocardial contractility. Treatment of SVT, atrial flutter, and atrial fibrillation.

Monitoring

Follow heart rate and rhythm closely. Periodic EKGs to assess both desired effects and signs of toxicity. Follow closely (especially in patients receiving diuretics or amphotericin B) for decreased serum potassium and magnesium, or increased calcium and magnesium, all of which predispose to digoxin toxicity. Assess renal function. Be aware of drug interactions. May follow serum drug concentrations if assay is available that excludes endogenous digoxin-like substances. Therapeutic serum concentration is 1 to 2 ng/mL.

Pharmacology

Digitalis glycoside with positive inotropic and negative chronotropic actions. Increases myocardial catecholamine levels (low doses) and inhibits sarcolemmal sodium-potassium-ATPase (higher doses) to enhance contractility by increasing systolic intracellular calcium-ion concentrations. Indirectly increases vagal activity, thereby slowing S-A node firing and A-V node conduction. Other effects include peripheral, splanchnic, and perhaps, pulmonary vasoconstriction, and reduced CSF production. Serum concentration peaks 30 to 90 minutes after an oral dose, with myocardial peak occurring in 4 to 6 hours. Large volume of distribution that increases with age during infancy. Rapid absorption of oral dose from small intestine; reduced by antacids and rapid transit times. 20% protein bound. Probably not significantly metabolized. Glomerular filtration and tubular secretion account for most of the total body clearance of digoxin, although significant nonrenal elimination has been proposed.

continued...

Sidebar: CARDIOVASCULAR

Adverse Effects/Precautions

Nontoxic Cardiac Effects
- Shortening of QTc interval
- Sagging ST segment
- Diminished T-wave amplitude
- Slowing of heart rate

Toxic Cardiac Effects
- Prolongation of PR interval
- Sinus bradycardia or S-A block
- Atrial or nodal ectopic beats
- Ventricular arrhythmias

Other Effects: Feeding intolerance, vomiting, diarrhea, and lethargy.

Treatment of Life-Threatening Digoxin Toxicity: Digibind® Digoxin Immune Fab, IV over 30 minutes through 0.22 micron filter.

$$\text{Dose (\# of vials)} = \frac{\text{(serum digoxin concentration) x (weight [kg])}}{100}$$

Each vial contains 38 mg (enough to bind 0.5 mg Digoxin).

Special Considerations/Preparation
Pediatric dosage forms: Injectable (100 mcg/mL) and elixir (50 mcg/mL). Store at room temperature and protect from light.
Dilute injectable as follows:
1) Draw up digoxin into syringe.
2) Inject desired amount of drug into second syringe containing a fourfold or greater volume of solution-compatible diluent. Use diluted product immediately.

Drug interactions: Amiodarone, indomethacin, spironolactone, quinidine, and verapamil decrease digoxin clearance. Cisapride and metoclopramide decrease digoxin absorption. Spironolactone interferes with radioimmunoassay. Erythromycin may increase digoxin absorption.

Solution compatibility (only when diluted fourfold or greater): D_5W, $D_{10}W$, NS, and sterile water for injection.

Terminal Injection Site Compatibility: Dex/AA and fat emulsion. Cimetidine, famotidine, furosemide, heparin, hydrocortisone succinate, insulin, lidocaine, linezolid, meropenem, midazolam, morphine, potassium chloride, propofol, prostaglandin E_1, ranitidine, and remifentanil.

Incompatibility: Dobutamine and fluconazole.

Selected References
◆ Product Information, GlaxoSmithKline: *Physicians' Desk Reference,* ed 57. Montvale, NJ: Medical Economics Data, 2003, p 1572.
◆ Smith TW: Digitalis: Mechanisms of action and clinical use. *N Engl J Med* 1988;318:358.
◆ Roberts RJ: *Drug Therapy in Infants.* Philadelphia: WB Saunders Co, 1984, p 138.
◆ Johnson GL, Desai NS, Pauly TH, Cunningham MD: Complications associated with digoxin in low-birth-weight infants. *Pediatrics* 1982;69:463.
◆ Nyberg L, Wettrell G: Pharmacokinetics and dosage of digoxin in neonates and infants. *Eur J Clin Pharmacol* 1980;18:69.
◆ Pinsky WW, Jacobsen JR, Gillette PC, et al: Dosage of digoxin in premature infants. *J Pediatr* 1979;96:639.

Special Considerations updated 3/2002
Compatibilities updated 3/2003

Dobutamine

Dose & Administration

2 to 25 mcg/kg per minute continuous IV infusion. Begin at a low dose and titrate by monitoring effects. Use a large vein for IV.

Uses

Treatment of hypoperfusion and hypotension.

Monitoring

Continuous heart rate and intra-arterial blood pressure monitoring preferable. Observe IV site for signs of extravasation.

Adverse Effects/Precautions

May cause hypotension if patient is hypovolemic. Volume loading is recommended before starting dobutamine therapy. Tachycardia occurs at high dosage. Arrhythmias, hypertension, and cutaneous vasodilation. Increases myocardial oxygen consumption. Tissue ischemia occurs with infiltration.

Pharmacology

Synthetic catecholamine with primarily β_1-adrenergic activity. Inotropic vasopressor. Increases myocardial contractility, cardiac index, oxygen delivery, and oxygen consumption. Decreases systemic and pulmonary vascular resistance (adults). Dobutamine has a more prominent effect on cardiac output than dopamine but less of an effect on blood pressure. Onset of action is 1 to 2 minutes after IV administration, with peak effect in 10 minutes. Must be administered by continuous IV infusion because of rapid metabolism of drug. Serum half-life is several minutes. Metabolized in the liver by sulfoconjugation to an inactive compound. There is wide interpatient variability in plasma clearance due to differences in metabolism and renal excretion.

Special Considerations/Preparation

Supplied as 250 mg per 20 mL vial (12.5 mg/mL). Reconstituted solution stable for 6 hours at room temperature and 48 hours refrigerated. Diluted solutions for infusion are stable for 24 hours. Slight discoloration does not indicate loss of potency.

Solution Compatibility: D_5W, D_5NS, and NS.

Terminal Injection Site Compatibility: Dex/AA and fat emulsion. Atropine, amiodarone, aztreonam, calcium chloride, calcium gluconate, dopamine, enalaprilat, epinephrine, famotidine, fentanyl, fluconazole, flumazenil, heparin, hydralazine, insulin, isoproterenol, lidocaine, linezolid, lorazepam, magnesium sulfate, meropenem, midazolam, morphine, nitroglycerin, nitroprusside, pancuronium bromide, potassium chloride, propofol, propranolol, phytonadione, ranitidine, remifentanil, tolazoline, vecuronium, and zidovudine.

Incompatibility: Acyclovir, alteplase, aminophylline, cefepime, bumetanide, diazepam, digoxin, furosemide, indomethacin, phenytoin, piperacillin-tazobactam, and sodium bicarbonate.

continued...

CARDIOVASCULAR

Administration Calculations

To calculate the **AMOUNT** of drug needed per **50 mL** infusion solution:

$$3 \times \frac{\text{desired dose (mcg/kg/min)}}{\text{desired fluid rate (mL/hr)}} \times \text{weight (kg)} = \text{mg of dobutamine}$$

To calculate the **VOLUME** of drug needed per **50 mL** infusion solution:

$$\frac{\text{mg of drug (found using equation above)}}{\text{concentration of drug (mg/mL)}} = \text{mL of dobutamine}$$

Example: 2-kg infant to receive dobutamine 5 mcg/kg per minute at infusion rate of 0.5 mL per hour. Concentration of dobutamine is 12.5 mg/mL.

$$3 \times \frac{5 \text{ mcg/kg/min}}{0.5 \text{ mL/hr}} \times 2 \text{ kg} = 60 \text{ mg of dobutamine in } 50 \text{ mL of infusion solution}$$

$$\frac{60 \text{ mg of dobutamine}}{12.5 \text{ mg/mL}} = 4.8 \text{ mL of dobutamine in } 50 \text{ mL of infusion solution}$$

Add 4.8mL dobutamine (12.5mg/mL) to 45.2 mL of compatible solution (e.g. D_5W) to yield 50 mL of dobutamine infusion with a concentration of 1200 mcg/mL.

Maximum concentration is 5000 mcg/mL.

Selected References

♦ Berg RA, Donnerstein RL, Padbury JF: Dobutamine infusion in stable, critically ill children: pharmacokinetics and hemodynamic actions. *Crit Care Med* 1993;21:678-86.
♦ Martinez AM, Padbury JF, Thio S: Dobutamine pharmacokinetics and cardiovascular responses in critically ill neonates. *Pediatrics* 1992;89:47.
♦ Leier CV, Unverferth DV: Dobutamine. *Ann Intern Med* 1983;99:490.
♦ Perkin RM, Levin DL, Webb R, et al: Dobutamine: A hemodynamic evaluation in children with shock. *J Pediatr* 1982;100:977.

Text updated 3/98
Compatibilities updated 3/2003

CARDIOVASCULAR

Dopamine

Dose & Administration

2 to 20 mcg/kg per minute continuous IV infusion. Begin at a low dose and titrate by monitoring effects. Use a large vein for IV.

Uses

Treatment of hypotension.

Monitoring

Continuous heart rate and intra-arterial blood pressure monitoring is preferable. Assess urine output and peripheral perfusion frequently. Observe IV site closely for blanching and infiltration.

Adverse Effects/Precautions

Tachycardia and arrhythmias. May increase pulmonary artery pressure. Reversible suppression of prolactin and thyrotropin secretion.

Tissue sloughing may occur with IV infiltration.

Suggested treatment: Inject a 1 mg/mL solution of phentolamine into the affected area. The usual amount needed is 1 to 5 mL, depending on the size of the infiltrate.

Pharmacology

Catecholamine. Metabolized rapidly. Serum half-life is 2 to 5 minutes, but clearance is quite variable.

Dopamine increases blood pressure primarily by increasing systemic vascular resistance via alpha-adrenergic effects. Effects on cardiac output vary with gestational age and baseline stroke volume. Selective renal vasodilation associated with increases in urine output has been noted in preterm neonates at doses of 2.5 to 7.5 mcg/kg/minute. No changes in mesenteric or cerebral blood flow were observed. Mechanism of action in neonates is controversial. Relative effects of dopamine at different doses are uncertain because of developmental differences in 1) endogenous norepinephrine stores, 2) α-adrenergic, β-adrenergic, and dopaminergic receptor functions, and 3) the ability of the neonatal heart to increase stroke volume. Responses tend to be individualized. Use higher doses with caution in patients with persistent pulmonary hypertension of the newborn.

Special Considerations/Preparation

Available in 40-mg/mL, 80-mg/mL, and 160-mg/mL vials for injection and premixed bags in concentrations of 800-, 1600-, and 3200-mcg/mL. Refrigerate open vial and use within 24 hours. **Admixtures exhibiting a color change should not be used.**

Solution Compatibility: D_5W and NS.

Terminal Injection Site Compatibility: Dex/AA and fat emulsion. Aminophylline, ampicillin, amiodarone, aztreonam, caffeine citrate, calcium chloride, chloramphenicol, dobutamine, enalaprilat, epinephrine, esmolol, famotidine, fentanyl, flumazenil, fluconazole, gentamicin, heparin, hydrocortisone succinate, lidocaine, lorazepam, linezolid, meropenem, metronidazole, midazolam, morphine, nitroglycerin, nitroprusside, oxacillin, pancuronium bromide, penicillin G, piperacillin-tazobactam, potassium chloride, propofol, prostaglandin E_1, ranitidine, tobramycin, tolazoline, vecuronium, and zidovudine.

Incompatibility: Acyclovir, alteplase, amphotericin B, cefepime, furosemide, indomethacin, insulin, and sodium bicarbonate.

continued...

Administration Calculations

To calculate the **AMOUNT** of drug needed per **50 mL** infusion solution:

$$3 \times \frac{\text{desired dose (mcg/kg/min)}}{\text{desired fluid rate (mL/hr)}} \times \text{weight (kg)} = \text{mg of dopamine}$$

To calculate the **VOLUME** of drug needed per **50 mL** infusion solution:

$$\frac{\text{mg of drug (found using equation above)}}{\text{concentration of drug (mg/mL)}} = \text{mL of dopamine}$$

Example: 2-kg infant to receive dopamine 5 mcg/kg per minute at infusion rate of 0.5 mL per hour. Concentration of dopamine is 40 mg/mL.

$$3 \times \frac{5 \text{ mcg/kg/min}}{0.5 \text{ mL/hr}} \times 2 \text{ kg} = 60 \text{ mg of dopamine needed per } 50 \text{ mL of infusion solution}$$

$$\frac{60 \text{ mg of dopamine}}{40 \text{ mg/mL}} = 1.5 \text{ mL of dopamine needed per } 50 \text{ mL of infusion solution}$$

Add 1.5 mL dopamine (40 mg/mL) to 48.5 mL of compatible solution (e.g. D_5W) to yield 50 mL of dopamine infusion with a concentration of 1200 mcg/mL.

Maximum concentration is 3200 mcg/mL.

Selected References

♦ Seri I, Abbasi S, Wood DC, Gerdes JS: Regional hemodynamic effects of dopamine in the sick preterm neonate. *J Pediatr* 1998;133:728-734.

♦ Seri I: Cardiovascular, renal, and endocrine actions of dopamine in neonates and children. *J Pediatr* 1995;126:333.

♦ Van den Berghe G, de Zegher F, Lauwers P: Dopamine suppresses pituitary function in infants and children. *Crit Care Med* 1994;22:1747.

♦ Roze JC, Tohier C, Maingueneau C, et al : Response to dobutamine and dopamine in the hypotensive very preterm infant. *Arch Dis Child* 1993;69:59-63.

♦ Padbury JF, Agata Y, Baylen BG, et al: Dopamine pharmacokinetics in critically ill newborn infants. *J Pediatr* 1987;110:293.

♦ DiSessa TG, Leitner M, Ti CC, et al: The cardiovascular effects of dopamine in the severely asphyxiated neonate. *J Pediatr* 1981;99:772.

Text updated 3/2000
Compatibilities updated 3/2003

CARDIOVASCULAR

Enalaprilat & Enalapril

Dose & Administration

Enalaprilat: Begin with 10 mcg/kg per dose (0.01 mg/kg per dose) IV over 5 minutes Q24 hours.

Enalapril maleate: Begin with 40 mcg/kg per dose (0.04 mg/kg per dose) given PO Q24 hours. Usual maximum dose 150 mcg/kg per dose (0.15 mg/kg per dose), as frequently as Q6 hours.

For both drugs, titrate subsequent doses and interval based on amount and duration of response. Dosage may need to be increased every few days.

Uses

Treatment of moderate to severe hypertension. Afterload reduction in patients with congestive heart failure.

Monitoring

Frequent assessment of blood pressure, particularly after the first dose. Periodic assessment of renal function and serum potassium.

Adverse Effects/Precautions

Use with extreme caution in patients with impaired renal function: oliguria and increased serum creatinine occur frequently.

Hypotension occurs primarily in patients who are volume-depleted.

Hyperkalemia occurs primarily in patients receiving potassium-sparing diuretics or potassium supplements. Cough has been reported frequently in adults.

Pharmacology

Enalapril is a prodrug that is hydrolyzed in the liver to form the active angiotensin-converting enzyme (ACE) inhibitor enalaprilat, which blocks the conversion of angiotensin I to angiotensin II, a potent vasoconstrictor. It thereby decreases plasma and tissue concentrations of angiotensin II and aldosterone, and increases plasma and tissue renin activity. Enalaprilat also prevents the breakdown of bradykinin, a potent vasodilator. Vascular resistance is reduced without reflex tachycardia. Beneficial effects are thought to be caused by a combination of afterload reduction and long-term inhibition of salt and water retention. Bioavailability of oral dosage form is uncertain in neonates, but is significantly less than the 60% reported in adults. Onset of action after oral dose is 1 to 2 hours. Duration of action is quite variable in neonates, ranging from 8 to 24 hours.

continued...

Special Considerations/Preparation

Enalaprilat is supplied as a 1.25 mg/mL solution for injection in 1 mL and 2 mL vials. Benzyl alcohol content is 9 mg/mL. To make a dilution for IV use, take 1 mL (1.25 mg) of solution and add 49 mL NS to make a final concentration of 25 mcg/mL (0.025 mg/mL).

Solution Compatibility: D_5W, D_5NS, and NS.

Terminal Injection Site Compatibility: Fat emulsion. Amikacin, aminophylline, ampicillin, aztreonam, calcium gluconate, cefazolin, ceftazidime, chloramphenicol, cimetidine, clindamycin, dobutamine, dopamine, erythromycin lactobionate, esmolol, famotidine, fentanyl, gentamicin, heparin, hydrocortisone succinate, lidocaine, linezolid, magnesium sulfate, meropenem, metronidazole, morphine, nafcillin, nitroprusside, penicillin G, phenobarbital, piperacillin, piperacillin-tazobactam, potassium chloride, propofol, ranitidine, remifentanil, tobramycin, trimethoprim-sulfamethoxazole, and vancomycin.

Incompatibility: Amphotericin B, cefepime, and phenytoin.

Enalapril maleate oral suspension can be prepared by crushing a 2.5 mg tablet and adding to 25 mL of isotonic citrate buffer, yielding a final concentration of 100 mcg/mL (0.1 mg/mL). Suspension is stable for 30 days refrigerated.

Selected References

♦ Schilder JLAM, Van den Anker JN: Use of enalapril in neonatal hypertension. *Acta Paediatr* 1995;84:1426.

♦ Mason T, Polak MJ, Pyles L, et al: Treatment of neonatal renovascular hypertension with intravenous enalapril. *Am J Perinatol* 1992;9:254.

♦ Rasoulpour M, Marinelli KA: Systemic hypertension. *Clin Perinatol* 1992;19:121.

♦ Wells TG, Bunchman TE, Kearns GL: Treatment of neonatal hypertension with enalaprilat. *J Pediatr* 1990;117:665.

♦ Frenneaux M, Stewart RAH, Newman CMH, Hallidie-Smith KA: Enalapril for severe heart failure in infancy. *Arch Dis Child* 1989;64:219.

Text updated 3/97
Compatibilities updated 3/2003

CARDIOVASCULAR

Epinephrine

Dose & Administration

Severe bradycardia and hypotension: 0.1 to 0.3 mL/kg 1:10,000 concentration; equal to 0.01 to 0.03 mg/kg, or 10 to 30 mcg/kg).

IV push, or IC.

May be given ET, immediately followed by 1 mL NS.

IV continuous infusion: Start at 0.1 mcg/kg per minute and adjust to desired response, to a maximum of 1 mcg/kg per minute.

If possible, correct acidosis before administration of epinephrine to enhance the effectiveness of the drug.

Uses

Acute cardiovascular collapse. Short-term use for cardiac failure resistant to other drug management. In older infants, may be used subcutaneously for relief of bronchospasm.

Monitoring

Monitor heart rate and blood pressure continuously. Observe IV site for signs of infiltration.

Adverse Effects/Precautions

Cardiac arrhythmias (PVCs and ventricular tachycardia). Renal vascular ischemia. Severe hypertension with intracranial hemorrhage. Increases myocardial oxygen requirements. Therapeutic doses may cause hypokalemia. IV infiltration may cause tissue ischemia and necrosis.

Pharmacology

Stimulates alpha and beta adrenergic receptors—increases heart rate; increases myocardial contractility, automaticity, and conduction velocity; increases systemic vascular resistance (via constriction of arterioles); increases blood flow to skeletal muscle, brain, liver, and myocardium; decreases renal blood flow by 40%.

Special Considerations/Preparation

Always use as a 1:10,000 concentration (0.1 mg/mL) for individual doses. Use 1:1000 (1 mg/mL) concentration to prepare continuous infusion solution.

Protect from light.

Solution Compatibility: D_5W, $D_{10}W$, and NS.

Terminal Injection Site Compatibility: Dex/AA. Amikacin, ampicillin, calcium chloride, calcium gluconate, cimetidine, dobutamine, dopamine, famotidine, fentanyl, furosemide, heparin, hydrocortisone succinate, lorazepam, midazolam, morphine, nitroglycerin, nitroprusside, pancuronium bromide, potassium chloride, propofol, prostaglandin E_1, ranitidine, remifentanil, vecuronium, and vitamin K_1.

Incompatibility: Aminophylline, hyaluronidase, and sodium bicarbonate.

continued...

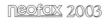

Administration Calculations

To calculate the **AMOUNT** of drug needed per **50 mL** infusion solution:

$$3 \times \frac{\text{desired dose (mcg/kg/min)}}{\text{desired fluid rate (mL/hr)}} \times \text{weight (kg)} = \text{mg of epinephrine}$$

To calculate the **VOLUME** of drug needed per **50 mL** of infusion solution:

$$\frac{\text{mg of drug (found using equation above)}}{\text{concentration of drug (mg/mL)}} = \text{mL of epinephrine}$$

Example: 2-kg infant to receive epinephrine 0.1 mcg/kg per minute at infusion rate of 0.5 mL per hour. Concentration of the 1:1000 epinephrine solution is 1 mg/mL.

$$3 \times \frac{0.1 \text{ mcg/kg/min}}{0.5 \text{ mL/hr}} \times 2 \text{ kg} = 1.2 \text{ mg of epinephrine needed per } 50 \text{ mL of infusion solution}$$

$$\frac{1.2 \text{ mg of epinephrine}}{1 \text{ mg/mL}} = 1.2 \text{ mL of epinephrine needed per } 50 \text{ mL of infusion solution}$$

Add 1.2 mL of epinephrine (1:1000) to 48.8 mL of compatible solution (e.g. D_5W) to yield 50 mL of epinephrine infusion with a concentration of 24 mcg/mL.

Maximum concentration is 64 mcg/mL.

Selected References

♦ Kattwinkel J, Niermeyer S, Nadkarni V, et al: ILCOR advisory statement: Resuscitation of the newly born infant. *Pediatrics* 1999;103(4).
URL: http://www.pediatrics.org/cgi/content/full/103/4/e56.

♦ Burchfield DJ: Medication use in neonatal resuscitation. *Clin Perinatol* 1999;26:683-691.

♦ Bloom RS, Cropley C: *Textbook of Neonatal Resuscitation*. American Heart Association, 1994, p 6-9.

♦ Zaritsky A, Chernow B: Use of catecholamines in pediatrics. *J Pediatr* 1984;105:341.

Updated 3/2000
Compatibilities updated 3/2003

CARDIOVASCULAR

Enoxaparin

(Low Molecular Weight Heparin)

Dose and Administration

Initial treatment of thrombosis: 1.5 mg/kg per dose SC every 12 hours.
Infants older than 2 months of age: 1 mg/kg per dose SC every 12 hours.
Preterm infants may initially be dosed 1 mg/kg per dose IV every 8 hours.
Adjust dosage to maintain anti-factor X_a level between 0.5 and 1.0 U/mL.
Call 1-800-NOCLOTS for case reporting and treatment guidance.
Low-risk prophylaxis: 0.75 mg/kg per dose SC every 12 hours.
Infants older than 2 months of age: 0.5 mg/kg per dose SC every 12 hours.
Adjust dosage to maintain anti-factor X_a level between 0.1 and 0.4 U/mL.

Uses

Anticoagulation. Advantages over standard unfractionated heparin:
(1) may be given subcutaneously, (2) more predictable pharmacokinetics,
(3) dosing every 8 to 12 hours, (4) less frequent bleeding complications.

Monitoring

Measure anti-factor X_a concentrations 4 hours after a dose (See above for desired range). Assess for signs of bleeding and thrombosis.

Adverse Effects/Precautions

Limited data are available in neonates. In the prospective cohort study (Dix, et al) mortality attributed to enoxaparin therapy was 1%, major bleeding 4%, and minor bleeding 17%.

Pharmacology

Enoxaparin has considerably less activity against thrombin than does standard heparin. Activates antithrombin III, which progressively inactivates both thrombin and factor X_a, key proteolytic enzymes in the formation of fibrinogen and activation of prothrombin. Efficacy in neonates is decreased due to low antithrombin plasma concentrations. Metabolized by liver. Renal excretion should occur within 6 hours, but may be delayed. Clearance in neonates is more rapid than in older infants, children or adults. Half-life is dose-dependent, but averages 1 to 3 hours.

Special Considerations/Preparation

Available as 100 mg/mL concentration in prefilled syringes and ampules.
Solution compatibility: NS and sterile water.
Terminal injection site compatibility: No data are currently available.

Selected References

♦ Monagle P, Michelson AD, Bovill E, Andrew M : Antithrombotic therapy in children. *Chest* 2001;119:344-370S.

♦ Edstrom CS, Christensen RD: Evaluation and treatment of thrombosis in the neonatal intensive care unit. *Clin Perinatol* 2000;27:623-41.

♦ Dix D, Andrew M, Marzinotto V, et al: The use of low molecular heparin in pediatric patients: A prospective cohort study. *J Pediatr* 2000;136:439-45.

♦ Dunaway KK, Gal P, Ransom JL: Use of enoxaparin in a preterm infant. *Ann Pharmacother* 2000;34:1410-3.

♦ Klinger G, Hellmann J, Daneman A: Severe aortic thrombosis in the neonate - successful treatment with low-molecular-weight heparin: Two case reports and review of the literature. *Am J Perinatol* 2000;17:151-8.

♦ Massicotte P, Adams M, Marzinotto V, et al: Low-molecular-weight heparin in pediatric patients with thrombotic disease: A dose finding study. *J Pediatr* 1996;128:313-8.

Added 3/2001

CARDIOVASCULAR

Flecainide

Dose & Administration

Begin at 2 mg/kg per dose Q12 hours PO. Adjust dose based on response and serum concentrations to a maximum of 4 mg/kg per dose Q12 hours. Correct preexisting hypokalemia or hyperkalemia before administration.

Uses

Treatment of supraventricular arrhythmias not responsive to conventional therapies. Contraindicated in patients with structurally abnormal hearts.

Monitoring

Continuous EKG during initiation of therapy, as this is the most common time to see drug-induced arrhythmias. Follow trough serum concentrations closely at initiation, 3 to 5 days after any dose change, and with any significant change in clinical status or diet. Therapeutic trough levels are 200 to 800 nanograms/mL.

Adverse Effects/Precautions

Flecainide can cause new or worsened arrhythmias, including AV block, bradycardia, ventricular tachycardia, torsades de pointes. There is also a negative inotropic effect. Dizziness, blurred vision, and headache have been reported in children.

Pharmacology

Flecainide is a Class I-C antiarrhythmic that produces a dose-related decrease in intracardiac conduction in all parts of the heart, thereby increasing PR, QRS and QT intervals. Effects upon atrioventricular (AV) nodal conduction time and intra-atrial conduction times are less pronounced than those on the ventricle. Peak serum concentrations occur 2 to 3 hours after an oral dose. Infant formula and milk products interfere with drug absorption. Plasma protein binding is about 40% in adults and is independent of plasma drug level. Children under 1 year of age have elimination half-life values of 11 to 12 hours. Elimination half-life in newborns after maternal administration is as long as 29 hours. Steady-state plasma levels in normal renal and hepatic function may not be achieved until 3 to 5 days of therapy at a given dose. Therefore, do not increase dosage more frequently than once every 4 days, since optimal effect may not be achieved during the first 2 to 3 days of therapy.

continued...

Special Considerations/Preparation

Supplied in 50-mg, 100-mg, and 150-mg tablets. An oral suspension with a final concentration of 5 mg/mL can be made as follows: crush 6 (six) 100-mg tablets, slowly mix in 20 mL of a 1:1 mixture of Ora-Sweet® and Ora-Plus®, or cherry syrup (cherry syrup concentrate diluted 1:4 with simple syrup) to form a uniform paste, then add to this mixture enough vehicle to make a final volume of 120 mL. Shake well and protect from light. Stable for 45 days refrigerated and at room temperature when stored in amber glass or plastic.

Selected References

♦ O'Sullivan JJ, Gardiner HM, Wren C: Digoxin or flecainide for prophylaxis of supraventricular tachycardia in infants? *J Am Coll Cardiol* 1995;26:991-994.

♦ Luedtke SA, Kuhn RJ, McCaffrey FM: Pharmacologic management of supraventricular tachycardia in children. *Ann Pharmacother* 1997;31:1227-43.

♦ Perry JC, Garson A: Flecainide acetate for treatment of tachyarrhythmias in children: Review of world literature on efficacy, safety, and dosing. *Am Heart J* 1992;124:1614-21.

♦ Wiest DB, Garner SS, Pagacz LR, et al: Stability of flecainide acetate in an extemporaneously compounded oral suspension. *Am J Hosp Pharm* 1992;49:1467-70.

CARDIOVASCULAR

Heparin

Dose & Administration

Maintaining patency of peripheral and central vascular catheters: 0.5 to 1 U/mL of IV fluid.

Treatment of thrombosis: 75 U/kg bolus, followed by 28 U/kg per hour continuous infusion. Four hours after initiating therapy, measure aPTT, then adjust dose to achieve an aPTT that corresponds to an anti-factor X_a level of 0.3 to 0.7 (this is usually equivalent to an aPTT of 60 to 85 seconds). Treatment should be limited to 10 to 14 days.

Make certain correct concentration is used.

Uses

See above. Only continuous infusions (rather than intermittent flushes) have been demonstrated to maintain catheter patency. Treatment of renal vein thromboses is limited to those that are bilateral or extend into the IVC. Although data are limited, enoxaparin may be preferable to heparin for treatment of thromboses.

Call 1-800-NOCLOTS for case reporting and treatment guidance.

Monitoring

Follow platelet counts every 2 to 3 days. When treating thromboses, maintain a prolonged aPTT in a range corresponding to an anti-factor X_a level of 0.3 to 0.7 units/mL. Assess for signs of bleeding and thrombosis.

Adverse Effects/Precautions

Data are insufficient to make specific recommendations regarding anticoagulation therapy. Heparin-induced thrombocytopenia (HIT) has been reported to occur in approximately 1% of newborns exposed to heparin. Heparin-associated antiplatelet antibodies were found in half of the newborns who were both thrombocytopenic and heparin-exposed. Although the thrombocytopenia resolved spontaneously in most patients upon stopping the heparin, a high incidence of ultrasonographic-documented aortic thrombosis was seen. Contraindicated in infants with evidence of intracranial or GI bleeding or thrombocytopenia (below 50,000/mm³). Long term use of therapeutic doses of heparin can lead to osteoporosis.

Pharmacology

Activates antithrombin III, which progressively inactivates both thrombin and factor X_a, key proteolytic enzymes in the formation of fibrinogen and activation of prothrombin. Efficacy in neonates is decreased due to low antithrombin plasma concentrations. Metabolized by liver. Renal excretion should occur within 6 hours, but may be delayed. Clearance in neonates is more rapid than in children or adults. Half-life is dose-dependent, but averages 1 to 3 hours.

continued...

Special Considerations/Preparation

Keep protamine sulfate on hand to manage hemorrhage (1 mg for each 100 U of heparin given in last 4 hours). Available in 10 U/mL (for IV reservoirs); 100 U/mL; 1000 U/mL (for central catheters); and 10,000 U/mL.

Solution Compatibility: D_5W, $D_{10}W$, and NS.

Terminal Injection Site Compatibility: Dex/AA and fat emulsion. Acyclovir, aminophylline, ampicillin, amphotericin B, atropine, aztreonam, caffeine citrate, calcium gluconate, cefazolin, cefepime, cefotaxime, cefoxitin, ceftazidime, ceftriaxone, chloramphenicol, cimetidine, clindamycin, dexamethasone, digoxin, dobutamine, dopamine, enalaprilat, epinephrine, erythromycin lactobionate, esmolol, famotidine, fentanyl, flecainide, fluconazole, furosemide, hydralazine, hydrocortisone succinate, insulin, isoproterenol, lidocaine, linezolid, lorazepam, meropenem, methicillin, metoclopramide, metronidazole, mezlocillin, midazolam, morphine, nafcillin, naloxone, netilmicin, neostigmine, nitroglycerin, oxacillin, pancuronium bromide, penicillin G, phenobarbital, phytonadione, piperacillin, piperacillin-tazobactam, potassium chloride, propofol, propranolol, prostaglandin E_1, ranitidine, remifentanil, sodium bicarbonate, sodium nitroprusside, ticarcillin/clavulanate, trimethoprim-sulfamethoxazole, vecuronium, and zidovudine.

Incompatibility: Alteplase, amikacin, amiodarone, diazepam, gentamicin, methadone, phenytoin, tobramycin, and vancomycin.

Selected References

♦ Schmugge M, Risch L, Huber AR, et al: Heparin-induced thromobocytopenia-associated thrombosis in pediatric intensive care patients. *Pediatrics* 2002;109(1). URL:http://www.pediatrics.org/cgi/content/full/109/1/e10.

♦ Monagle P, Michelson AD, Bovill E, Andrew M : Antithrombotic therapy in children. *Chest* 2001;119:344-370S.

♦ Edstrom CS, Christensen RD: Evaluation and treatment of thrombosis in the neonatal intensive care unit. *Clin Perinatol* 2000;27:623-41.

♦ Sutor AH, Massicotte P, Leaker M, Andrew M: Heparin therapy in pediatric patients. *Semin Thromb Hemostas* 1997;23:303-19.

♦ Chang GY, Leuder FL, DiMichele DM, et al: Heparin and the risk of intraventricular hemorrhage in premature infants. *J Pediatr* 1997;131:362-66.

♦ Paisley MK, Stamper M, Brown J, et al: The use of heparin and normal saline flushes in neonatal intravenous catheters. *Pediatr Nurs* 1997;23:521-27.

♦ Kotter RW: Heparin vs saline for intermittent intravenous device maintenance in neonates. *Neonat Network* 1996;15:43-47.

♦ Moclair A, Bates I: The efficacy of heparin in maintaining peripheral infusions in neonates. *Eur J Pediatr* 1995;154:567-70.

♦ Spadone D, Clark F, James E, et al: Heparin-induced thrombocytopenia in the newborn. *J Vasc Surg* 1992;15:306.

References updated 3/2002
Compatibilities updated 3/2003

Dose and Administration

IV (if available): Begin with 0.1 to 0.5 mg/kg per dose Q6 to 8 hours. Dose may be gradually increased as required for blood pressure control to a maximum of 2 mg/kg per dose Q6 hours.

PO: 0.25 to 1 mg/kg per dose Q6 to 8 hours, or approximately twice the required IV dose. Administer with food to enhance absorption.

Note: Use with a ß-blocking agent is often recommended to enhance the antihypertensive effect and decrease the magnitude of the reflex tachycardia. This is expected to reduce hydralazine IV dosage requirements to less than 0.15 mg/kg per dose.

Uses

Treatment of mild to moderate neonatal hypertension by vasodilation. Afterload reduction in patients with congestive heart failure.

Monitoring

Frequent assessment of blood pressure and heart rate. Guaiac stools. Periodic CBC during long-term use.

Adverse Effects/Precautions

Diarrhea, emesis, and temporary agranulocytosis have been reported in neonates. Tachycardia, postural hypotension, headache, nausea, and a lupus-like syndrome occur in 10% to 20% of adults. Uncommon reactions in adults include GI irritation and bleeding, drug fever, rash, conjunctivitis, and bone marrow suppression.

Pharmacology

Causes direct relaxation of smooth muscle in the arteriolar resistance vessels. Major hemodynamic effects: Decrease in systemic vascular resistance and a resultant increase in cardiac output. Increases renal, coronary, cerebral, and splanchnic blood flow. When administered orally, hydralazine has low bioavailability because of extensive first-pass metabolism by the liver and intestines. The rate of enzymatic metabolism is genetically determined by the acetylator phenotype—slow acetylators have higher plasma concentrations and a higher incidence of adverse effects.

continued...

Hydralazine

Special Considerations/Preparation

Hydralazine hydrochloride injection for IV use (20 mg/mL) is available in 1 mL and 2 mL vials from SoloPak Laboratories. A 1 mg/mL dilution may be made by diluting 0.5 mL of the 20 mg/mL concentrate with 9.5 mL of preservative-free normal saline for injection. Dilution is stable for 24 hours.

Only 10-, 20-, 50-, and 100-mg tablets are manufactured for oral use. Oral formulations using simple syrups containing dextrose, fructose, or sucrose are unstable. To prepare an oral suspension, crush a 50 mg tablet and dissolve in 4 mL of 5% mannitol, then add 46 mL of sterile water to make a final concentration of 1 mg/mL. Protect from light. Stable for 7 days refrigerated.

Solution compatibility: D_5W, $D_{10}W$, and NS.

Terminal injection site compatibility: Dex/AA. Dobutamine, heparin, hydrocortisone succinate, potassium chloride, and prostaglandin E_1.

Incompatibility: Aminophylline, ampicillin, furosemide, and phenobarbital.

Selected References

♦ Artman M, Graham TP Jr: Guidelines for vasodilator therapy of congestive heart failure in infants and children. *Am Heart J* 1987;113:995.

♦ Gupta VD, Stewart KR, Bethea C: Stability of hydralazine hydrochloride in aqueous vehicles. *J Clin Hosp Pharm* 1986;11:215.

♦ Beekman RH, Rocchini AP, Rosenthal A: Hemodynamic effects of hydralazine in infants with a large ventricular septal defect. *Circulation* 1982;65:523.

♦ Fried R, Steinherz LJ, Levin AR, et al: Use of hydralazine for intractable cardiac failure in childhood. *J Pediatr* 1980;97:1009.

Text updated 3/96
Compatibilities updated 3/97

Indomethacin

Dose & Administration

PDA Closure Dose (mg/kg)

Age at 1st dose	1st	2nd	3rd
< 48 h	0.2	0.1	0.1
2 to 7 d	0.2	0.2	0.2
> 7 d	0.2	0.25	0.25

IV infusion by syringe pump over at least 30 minutes to minimize adverse effects on cerebral, GI, and renal blood flow velocities. Usually three doses per course, maximum two courses. Give at 12- to 24-hour intervals with close monitoring of urine output. If anuria or severe oliguria occurs, subsequent doses should be delayed.

Longer treatment courses may be used to decrease likelyhood of reopening: 0.2 mg/kg Q24 hours for a total of 5 to 7 days.

Prevention of IVH: 0.1 mg/kg Q24 hours for 3 doses, beginning at 6 to 12 hours of age.

Uses

Closure of ductus arteriosus. Prevention of intraventricular hemorrhage.

Monitoring

Monitor urine output, serum electrolytes, glucose, creatinine and BUN, and platelet counts. Assess murmur, pulse pressure. Assess for GI bleeding by guaiacing stools and gastric aspirate. Observe for prolonged bleeding from puncture sites.

Adverse Effects/Precautions

If oliguria occurs, observe for hyponatremia and hypokalemia, and consider prolonging the dosing interval of renally excreted drugs (e.g. gentamicin). Consider withholding feedings. Hypoglycemia is common, usually preventable by increasing the glucose infusion rate by 2 mg/kg per minute. Causes platelet dysfunction. Contraindicated in active bleeding, significant thrombocytopenia or coagulation defects, necrotizing enterocolitis, and/or significantly impaired renal function. Rapid (<5-minute) infusions are associated with reductions in organ blood flow.

Pharmacology

Inhibitor of prostaglandin synthesis. Decreases cerebral, renal and GI blood flow. Metabolized in the liver to inactive compounds and excreted in the urine and feces. Serum half-life is approximately 30 hours, with a range of 15 to 50 hours, partially dependent on postnatal age. In most studies, the response of the ductus and adverse effects of indomethacin are only weakly correlated with plasma concentration.

continued...

Special Considerations/Preparation

Supplied as a lyophilized powder in 1-mg single dose vials.

Indomethacin sodium trihydrate salt is not buffered, and is insoluble in solutions with pH <6.0; the manufacturer therefore recommends against continuous infusion in typical IV solutions. Reconstitute using 1 to 2 mL of preservative-free NS or sterile water for injection. Reconstituted indomethacin is stable in polypropylene syringes and glass vials for 12 days when stored at room temperature or refrigerated. Observe for precipitation.

Solution Compatibility: Sterile water for injection.
(No visual precipitation in 24 hours): $D_{2.5}W$, D_5W, and NS.

Terminal Injection Site Compatibility: Furosemide, insulin, nitroprusside, potassium chloride, and sodium bicarbonate.

Incompatibility: $D_{7.5}W$, $D_{10}W$, Dex/AA. Calcium gluconate, cimetidine, dobutamine, dopamine, gentamicin, tobramycin, and tolazoline.

Selected References

♦ Clyman RI: Recommendations for the postnatal use of indomethacin: an analysis of four separate treatment strategies. *J Pediatr* 1996;128:601.

♦ Hammerman C, Aramburo MJ: Prolonged indomethacin therapy for the prevention of recurrences of patent ductus arteriosus. *J Pediatr* 1990;117:771.

♦ Hosono S, Ohono T, Kimoto H: Preventative management of hypoglycemia in very low-birthweight infants following indomethacin therapy for patent ductus arteriosus. *Pediatr Internat* 2001;43:465-468.

♦ Coombs RC, Morgan MEI, Durbin GM, et al: Gut blood flow velocities in the newborn: Effects of patent ductus arteriosus and parenteral indomethacin. *Arch Dis Child* 1990;65:1067.

♦ Colditz P, Murphy D, Rolfe P, Wilkinson AR: Effect of infusion rate of indomethacin on cerebrovascular responses in preterm infants. *Arch Dis Child* 1989;64:8.

♦ Walker SE, Gray S, Schmidt B: Stability of reconstituted indomethacin sodium trihydrate in original vials and polypropylene syringes. *Am J Health Syst Pharm* 1998;15:154.

♦ Ishisaka DY, Van Vleet J, Marquardt E: Visual compatibility of indomethacin sodium trihydrate with drugs given to neonates by continuous infusion. *Am J Hosp Pharm* 1991;48:2442.

♦ Gersony WM, Peckham GJ, Ellison RC, et al: Effects of indomethacin in premature infants with patent ductus arteriosus: Results of a national collaborative study. *J Pediatr* 1983;102:895.

♦ Brash AR, Hickey DE, Graham TP, et al: Pharmacokinetics of indomethacin in the neonate: Relation of plasma indomethacin levels to response of the ductus arteriosus. *N Engl J Med* 1981;305:67.

♦ Yaffe SJ, Friedmann WF, Rogers D, et al: The disposition of indomethacin in preterm babies. *J Pediatr* 1980;97:1001.

♦ Schmidt B, Davis P, Moddeman D, et al: Long-term effects of indomethacin prophylaxis in extremely-low-birth-weight infants. *N Engl J Med* 2001; 344:1966-1972.

♦ Fowlie PW: Prophylactic indomethacin: systematic review and meta-analysis. *Arch Dis Child* 1996;74:F81.

♦ Ment LR, Oh W, Ehrenkranz RA, et al: Low-dose indomethacin and prevention of intraventricular hemorrhage: A multicenter randomized trial. *Pediatrics* 1994;93:543.

Updated 3/2003
Compatibilities updated 3/2001

Isoproterenol

CARDIOVASCULAR

Dose & Administration

0.05 to 0.5 mcg/kg per minute continuous IV infusion.
Maximum dose 2 mcg/kg per minute.
Dosage often titrated according to heart rate.
Acidosis should be corrected before infusion.

Uses

Increases cardiac output in patients with cardiovascular shock. Pulmonary vasodilator (older infants).

Monitoring

Continuous vital signs, intra-arterial blood pressure, CVP monitoring preferable. Periodic blood glucose reagent strips.

Adverse Effects/Precautions

Cardiac arrhythmias. Tachycardia severe enough to cause CHF. Decreases venous return to heart. Systemic vasodilation. May cause hypoxemia by increasing intrapulmonary shunt. Hypoglycemia.

Pharmacology

β-receptor stimulant, sympathomimetic. Increases cardiac output by 1) increasing rate (major) and 2) increasing strength of contractions (minor). Insulin secretion is stimulated. Afterload reduction via β_2 effects on arterioles.

Special Considerations/Preparation

Supplied as 0.2-mg/mL solution in 5-mL and 10-mL vials.

Solution Compatibility: D_5W, $D_{10}W$, and NS.

Terminal Injection Site Compatibility: Dex/AA and fat emulsion. Aminophylline, amiodarone, calcium chloride, calcium gluceptate, calcium gluconate, cimetidine, dobutamine, famotidine, heparin, hydrocortisone succinate, netilmicin, nitroprusside, pancuronium bromide, potassium chloride, propofol, prostaglandin E_1, ranitidine, remifentanil, and vecuronium.

Incompatibility: Furosemide and sodium bicarbonate.

continued...

Administration Calculations

To calculate the **AMOUNT** of drug needed per **50 mL** infusion solution:

$$3 \times \frac{\text{desired dose (mcg/kg/min)}}{\text{desired fluid rate (mL/hr)}} \times \text{weight (kg)} = \text{mg of isoproterenol}$$

To calculate the **VOLUME** of drug needed per **50 mL** infusion solution:

$$\frac{\text{mg of drug (found using equation above)}}{\text{concentration of drug (mg/mL)}} = \text{mL of isoproterenol}$$

Example: 2-kg infant to receive isoproterenol 0.1 mcg/kg per minute at infusion rate of 1 mL per hour. Concentration of isoproterenol solution is 0.2 mg/mL.

$$3 \times \frac{0.1 \text{ mcg/kg/min}}{1 \text{ mL/hr}} \times 2 \text{ kg} = 0.6 \text{ mg of isoproterenol per } 50 \text{ mL of infusion solution}$$

$$\frac{0.6 \text{ mg of isoproterenol}}{0.2 \text{ mg/mL}} = 3 \text{ mL of isoproterenol per } 50 \text{ mL of infusion solution}$$

Add 3 mL of isoproterenol (0.2 mg/mL) to 47 mL of compatible solution (e.g. D_5W) to yield 50 mL of isoproterenol infusion with a concentration of 12 mcg/mL.

Maximum concentration 20 mcg/mL.

Selected References

♦ Cabal LA, Devaskar U, Siassi B, et al: Cardiogenic shock associated with perinatal asphyxia in preterm infants. *J Pediatr* 1980;96:705.

♦ Daoud FS, Reeves JT, Kelly DB: Isoproterenol as a potential pulmonary vasodilator in primary pulmonary hypertension. *Am J Cardiol* 1978;42:817.

Text updated 1/91
Compatibilities updated 3/2003

CARDIOVASCULAR

Lidocaine

Dose & Administration

Initial bolus dose: 0.5 to 1 mg/kg IV push over 5 minutes.
Repeat Q10 minutes as necessary to control arrhythmia. Maximum total bolus dose should not exceed 5 mg/kg.

Maintenance IV infusion: 10 to 50 mcg/kg per minute. Premature neonates should receive lowest dosage.

Uses

Short-term control of ventricular arrhythmias, including ventricular tachycardia, premature ventricular contractions, and arrhythmias resulting from digitalis intoxication.

Monitoring

Continuous monitoring of EKG, heart rate, and blood pressure. Assess level of consciousness. Observe for seizure activity. Therapeutic total lidocaine serum concentrations are 1 to 5 mcg/mL.

Adverse Effects/Precautions

Early signs of CNS toxicity are drowsiness, agitation, vomiting, and muscle twitching. Later signs include seizures, loss of consciousness, respiratory depression, and apnea. Cardiac toxicity is associated with excessive doses and includes bradycardia, hypotension, heart block, and cardiovascular collapse.

Contraindicated in infants with cardiac failure and heart block. Serum lidocaine concentrations increase when using either cimetidine or propranolol in combination.

Pharmacology

Lidocaine is a Type 1b antiarrhythmic agent used intravenously. Onset of action is 1 to 2 minutes after bolus administration. Plasma half-life in neonates is 3 hours. Free drug fraction in both term and premature neonates is approximately twice that found in older children because of significantly reduced protein binding by α_1-acid glycoprotein. Transformed in the liver to metabolites with antiarrhythmic activity; approximately 30% is excreted unchanged in neonates.

Special Considerations/Preparation

Use only preservative-free lidocaine without epinephrine.
Available in multiple concentrations ranging from 1% to 20%. To make a dilution for bolus dosing, dilute 10 mg lidocaine (0.5 mL of 2% solution) in 9.5 mL NS or D_5W, yielding a 1 mg/mL final concentration.

Solution Compatibility: D_5W, $D_{10}W$, and NS.

Terminal Injection Site Compatibility: Dex/AA and fat emulsion. Alteplase, aminophylline, amiodarone, ampicillin, calcium chloride, calcium gluconate, cefazolin, cefoxitin, ceftriaxone, chloramphenicol, cimetidine, dexamethasone, digoxin, dobutamine, dopamine, enalaprilat, erythromycin lactobionate, famotidine, fentanyl, flumazenil, furosemide, glycopyrrolate, heparin, hydrocortisone succinate, insulin, linezolid, methicillin, metoclopramide, morphine, nafcillin, nitroglycerin, penicillin G, pentobarbital, potassium chloride, procainamide, prostaglandin E_1, ranitidine, sodium bicarbonate, and sodium nitroprusside.

Incompatibility: Phenytoin.

continued...

Administration Calculations

To calculate the **AMOUNT** of drug needed per **50 mL** infusion solution:

$$3 \times \frac{\text{desired dose (mcg/kg/min)}}{\text{desired fluid rate (mL/hr)}} \times \text{weight (kg)} = \text{mg of lidocaine}$$

To calculate the **VOLUME** of drug needed per **50 mL** infusion solution:

$$\frac{\text{mg of drug (found using equation above)}}{\text{concentration of drug (mg/mL)}} = \text{mL of lidocaine}$$

Example: 2-kg infant to receive 10 mcg/kg per minute of lidocaine at infusion rate of 0.5 mL per hour. Concentration of the 2% lidocaine solution is 20 mg/mL.

$$3 \times \frac{10 \text{ mcg/kg/min}}{0.5 \text{ mL/hr}} \times 2 \text{ kg} = 120 \text{ mg of lidocaine needed per } 50 \text{ mL of infusion solution}$$

$$\frac{120 \text{ mg of lidocaine}}{20 \text{ mg/mL}} = 6 \text{ mL of lidocaine needed per } 50 \text{ mL of infusion solution}$$

Add 6 mL of lidocaine (20 mg/mL) to 44 mL of compatible solution (e.g. D_5W) to yield 50 mL of lidocaine infusion with a concentration of 2.4 mg/mL.

Maximum infusion concentration 4 mg/mL.

Selected References

♦ Lerman J, Strong A, LeDez KM, et al: Effects of age on the serum concentration of α_1-acid glycoprotein and the binding of lidocaine in pediatric patients. *Clin Pharmacol Ther* 1989;46:219.

♦ Mihaly GW, Moore RG, Thomas J: The pharmacokinetics and metabolism of the anilide local anesthetics in neonates. I. Lignocaine. *Eur J Clin Pharmacol* 1978;13:143.

♦ Gelband H, Rosen MR: Pharmacologic basis for the treatment of cardiac arrhythmias. *Pediatrics* 1975;55:59.

Added 1/94
Compatibilities updated 3/2003

Phentolamine

Dose and Administration

Inject a 1-mg/mL solution of phentolamine subcutaneously into the affected area. Usual amount needed is 1 to 5 mL, depending on the size of the infiltrate. May be repeated if necessary.

Uses

Prevention of dermal necrosis and sloughing caused by extravasation of vasoconstrictive agents, e.g. dopamine.

Monitoring

Assess affected area for reversal of ischemia. Monitor blood pressure.

Adverse Effects/Precautions

Hypotension could potentially occur if a very large dose is administered. Consider using topical 2% nitroglycerin ointment if affected extremity is significantly swollen.

Pharmacology

Alpha-adrenergic blocking agent that produces peripheral vasodilation, thereby reversing ischemia produced by vasopressor infiltration. The effect should be seen almost immediately. Biological half-life when injected subcutaneously is less than 20 minutes.

Special Considerations/Preparation

Available in 5-mg vial as a lyophylized powder.
To prepare:
1) Reconstitute one vial with 1 mL of NS.
2) Dilute to a concentration of 1 mg/mL with 4 mL NS. Use immediately.
Do not use if solution is discolored or contains particulate contamination.

Selected References

♦ Denkler KA, Cohen BE: Reversal of dopamine extravasation injury with topical nitroglycerin ointment. *Plast Reconstr Surg* 1989;84:811.
♦ Siwy BK, Sadove AM: Acute management of dopamine infiltration injury with Regitine. *Plast Reconstr Surg* 1987;80:610.

Added 1/92

CARDIOVASCULAR

Dose and Administration

Starting oral dose: 0.25 mg/kg per dose Q6 hours.
Increase as needed to maximum of 3.5 mg/kg per dose Q6 hours.

Starting IV dose: 0.01 mg/kg Q6 hours over 10 minutes.
Increase as needed to maximum of 0.15 mg/kg per dose Q6 hours.
Effective dosage requirements will vary significantly.

Uses

Treatment of tachyarrhythmias and hypertension. Preferred therapy for SVT if associated with Wolff-Parkinson-White syndrome. Palliation of tetralogy of Fallot and hypertrophic obstructive cardiomyopathy. Adjunctive treatment of neonatal thyrotoxicosis.

Monitoring

Continuous EKG monitoring during acute treatment of arrhythmias and during IV therapy. Measure systemic blood pressure frequently. Measure blood glucose during initiation of treatment and after dosage changes. Assess for increased airway resistance.

Adverse Effects/Precautions

Adverse effects are related to ß-receptor blockade: Bradycardia, bronchospasm, and hypoglycemia are most frequently reported. Hypotension occurs in patients with underlying myocardial dysfunction. Contraindicated in patients with reactive airway disease or diminished myocardial contractility. A withdrawal syndrome (nervousness, tachycardia, sweating, hypertension) has been associated with sudden cessation of the drug.

Pharmacology

Propranolol is the most widely used nonselective ß-adrenergic-receptor blocking agent. Peak serum concentration is reached approximately 2 hours after an oral dose. Propranolol undergoes significant first-pass hepatic metabolism, resulting in 30% to 40% bioavailability. Protein binding is 70% in neonates. Serum half-life is prolonged in patients with liver disease. Elimination is by renal excretion of metabolites.

Special Considerations/Preparation

Oral solutions are available in concentrations of 4 mg/mL and 8 mg/mL and are stable for 6 months at room temperature. Injectable form is available in 1-mL ampules containing 1 mg.
Make a 0.1 mg/mL dilution by adding 1 ampul to 9 mL preservative-free normal saline. **Protect from light.** Store at room temperature.

Solution compatibility: D_5W and NS.

Terminal injection site compatibility: Alteplase, dobutamine, heparin, hydrocortisone succinate, linezolid, morphine, potassium chloride, and propofol.

Selected References

♦ Schneeweiss A: Neonatal cardiovascular pharmacology, in Long WA (ed): *Fetal and Neonatal Cardiology*. Baltimore: WB Saunders Co, 1990, p 675.
♦ Pickoff AS, Zies L, Ferrer PL, et al: High-dose propranolol therapy in the management of supraventricular tachycardia. *J Pediatr* 1979;94:144.
♦ Gillette P, Garson A, Eterovic E, et al: Oral propranolol treatment in infants and children. *J Pediatr* 1978;92:141.

Compatibilities updated 3/2002

CARDIOVASCULAR

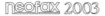

Prostaglandin E$_1$ (Alprostadil)

Dose & Administration

Initial dose: 0.05 to 0.1 mcg/kg per minute by continuous IV infusion. Titrate to infant's response—oxygenation *versus* adverse effects.

Maintenance dose: May be as low as 0.01 mcg/kg per minute. Higher initial doses are usually no more effective and have a high incidence of adverse effects.

May also be given via UAC positioned near ductus arteriosus.

Uses

To promote dilation of ductus arteriosus in infants with congenital heart disease dependent on ductal shunting for oxygenation/perfusion.

Monitoring

Closely monitor respiratory and cardiovascular status. Assess for improvement in oxygenation. Closely monitor infant's temperature. Ensure reliable IV access: duration of effect is short.

Adverse Effects/Precautions

Be prepared to intubate/resuscitate.

Common (6% to 15%): Apnea, fever, leukocytosis, cutaneous flushing, and bradycardia. Gastric outlet obstruction and reversible cortical proliferation of the long bones after prolonged treatment (>120 hours).

Uncommon (1% to 5%): Seizures, hypoventilation, hypotension, tachycardia, cardiac arrest, edema, sepsis, diarrhea, and disseminated intravascular coagulation.

Rare (<1%): Urticaria, bronchospasm, hemorrhage, hypoglycemia, and hypocalcemia.

Musculoskeletal changes: Widened fontanels, pretibial and soft tissue swelling, and swelling of the extremities may occur after 9 days of therapy. Cortical hyperostosis and periostitis may occur with long-term (>3 months) therapy. These changes resolve over weeks after discontinuation of therapy.

Pharmacology

Vasodilation of **all** arterioles. Inhibition of platelet aggregation. Stimulation of uterine and intestinal smooth muscle. Maximal drug effect usually seen within 30 minutes in cyanotic lesion; may take several hours in acyanotic lesions.

continued...

Special Considerations/Preparation

Supplied a 1 mL (500 mcg) ampules that must be refrigerated. **Dilute before administration to a concentration less than 20 mcg/mL.** Prepare fresh infusion solutions every 24 hours. Osmolality of undiluted (500 mcg/mL) is 23,250 mOsm/kg. Extravasation may cause tissue sloughing and necrosis.

Solution Compatibility: D$_5$W and NS. No data are currently available on Dex/AA.

Terminal Injection Site Compatibility: Aminophylline, atropine, calcium chloride, cefazolin, cimetidine, clindamycin, dexamethasone, digoxin, dopamine, epinephrine, furosemide, gentamicin, glycopyrolate, heparin, hydralazine, hydrocortisone succinate, isoproterenol, lidocaine, metoclopramide, metronidazole, midazolam, morphine, nitroglycerine, nitroprusside, pancuronium, phenobarbital, potassium chloride, penicillin G, and ranitidine.

Sample Dilution and Infusion Rate: Mix 1 ampule (500 mcg) in 49 mL of compatible solution (e.g.,D$_5$W) yielding a concentration of 10 mcg/mL. Infuse at a rate of 0.6 mL/kg per hour to provide a dose of 0.1 mcg/kg per minute.

Selected References

♦ Arav-Boger R, Baggett HC, Spevak PJ, Willoughby RE: Leukocytosis caused by prostaglandin E$_1$ in neonates. *J Pediatr* 2001;138:263-265.

♦ Kaufman MB, El-Chaar GM: Bone and tissue changes following prostaglandin therapy in neonates. *Ann Pharmacother* 1996;30:269.

♦ Peled N, Dagan O, Babyn P, et al: Gastric-outlet obstruction induced by prostaglandin therapy in neonates. *N Engl J Med* 1992;327:505.

♦ Gannaway WI, et al: Chemical stability of alprostadil (PGE-1) in combination with common injectable medications (abstract #P-152E). *American Society of Hospital Pharmacists Midyear Clinical Meeting Abstracts* 1989;24:75A.

♦ Roberts RJ: *Drug Therapy in Infants.* Philadelphia: WB Saunders Co, 1984, p 250.

♦ Lewis AB, Freed MD, Heymann MA, et al: Side effects of therapy with prostaglandin E$_1$ in infants with congenital heart disease. *Circulation* 1981;64:893.

♦ Heymann MA: Pharmacologic use of prostaglandin E$_1$ in infants with congenital heart disease. *Am Heart J* 1981;101:837.

Updated 3/2003
Compatibilities updated 3/2001

Protamine

Dose and Administration

1 mg protamine sulfate/100 U of heparin given in last 4 hours.
Slow IV push, or IM.

Use

Heparin antagonist.

Monitoring

Monitor vital signs, clotting functions, and blood pressure continuously. Observe for bleeding.

Adverse Effects/Precautions

Excessive doses can cause serious bleeding problems. Hypotension, bradycardia, dyspnea, and transitory flushing have been reported in adults.

Pharmacology

Anticoagulant when given alone. Combines ionically with heparin to form a stable complex devoid of anticoagulant activity. Rapid action after IV use (5 minutes).

Special Considerations/Preparation

Available as a 10-mg/mL concentration in 5-, and 25-mL ampules, and 5-, 1 and 25-mL vials. **Keep refrigerated.**

Solution compatibility: D_5W and NS. No data are currently available on Dex/AA.

Terminal injection site compatibility: Cimetidine and ranitidine. No data are currently available on heparin, potassium chloride, or other medications.

Selected Reference

♦ Roberts RJ: *Drug Therapy in Infants.* Philadelphia: WB Saunders Co, 1984, p 301.

Updated 3/97

Dose and Administration
Initial dose: 1 mg/kg per dose PO Q12 hours.
Gradually increase as needed every 3 to 5 days until stable rhythm is maintained.
Maximum dose: 4 mg/kg per dose PO Q12 hours.

Uses
Treatment of refractory ventricular and supraventricular tachyarrhythmias.

Monitoring
Frequent EKG during initiation of therapy.

Adverse Effects/Precautions
Proarrhythmic effects occur in 10% of pediatric patients: sinoatrial block, A-V block, torsades de pointes and ventricular ectopic activity. These effects usually occur in the first few days of treatment. Prolongation of the QT interval is dose-dependent. Other adverse effects include fatigue, dyspnea, and hypotension.

Pharmacology
Sotalol is an antiarrhythmic agent that combines Class II beta-blocking properties with Class III prolongation of cardiac action potential duration. Betapace® is a racemic mixture of *d*- and *l*-sotalol. Oral bioavailability is good, but absorption is decreased by 20 to 30% by food, especially milk. Sotalol does not bind to plasma proteins, is not metabolized, and is renally excreted as unchanged drug. Limited pharmacokinetic data in infants show a half-life of 8 hours, increasing significantly in elderly patients and those with renal dysfunction.

Special Considerations/Preparation
Supplied in 80-mg, 120-mg, 160-mg, and 240-mg tablets. A 5 mg/mL oral suspension may be made as follows: crush 5 (five) 120-mg tablets, slowly mix in 84 mL of 1% methylcellulose, then add enough simple syrup to make a total volume of 120 mL. Stable for 60 days when kept refrigerated.

Selected References
♦ Saul JP, Schaffer MS, Karpawich PP, et al: Single dose pharmacokinetics of sotalol in a pediatric population with supraventricular and/or ventricular tachyarrhythmia. *J Clin Pharmacol* 2001;41:35-43.

♦ Pfammatter JP, Paul T, Lehmann C, Kallfelz HC: Efficacy and proarrhythmia of oral sotalol in pediatric patients. *J Am Coll Cardiol* 1995;26:1002.

♦ Tanel RE, Walsh EP, Lulu JA, and Saul JP: Sotalol for refractory arrhythmias in pediatric and young adult patients: Initial efficacy and long-term outcome. *Am Heart J* 1995;130:791.

♦ Hohnloser SH, Woosley RL: Sotalol. *N Engl J Med* 1994;331:31.

♦ Nappi JM, McCollam PL: Sotalol: A breakthrough antiarrhythmic? *Ann Pharmacother* 1993;27:1359.

♦ Maragnes P, Tipple M, Fournier A: Effectiveness of oral sotalol for treatment of pediatric arrhythmias. *Am J Cardiol* 1992;69:751.

References and Pharmacology updated 3/2001

CARDIOVASCULAR

Sodium Nitroprusside

Dose and Administration

Initial Dose: 0.25 to 0.5 mcg/kg per minute continuous IV infusion by syringe pump. Use a large vein for IV.

Titrate dose upward Q20 minutes until desired response is attained.

Usual maintenance dose is < 2 mcg/kg per minute.

For hypertensive crisis, may use up to 10 mcg/kg per minute, but for no longer than 10 minutes.

Consider administering in a 1:10 mixture with sodium thiosulfate to minimize cyanide accumulation.

Uses

Acute treatment of hypertensive emergencies. Acute afterload reduction in patients with refractory congestive heart failure.

Monitoring

Continuous heart rate and intra-arterial blood pressure monitoring is mandatory. Daily measurement of RBC cyanide (should be less than 200 ng/mL) and serum thiocyanate (should be less than 50 mcg/mL) concentrations. Assess frequently for development of metabolic acidosis. Daily assessment of renal and hepatic function.

Monitor IV site closely.

Adverse Effects/Precautions

Severe hypotension and tachycardia. Cyanide toxicity may occur with prolonged treatment (> 3 days) and high (>3 mcg/kg per minute) doses. Use with caution in liver and renal failure patients due to possible impairment of the metabolism of cyanide to thiocyanate. Extravasation can cause tissue sloughing and necrosis.

Pharmacology

Direct-acting nonselective (arterial and venous) vasodilator. Immediately interacts with RBC oxyhemoglobin, dissociating and forming methemoglobin with release of cyanide and nitric oxide. Rapid onset of action with a serum half-life of 3 to 4 minutes in adults. Further metabolized to thiocyanate in the liver and kidney. Thiocyanate is renally eliminated with a half-life of 4 to 7 days.

continued...

Special Considerations/Preparation

Available as powder for injection in 2 mL and 5 mL single-dose 50 mg vials. Reconstitute contents of vial with 2 to 3 mL of D_5W or NS. **Do not administer reconstituted drug directly from vial.**

Dilute entire vial contents to a final concentration less than 200 mcg/mL (0.2 mg/mL) in D_5W or NS. Then prepare a 1:10 (by weight) solution of sodium nitroprusside and sodium thiosulfate. Use within 24 hours of preparation. Protect from light with aluminum foil or other opaque material. Blue, green or deep red discoloration indicates nitroprusside inactivation. Slight brownish discoloration is common and not significant.

> **Example:** Mix 50 mg (1 vial) of sodium nitroprusside in 250 mL D_5W. Add 500 mg sodium thiosulfate (5mL of 10% solution). Mixture is stable for 7 days. **Protect from light.**

Solution compatibility: D_5W and NS only.

Terminal injection site compatibility: Fat emulsion. Aminophylline, calcium chloride, cimetidine, dobutamine, dopamine, enalaprilat, epinephrine, esmolol, famotidine, furosemide, heparin, indomethacin, insulin, isoproterenol, lidocaine, magnesium, midazolam, morphine, nitroglycerin, pancuronium, potassium chloride, procainamide, propofol, prostaglandin E_1, ranitidine, and vecuronium.

Incompatibility: Amiodarone.

Selected References

♦ Friederich JA, Butterworth JF: Sodium nitroprusside: Twenty years and counting. *Anesth Analg* 1995;81:152.

♦ Benitz WE, Malachowski N, Cohen RS, et al: Use of sodium nitroprusside in neonates: Efficacy and safety. *J Pediatr* 1985;106:102.

♦ Roberts RJ: *Drug Therapy in Infants.* Philadelphia: WB Saunders Co, 1984, p 184.

♦ Dillon TR, Janos GG, Meyer RA, et al: Vasodilator therapy for congestive heart failure. *J Pediatr* 1980;96:623.

♦ Seto W, Trope A, Carfrae L, et al: Visual compatibility of sodium nitroprusside with other injectable medications given to pediatric patients. *Am J Health-Syst Pharm* 2001;58:1422-6.

Added 3/96
Compatibilities updated 3/2002

CNS Drugs

Acetaminophen

Dose & Administration

Oral Loading dose: 20 to 25 mg/kg. Maintenance: 12 to 15 mg/kg per dose.
Rectal Loading dose: 30 mg/kg. Maintenance: 12 to 18 mg/kg per dose.

Maintenance intervals: Term infants: Q6 hours;
  Preterm infants > 32 weeks GA: Q8 hours;
  Preterm infants < 32 weeks GA: Q12 hours;

Uses

Fever reduction and treatment of mild to moderate pain.

Monitoring

Assess for signs of pain. Monitor temperature. Assess liver function. Serum acetaminophen concentration is obtained only to assess toxicity.

Adverse Effects/Precautions

Liver toxicity occurs with excessive doses or after prolonged administration (>48 hours) of therapeutic doses. Rash, fever, thrombocytopenia, leukopenia, and neutropenia have been reported in children.

Pharmacology

Nonnarcotic analgesic and antipyretic. Peak serum concentration occurs approximately 60 minutes after an oral dose. Absorption after rectal administration is variable and prolonged. Extensively metabolized in the liver, primarily by sulfation with a small amount by glucuronidation. Metabolites and unchanged drug are excreted by the kidney. Elimination half-life is approximately 3 hours in term neonates, 5 hours in preterm neonates > 32 weeks gestation, and up to 11 hours in more immature neonates. Elimination is prolonged in patients with liver dysfunction.

Special Considerations/Preparation

Dosage forms: Drops: 100 mg/mL, 48 mg/mL (alcohol-free).
Elixir: 16 mg/mL, 24 mg/mL, 32 mg/mL.
Liquid: 32 mg/mL (alcohol-free). Liquid: 33.33 mg/mL (7% alcohol).
Suppositories: 80,120, 325, 600, and 650 mg.
Inaccurate dosing may occur with rectal administration because of unequal distribution of acetaminophen in the suppositories.

Treatment of Serious Acetaminophen Toxicity: N-acetylcysteine, 150 mg/kg, in 5% dextrose given IV over 30 minutes (loading dose), followed by 50 mg/kg over 4 hours, then 100 mg/kg per 24 hours until the International Normalized Prothrombin (INR) normalizes.

Selected References

♦ Anderson BJ, van Lingen RA, Hansen TG, et al: Acetaminophen developmental pharmacokinetics in premature neonates and infants. *Anesthesiology* 2002;96: 1336-45.

♦ Isbister GK, Bucens IK, Whyte IM: Paracetamol overdose in a preterm neonate. *Arch Dis Child Fetal Neonatal Ed* 2001;85:F70-F72.

♦ Arana A, Morton NS, Hansen TG: Treatment with paracetamol in infants. *Acta Anaesthesiol Scand* 2001;45:20-29.

♦ Levy G, Khanna NN, Soda DM, et al: Pharmacokinetics of acetaminophen in the human neonate: Formation of acetaminophen glucuronide and sulfate in relation to plasma bilirubin concentration and D-glucaric acid excretion. *Pediatrics* 1975;55:818.

Updated 3/2003

Dose and Administration

25 to 75 mg/kg per dose PO or PR. Oral preparation should be diluted or administered after a feeding to reduce gastric irritation.

Uses

Sedative/hypnotic for short-term use only. Chloral hydrate has no analgesic properties; excitement may occur in patients with pain.

Monitoring

Assess level of sedation.

Adverse Effects/Precautions

Gastric irritation and paradoxical excitement may occur after a single dose. Toxic effects have generally been reported in patients who received either repeated doses at regular intervals or acute overdoses. These effects may persist for days and include CNS, respiratory, and myocardial depression; cardiac arrhythmias; and ileus and bladder atony. Indirect hyperbilirubinemia may occur because TCE and bilirubin compete for hepatic conjugation.

Do not use in patients with significant hepatic and/or renal disease.

Pharmacology

Well absorbed from the oral route, with the onset of action in 10 to 15 minutes. Chloral hydrate is rapidly converted by alcohol dehydrogenase to the active and potentially toxic metabolite trichloroethanol (TCE), which is excreted renally after glucuronidation in the liver. It is also metabolized to trichloroacetic acid (TCA), which is carcinogenic in mice when given in very high doses. Both TCE (8 to 64 hours) and TCA (days) have long serum half-lives in neonates and accumulate with repeated doses.

Special Considerations/Preparation

Chloral hydrate is available in syrup as 50-mg/mL and 100-mg/mL concentrations. Osmolality is 3285 mOsm/kg of water.

The preparations are light-sensitive: Store in a dark container.

Also available as 324- and 648-mg suppositories.

Selected References

♦ American Academy of Pediatrics, Committee on Drugs and Committee on Environmental Health: Use of chloral hydrate for sedation in children. *Pediatrics* 1993;92:471.

♦ Mayers DJ, Hindmarsh KW, Gorecki DKJ, Sankaran K: Sedative/hypnotic effects of chloral hydrate in the neonate: Trichloroethanol or parent drug? *Dev Pharmacol Ther* 1992;19:141.

♦ Anyebuno MA, Rosenfeld CR: Chloral hydrate toxicity in a term infant. *Dev Pharmacol Ther* 1991;17:116.

♦ Mayers DJ, Hindmarsh KW, Sankaran K, et al: Chloral hydrate disposition following single-dose administration to critically ill neonates and children. *Dev Pharmacol Ther* 1991;16:71.

♦ Reimche LD, Sankaran K, Hindmarsh KW, et al: Chloral hydrate sedation in neonates and infants: Clinical and pharmacologic considerations. *Dev Pharmacol Ther* 1989;12:57.

Updated 1/94

CNS DRUGS

Fentanyl

Dose & Administration

Sedation and analgesia: 1 to 4 mcg/kg per dose IV slow push. Repeat as required (usually Q2 to 4 hours).

Infusion rate: 1 to 5 mcg/kg per hour.
Tolerance may develop rapidly following constant infusion.

Anesthesia: 5 to 50 mcg/kg per dose.

Uses

Analgesia. Sedation. Anesthesia.

Monitoring

Monitor respiratory and cardiovascular status closely. Observe for abdominal distention, loss of bowel sounds, and muscle rigidity.

Adverse Effects/Precautions

Respiratory depression occurs when anesthetic doses (>5 mcg/kg) are used and may also occur unexpectedly because of redistribution. Chest wall rigidity has occurred in 4% of neonates who received 2.2 to 6.5 mcg/kg per dose, occasionally associated with laryngospasm. This was reversible with administration of naloxone. Tolerance may develop to analgesic doses with prolonged use. Urinary retention may occur during continuous infusions. Significant withdrawal symptoms have been reported in patients treated with continuous infusion for 5 days or longer.

Pharmacology

Synthetic opioid narcotic analgesic that is 50 to 100 times more potent than morphine on a weight basis. Extremely lipid soluble. Penetrates the CNS rapidly. Transient rebound in fentanyl serum concentration may reflect sequestration and subsequent release of fentanyl from body fat. Metabolized extensively in the liver by CYP 3A4 enzyme system and then excreted by the kidney. Serum half-life is prolonged in patients with liver failure. Highly protein bound. Wide variability in apparent volume of distribution (10 to 30 L/kg) and serum half-life (1 to 15 hours).

continued...

Special Considerations/Preparation

Naloxone should be readily available to reverse adverse effects.

Available in 2-, 5-, 10-, and 20-mL ampules in a concentration of 50 mcg/mL. A 4-mcg/mL dilution may be made by adding 0.8 mL of the 50 mcg/mL concentration to 9.2 mL preservative-free normal saline. Stable for 24 hours refrigerated. Protect from light.

Solution Compatibility: D_5W, $D_{10}W$, and NS.

Terminal Injection Site Compatibility: Dex/AA and fat emulsion. Atropine, caffeine citrate, cimetidine, dexamethasone, dobutamine, dopamine, enalaprilat, epinephrine, esmolol, furosemide, heparin, hydrocortisone succinate, lidocaine, linezolid, lorazepam, metoclopramide, midazolam, morphine, nafcillin, pancuronium bromide, potassium chloride, propofol, ranitidine, remifentanil, sodium bicarbonate, and vecuronium.

Incompatibility: Pentobarbital and phenytoin.

Selected References

♦ Fahnenstich H, Steffan J, Kau N, Bartmann P: Fentanyl-induced chest wall rigidity and laryngospasm in preterm and term infants. *Crit Care Med* 2000;28:836-839.

♦ Saarenmaa E, Neuvonen PJ, Fellman V: Gestational age and birth weight effects on plasma clearance of fentanyl in newborn infants. *J Pediatr* 2000;136:767-770.

♦ Muller P and Vogtmann C: Three cases with different presentation of fentanyl-induced muscle rigidity-A rare problem in intensive care of neonates. *Am J Perinatol* 2000;17:23-26.

♦ Santeiro mL, Christie J, Stromquist C, et al: Pharmacokinetics of continuous infusion fentanyl in newborns. *J Perinatol* 1997;17:135-139.

♦ Arnold JH, Truog RD, Orav EJ, et al: Tolerance and dependence in neonates sedated with fentanyl during extracorporeal membrane oxygenation. *Anesthesiology* 1990;73:1136.

♦ Koehntop DE, Rodman JH, Brundage DM, et al: Pharmacokinetics of fentanyl in neonates. *Anesth Analg* 1986;65:227.

♦ Johnson KL, Erickson JP, Holley Of, et al: Fentanyl pharmacokinetics in the pediatric population. *Anesthesiology* 1984;61:A441.

♦ Reilly CS, Wood AJ, Wood M: Variability of fentanyl pharmacokinetics in man. *Anaesthesia* 1984;40:837.

♦ Mather LE: Clinical pharmacokinetics of fentanyl and its newer derivatives. *Clin Pharmacokinet* 1983;8:422.

Text updated 3/2002
Compatibilities updated 3/2003

CNS DRUGS

Fosphenytoin

Dose and Administration

Note: Fosphenytoin dosing is expressed in phenytoin equivalents (PE). (Fosphenytoin 1 mg PE = phenytoin 1 mg)

Loading dose: 15 to 20 mg PE/kg IM or IV infusion over at least 10 minutes.

Maintenance dose: 4 to 8 mg PE/kg Q24 hours IM or IV slow push. Begin maintenance 24 hours after loading dose.

Maximum rate of infusion 1.5 mg PE/kg per minute. May be administered more rapidly than phenytoin due to less infusion-related toxicity. Flush IV with saline before and after administration.

Term infants older than 1 week of age may require up to 8 mg PE/kg per dose Q8 to 12 hours.

Uses

Anticonvulsant. Generally used to treat seizures that are refractory to phenobarbital. Can be administered with lorazepam for rapid onset of seizure control.

Monitoring

Monitor blood pressure closely during infusion. Measure trough serum phenytoin (**not** fosphenytoin) concentration; obtain 48 hours after IV loading dose. Therapeutic serum phenytoin concentration: Probably 6 to 15 mcg/mL (? 10 to 20). Collect blood samples in EDTA tubes to minimize fosphenytoin to phenytoin conversion in the tube.

Adverse Effects/Precautions

Clinical signs of toxicity, such as drowsiness, are difficult to identify in infants, but are dose and infusion rate dependent. Minor venous irritation upon IV administration. Fosphenytoin drug interactions are similar to phenytoin (i.e. carbamazepine, cimetidine, corticosteroids, digoxin, furosemide, phenobarbital, and valproate).

Use with caution in neonates with hyperbilirubinemia: both fosphenytoin and bilirubin displace phenytoin from protein-binding sites, resulting in increased serum free phenytoin concentration.

continued...

Pharmacology

Fosphenytoin is a water-soluble prodrug of phenytoin rapidly converted by phosphatases in blood and tissue. It has no known intrinsic pharmacologic activity before conversion to phenytoin. Each 1.5 mg of fosphenytoin is metabolically converted to 1 mg phenytoin. Conversion half-life of fosphenytoin administered intravenously to pediatric patients has been reported to be 7.1 minutes (range, 3.8 to 9.6 minutes). Data obtained using spiked blood samples from term and preterm neonates demonstrated similar conversion rates. No drugs have been identified to interfere with the conversion of fosphenytoin to phenytoin. Fosphenytoin is highly protein bound (adults 95% to 99%) and does not penetrate the blood-brain barrier. Serum half-life reflects that of phenytoin (18 to 60 hours) due to rapid conversion. The conversion of fosphenytoin to phenytoin yields very small amounts of formaldehyde and phosphate. This is only significant in cases of large overdosage. Phenytoin serum concentrations measured up to two hours after IV and four hours after IM dose may be falsely elevated due to fosphenytoin interaction with immunoanalytic methods (e.g. TDx fluorescence polarization).

Special Considerations/Preparation

Available as an injectable solution in a concentration equivalent to 50 mg PE/mL, in 2- and 10-mL vials. Administer IM undiluted. Administer IV after diluting in NS or D_5W to a concentration of 1.5 to 25 mg PE/mL. The pH is 8.6 to 9.0.

Store refrigerated. Stable for 48 hours at room temperature. Do not use vials containing particulate matter.

Solution compatibility: D_5W, $D_{10}W$ and NS.

Terminal injection site compatibility: Lorazepam, phenobarbital, and potassium chloride.

Incompatibility: Midazolam.

Selected References

♦ Takeoka M, Krishnamoorthy KS, Soman TB, et al: Fosphenytoin in infants. *J Child Neurol* 1998;13:537-540.

♦ Morton LD: Clinical experience with fosphenytoin in children. *J Child Neurol* 1998;13(Suppl 1):S19-S22.

♦ Hatzopoulus FK, Carlos MA, Fischer JH: Safety and pharmacokinetics of intramuscular fosphenytoin in neonates. *Pediatr Res* 1998; 43:60A.

♦ Boucher BA: Fosphenytoin: A novel phenytoin prodrug. *Pharmacother* 1996;16:777.

♦ Fischer JH, Cwik MJ, Luer MS, et al: Stability of fosphenytoin sodium with intravenous solutions in glass bottles, polyvinyl chloride bags, and polypropylene syringes. *Ann Pharmacother* 1997;31:553-559.

♦ English BA, Riggs RM, Webster AA, Benner KW: Y-site stability of fosphenytoin and sodium phenobarbital. *Int J Pharm Compound* 1999;3:64-66.

♦ Riggs RM, English BA, Webster AA, et al: Fosphenytoin Y-site stability studies with lorazepam and midazolam hydrochloride. *Int J Pharm Compound* 1999;3:235-238.

Added 3/2000

CNS DRUGS

Lorazepam

Dose & Administration
0.05 to 0.1 mg/kg per dose IV slow push. Repeat doses based on clinical response.

Uses
Anticonvulsant—acute management of patients with seizures refractory to conventional therapy.

Monitoring
Monitor respiratory status closely. Observe IV site for signs of phlebitis or extravasation.

Adverse Effects/Precautions
Respiratory depression. Rhythmic myoclonic jerking has occurred in premature neonates receiving lorazepam for sedation.

Pharmacology
Dose-dependent CNS depression. Onset of action within 5 minutes; peak serum concentration within 45 minutes. Duration of action is 3 to 24 hours. Mean half-life in term neonates is 40 hours. Metabolized to an inactive glucuronide, which is excreted by the kidneys. Highly lipid-soluble. Phenobarbital serum concentrations may increase after lorazepam administration.

Special Considerations/Preparation
Limited data are available for neonates. Available in 2 mg/mL and 4 mg/mL concentrations. Preparation contains 2% (20 mg/mL) benzyl alcohol and 18% polyethylene glycol 400 in propylene glycol. We recommend using the 4 mg/mL dosage strength diluted to 0.4 mg/mL with preservative-free sterile water for injection. This will make it easier to measure the dose and decrease the benzyl alcohol content to 0.5 mg/kg per dose.
Solutions should not be used if they are discolored or contain a precipitate.

Solution Compatibility: D_5W, NS, and sterile water for injection.

Terminal Injection Site Compatibility: Acyclovir, amikacin, bumetanide, cefepime, cefotaxime, cimetidine, dexamethasone, dobutamine, dopamine, epinephrine, erythromycin lactobionate, famotidine, fentanyl, fluconazole, fosphenytoin, furosemide, gentamicin, heparin, hydrocortisone succinate, labetalol, linezolid, metronidazole, midazolam, morphine, nitroglycerin, pancuronium bromide, piperacillin, piperacillin-tazobactam, potassium chloride, propofol, ranitidine, remifentanil, trimethoprim-sulfamethoxazole, vancomycin, vecuronium, and zidovudine.

Incompatibility: Fat emulsion. Aztreonam, imipenem/cilastatin, and omeprazole.

Selected References
♦ Sexson WR, Thigpen J, Stajich GV: Stereotypic movements after lorazepam administration in premature neonates: a series and review of the literature. *J Perinatol* 1995;15:146-49.
♦ McDermott CA, Kowalczyk AL, Schnitzler ER, et al: Pharmacokinetics of lorazepam in critically ill neonates with seizures. *J Pediatr* 1992;120:479.
♦ Deshmukh A, Wittert W, Schnitzler E, Mangurten HH: Lorazepam in the treatment of refractory neonatal seizures. *Am J Dis Child* 1986;140:1042.

Text updated 3/98
Compatibilities updated 3/2003

Dose & Administration

Initial dose: 0.05 to 0.2 mg/kg per dose Q12 to 24 hours, PO or IV slow push. Reduce dose by 10 to 20% per week over 4 to 6 weeks. Adjust weaning schedule based on signs and symptoms of withdrawal.

Uses

Treatment of opiate withdrawal.

Monitoring

Monitor respiratory and cardiac status closely. Assess for gastric residuals, abdominal distention, and loss of bowel sounds.

Adverse Effects/Precautions

Respiratory depression in excessive doses. Ileus and delayed gastric emptying.

Pharmacology

Long-acting narcotic analgesic. Oral bioavailability is 50%, with peak plasma levels obtained in 2 to 4 hours. Metabolized extensively via hepatic N-demethylation. Highly protein bound (90% adults). Serum half-life ranges from 16 to 25 hours in neonates and is prolonged in patients with renal failure. Rifampin and phenytoin accelerate the metabolism of methadone and can precipitate withdrawal symptoms.

Special Considerations/Preparation

Available as oral solutions in 1- and 2-mg/mL concentrations containing 8% alcohol, and a 10-mg/mL alcohol-free solution. May dilute 1 mL of the 10-mg/mL concentrated solution with 19 mL of sterile water to provide an oral dilution with a final concentration of 0.5-mg/mL. Stable for 24 hours refrigerated. IV form available in 1-mL ampules and 20-mL vials containing 10-mg/mL. Also available as 5- and 10-mg tablets.

Solution Compatibility: NS. No data currently available on D_5W, $D_{10}W$, or Dex/AA.

Terminal Injection Site Compatibility: Atropine, dexamethasone, lorazepam, methoclopramide, midazolam, and phenobarbital.

Incompatibility: Aminophylline, heparin, methicillin, phenytoin, secobarbital, and sodium bicarbonate.

Selected References

♦ Tobias JD, Schleien CL, Haun SE: Methadone as treatment for iatrogenic narcotic dependency in pediatric intensive care unit patients. *Crit Care Med* 1990;18:1292.

♦ Koren G, Maurice L: Pediatric uses of opioids. *Ped Clin North Am* 1989;36:1141.

♦ Rosen TS, Pippenger CE: Pharmacologic observations on the neonatal withdrawal syndrome. *J Pediatr* 1976;88:1044.

Added 1/95
Compatibilities updated 3/2003

CNS DRUGS

Midazolam

Dose & Administration

IV: 0.05 to 0.15 mg/kg **over at least 5 minutes.** Repeat as required, usually Q2 to 4 hours. May also be given IM. Dosage requirements are decreased by concurrent use of narcotics.

Continuous IV infusion: 0.01 to 0.06 mg/kg per hour.
(10 to 60 mcg/kg/hour). Dosage may need to be increased after several days of therapy because of development of tolerance and/or increased clearance.

Intranasal: 0.2 to 0.3 mg/kg per dose using 5 mg/mL injectable form.

Sublingual: 0.2 mg/kg per dose using 5 mg/mL injectable form mixed with a small amount of flavored syrup.

Oral: 0.25 mg/kg per dose using Versed® oral syrup. *

Uses

Sedative/hypnotic. Anesthesia induction. Treatment of refractory seizures.

Monitoring

Follow respiratory status and blood pressure closely, especially when used concurrently with narcotics. Assess hepatic function. Observe for signs of withdrawal after discontinuation of prolonged therapy.

Adverse Effects/Precautions

Respiratory depression and hypotension are common when used in conjunction with narcotics, or following rapid bolus administration. Seizure-like myoclonus has been reported in 8% of premature infants receiving continuous infusions - this also may occur following rapid bolus administration and in patients with underlying CNS disorders. Nasal administration may be uncomfortable because of a burning sensation.

Pharmacology

Relatively short-acting benzodiazepine with rapid onset of action. Sedative and anticonvulsant properties related to GABA accumulation and occupation of benzodiazepine receptor. Antianxiety properties related to increasing the glycine inhibitory neurotransmitter. Metabolized by hepatic CYP 3A4 to a less active hydroxylated metabolite, then glucuronidated before excretion in urine. Drug accumulation may occur with repeated doses, prolonged infusion therapy, or concurrent administration of cimetidine, erythromycin or fluconazole. Highly protein bound. Duration of action is 2 to 6 hours. Elimination half-life is approximately 4 to 6 hours in term neonates, and quite variable, up to 22 hours, in premature babies and those with impaired hepatic function. Bioavailability is approximately 36% with oral administration and 50% with sublingual and intranasal administration. Midazolam is water soluble in acidic solutions and becomes lipid soluble at physiologic pH.

continued...

CNS DRUGS

Special Considerations/Preparation

The injectable form is available as 5-mg/mL and 1-mg/mL concentrations in 1-, 2-, 5-, and 10-mL vials. Contains 1% (10 mg/mL) benzyl alcohol as a preservative: To decrease benzyl alcohol content, a 0.5-mg/mL dilution may be made by adding 1 mL of the 5-mg/mL concentration to 9 mL preservative-free sterile water for injection. Dilution stable for 24 hours refrigerated.

Versed® oral syrup is available in a 2 mg/mL concentration. Store at room temperature.

Solution Compatibility: D_5W, NS, and sterile water for injection.

Terminal Injection Site Compatibility: Dex/AA. Amiodarone, amikacin, atropine, calcium gluconate, cefazolin, cefotaxime, cimetidine, clindamycin, digoxin, dobutamine, dopamine, epinephrine, erythromycin lactobionate, esmolol, famotidine, fentanyl, fluconazole, gentamicin, glycopyrolate, heparin, imipenem/cilastatin, insulin, linezolid, lorazepam, methadone, metoclopramide, metronidazole, morphine, nitroglycerin, nitroprusside, pancuronium bromide, piperacillin, potassium chloride, propofol, prostaglandin E_1, ranitidine, remifentanil, sodium nitroprusside, theophylline, tobramycin, vancomycin, and vecuronium.

Incompatibility: Fat emulsion. Ampicillin, bumetanide, ceftazidime, dexamethasone, fosphenytoin, furosemide, hydrocortisone succinate, nafcillin, omeprazole, pentobarbital, phenobarbital, and sodium bicarbonate.

Selected References

♦ de Wildt SN, Kearns GL, Hop WCJ, et al: Pharmacokinetics and metabolism of intravenous midazolam in preterm infants. *Clin Pharmacol Ther* 2001;70:525-531.

♦ Coté CJ, Cohen IT, Suresh S, et al: A comparison of three doses of a commercially prepared oral midazolam syrup in children. *Anesth Analg* 2002;94:37-43.

♦ Sheth RD, Buckley DJ, Gutierrez AR: Midazolam in the treatment of refractory neonatal seizures. *Clin Neuropharmacol* 1996;2:165-70.

♦ Olkkola KT, Ahonen J, Neuvonen PJ: The effect of the systemic antimycotics, itraconazole and fluconazole, on the pharmacokinetics and pharmacodynamics of intravenous and oral midazolam. *Anesth Analg* 1996;82:511.

♦ Jacqz-Aigrain E, Daoud P, Burtin P, et al: Placebo-controlled trial of midazolam sedation in mechanically ventilated newborn babies. *Lancet* 1994;344:646-50.

♦ Magnyn JF, d'Allest AM, Nedelcoux H, et al: Midazolam and myoclonus in neonate. *Eur J Pediatr* 1994;153:389.

♦ Karl HW, Rosenberger JL, Larach mg, Ruffie JM: Transmucosal administration of midazolam for premedication of pediatric patients: Comparison of the nasal and sublingual routes. *Anesthesiology* 1993;78:885.

♦ Jacqz-Aigrain E, Daoud P, Burtin P, et al: Pharmacokinetics of midazolam during continuous infusion in critically ill neonates. *Eur J Clin Pharmacol* 1992;42:329.

♦ van Straaten HLM, Rademaker CMA, de Vries LS: Comparison of the effect of midazolam or vecuronium on blood pressure and cerebral blood flow velocity in the premature newborn. *Dev Pharmacol Ther* 1992;19:191.

Pharmacology updated 3/2003
Compatibilities updated 3/2003

CNS DRUGS

Morphine

Dose & Administration

0.05 to 0.2 mg/kg per dose IV over at least 5 minutes, IM, or SC. Repeat as required (usually Q4 hours).

Continuous infusion: Give a loading dose of 100 to 150 mcg/kg over 1 hour followed by 10 to 20 mcg/kg per hour.

Treatment of opioid dependence: Begin at most recent IV morphine dose equivalent. Taper 10 to 20% per day as tolerated. Oral dose is approximately 3 to 5 times IV dose.

Treatment of neonatal narcotic abstinence: 0.08 to 0.2 mg per dose PO Q3 to 4 hours.

Use a 0.4-mg/mL dilution made from either a concentrated oral morphine sulfate solution or deodorized tincture of opium (see Special Consideration/Preparation section).

Uses

Analgesia. Sedation. Treatment of opioid withdrawal and abstinence.

Monitoring

Monitor respiratory and cardiovascular status closely. Observe for abdominal distention and loss of bowel sounds. Consider urine retention if output is decreased.

Adverse Effects/Precautions

Naloxone should be readily available to reverse adverse effects. Marked respiratory depression (decreases the responsiveness of the respiratory center to CO_2 tension). Hypotension and bradycardia. Transient hypertonia. Ileus and delayed gastric emptying. Urine retention. Tolerance may develop after prolonged use—wean slowly. Seizures reported in two infants who received bolus plus infusion.

Pharmacology

Narcotic analgesic—stimulates brain opioid receptors. Increases venous capacitance, caused by release of histamine and central suppression of adrenergic tone. GI secretions and motility decreased. Increases smooth muscle tone. Morphine is converted in the liver to two glucuronide metabolites (morphine-6-glucuronide and morphine-3-glucuronide) that are renally excreted. Morphine-6-glucuronide (M6G) is a potent respiratory-depressant and analgesic. morphine-3-glucuronide (M3G) is an antagonist to the effects of morphine and morphine-6-glucuronide. Morphine is 20 to 40% bioavailable when administered orally. Pharmacokinetics are widely variable. Elimination half-life is approximately 9 hours for morphine and 18 hours for morphine-6-glucuronide. Steady state concentrations of morphine are reached by 24 to 48 hours.

continued...

Special Considerations/Preparation

Injectable solutions are available in dosage strengths ranging from 0.5 to 50 mg/mL. Alcohol-free, oral morphine-sulfate solutions are available in concentrations of 2, 4, and 20 mg/mL. Tincture of opium, 10% (10 mg/mL) contains 19% alcohol. Paregoric (camphorated tincture of opium) is not recommended; it contains alcohol (45%), camphor, anise oil, and benzoic acid.

A 0.4 mg/mL oral morphine dilution may be made by adding 1 mL of the 4 mg/mL injectable solution to 9 mL preservative-free normal saline. Stable for 7 days refrigerated. **Protect from light.**

Solution Compatibility: D_5W, $D_{10}W$, and NS.

For continuous infusions of morphine **containing heparin:** Use only NS; maximum morphine concentration 5 mg/mL.

Terminal Injection Site Compatibility: Dex/AA and fat emulsion. Acyclovir, alteplase, amikacin, aminophylline, amiodarone, ampicillin, atropine, aztreonam, bumetanide, calcium chloride, cefotaxime, cefoxitin, ceftazidime, ceftriaxone, chloramphenicol, cefazolin, cimetidine, clindamycin, dexamethasone, digoxin, dobutamine, dopamine, enalaprilat, epinephrine, erythromycin lactobionate, esmolol, famotidine, fentanyl, fluconazole, furosemide, gentamicin, glycopyrolate, heparin, hydrocortisone succinate, insulin, lidocaine, linezolid, lorazepam, meropenem, metoclopramide, metronidazole, mezlocillin, midazolam, nafcillin, nitroglycerine, oxacillin, pancuronium bromide, penicillin G, piperacillin, piperacillin-tazobactam, potassium chloride, propofol, propranolol, prostaglandin E_1, ranitidine, remifentanil, sodium bicarbonate, sodium nitroprusside, ticarcillin/clavulanate, tobramycin, trimethoprim-sulfamethoxazole, vancomycin, vecuronium, and zidovudine.

Incompatibility: Cefepime, pentobarbital, phenobarbital, and phenytoin.

Selected References

♦ Saarenmaa E, Neuvonen PJ, Rosenberg P, Fellman V: Morphine clearance and effects in newborn infants in relation to gestational age. *Clin Pharmacol Ther* 2000; 68:160-166.

♦ American Academy of Pediatrics Committee on Drugs: Neonatal drug withdrawal. *Pediatrics* 1998;101:1079-1088.

♦ Yaster M, Kost-Byerly S, Berde C, Billet C: The management of opioid and benzodiazepine dependence in infants, children, and adolescents. *Pediatrics* 1996;98:135-40.

♦ Barrett DA, Barker DP, Rutter N, et al: Morphine, morphine-6-glucuronide and morphine-3-glucuronide pharmacokinetics in newborn infants receiving diamorphine infusions. *Br J Clin Pharmacol* 1996;41:531.

♦ Hartley R, Green M, Quinn M, Levene MI: Pharmacokinetics of morphine infusion in premature neonates. *Arch Dis Child* 1993;69:55.

♦ Chay PCW, Duffy BJ, Walker JS: Pharmacokinetic-pharmacodynamic relationships of morphine in neonates. *Clin Pharmacol Ther* 1992;51:334.

♦ Koren G, Butt W, Chinyanga H, et al: Postoperative morphine infusion in newborn infants: Assessment of disposition characteristics and safety. *J Pediatr* 1985; 107:963.

References updated 3/2001
Compatibilities updated 3/2003

CNS DRUGS

Naloxone

Dose and Administration

0.1 mg/kg IV push, or ET. May give IM if adequate perfusion. May repeat in 3 to 5 minutes if no response during resuscitation. Do not use if maternal narcotic addiction is suspected – may precipitate withdrawal.

Uses

Narcotic antagonist. Adjuvant therapy to customary resuscitation efforts for narcotic-induced respiratory (CNS) depression.

Monitoring

Assess respiratory effort and neurologic status.

Adverse Effects/Precautions

No short-term toxicity observed. One case report of seizures secondary to acute opioid withdrawal after administration to an infant born to an opioid abuser. Long-term safety has not been investigated.

Pharmacology

Reverses respiratory depression by competing for CNS narcotic receptor sites. Onset of action within 1 to 2 minutes after IV administration, within 15 minutes of IM administration. Metabolized by the liver and excreted in the urine. Increases circulating catecholamines.

Special Considerations/Preparation

Do not mix in an alkaline solution. Available in 1 mg/mL and 0.4 mg/mL concentrations. **Store at room temperature and protect from light.**

Solution compatibility: No data are currently available on Dex/AA.

Terminal injection site compatibility: Heparin, linezolid, and propofol. No data are currently available on potassium chloride and other medications.

Selected References

♦ International Guidelines for Neonatal Resuscitation: An excerpt from the Guidelines 2000 for Cardiopulmonary Resuscitation and Emergency Cardiovascular Care: International Consensus on Science. Pediatrics 2000;106(3). URL:http://www.pediatrics.org/cgi/content/full/106/3/e29.

♦ Gibbs J, Newson T, Williams J, Davidson DC: Naloxone hazard in infant of opioid abuser. *Lancet* 1989;2:159.

♦ Gerhart T, Bancalari E, Cohen H, Rocha LF: Use of naloxone to reverse narcotic respiratory depression in the newborn infant. *J Pediatr* 1977;90:1009.

♦ Wiener PC, Hogg MIJ, Rosen M: Effects of naloxone on pethidine-induced neonatal depression. Part I: Intravenous naloxone. Part II: Intramuscular naloxone. *Br Med J* 1977;2:228.

Updated 3/2001
Compatibilities updated: 3/2002

Dose and Administration

Myasthenia gravis: 0.1 mg IM (give 30 minutes before feeding).
1 mg PO (give 2 hours before feeding). Dose may have to be increased and should be titrated.

Reversal of neuromuscular blockade: 0.04 to 0.08 mg/kg IV, in addition to atropine 0.02 mg/kg.

Uses

Neonatal transient myasthenia gravis. Neonatal persistent (congenital) myasthenia gravis. Reversing effects of neuromuscular blocking drugs.

Monitoring

Monitor respiratory and cardiovascular status closely.

Adverse Effects/Precautions

Contraindicated in presence of intestinal or urinary obstruction, bradycardia, or hypotension. Use cautiously in patients with bronchospasm or cardiac arrhythmia. Adverse effects include muscle weakness, tremors, bradycardia, hypotension, respiratory depression, bronchospasm, diarrhea, and excessive salivation.

Pharmacology

Inhibits acetylcholinesterase at the neuromuscular junction, allowing accumulation of acetylcholine and thus restoring activity.

Special Considerations/Preparation

Available as injectable solution in 1-mL ampules and 10-mL vials in concentrations of 1:1000 (1 mg/mL), 1:2000 (0.5 mg/mL), and 1:4000 (0.25 mg/mL). **Protect from light.**

Solution compatibility: No data.

Terminal injection site compatibility: Glycopyrolate, heparin, hydrocortisone succinate, netilmicin, pentobarbital and potassium chloride.

Selected References

♦ Fisher DM, Cronnelly R, Miller RD, Sharma M: The neuromuscular pharmacology of neostigmine in infants and children. *Anesthesiology* 1983;59:220.
♦ Goudsouzian NG, Crone RK, Todres ID: Recovery from pancuronium blockade in the neonatal intensive care unit. *Br J Anaesth* 1981;53:1303.
♦ Sarnat HB: Neuromuscular disorders in the neonatal period, in Korobken R, Guillemenault C (eds): *Advances in Perinatal Neurology.* New York: Spectrum Publications, 1979, p 153.

Text updated 3/2001
Compatibilities updated 3/2001

Pancuronium

Dose & Administration

0.1 mg/kg (0.04 to 0.15 mg/kg) IV push, as needed for paralysis. Usual dosing interval is 1 to 2 hours. Adjust dose as needed based on duration of paralysis.

Uses

Skeletal muscle relaxation/paralysis in infants requiring mechanical ventilation. Proposed desirable effects are improved oxygenation/ventilation, reduced barotrauma, and reduced fluctuations in cerebral blood flow.

Monitoring

Monitor vital signs frequently, blood pressure continuously. Use some form of eye lubrication.

Adverse Effects/Precautions

Hypoxemia may occur because of inadequate mechanical ventilation and deterioration in pulmonary mechanics. Tachycardia and blood pressure changes (both hypotension and hypertension) occur frequently. Increased salivation.

Pharmacology

Nondepolarizing muscle-relaxant that competitively antagonizes autonomic cholinergic receptors and also causes sympathetic stimulation. Partially hydroxylated by the liver, 40% excreted unchanged in urine. Onset of action is 1 to 2 minutes; duration varies with dose and age. Reversed by neostigmine and atropine.

Factors affecting duration of neuromuscular blockade:

Potentiation: Acidosis, hypothermia, renal failure, younger age, neuromuscular disease, hepatic disease, cardiovascular disease, aminoglycosides, hypermagnesemia, and hypokalemia.

Antagonism: Alkalosis, epinephrine, and hyperkalemia.

Sensation remains intact; analgesia should be used for painful procedures.

Special Considerations/Preparation

Available in 1 mg/mL and 2 mg/mL concentrations. Contains 1% (10 mg/mL) benzyl alcohol. **Refrigerate.**

Solution Compatibility: D_5W and NS.

Terminal Injection Site Compatibility: Dex/AA. Aminophylline, cefazolin, cimetidine, dobutamine, dopamine, epinephrine, esmolol, fentanyl, fluconazole, gentamicin, heparin, hydrocortisone succinate, isoproterenol, lorazepam, midazolam, morphine, netilmicin, nitroglycerin, nitroprusside, propofol, prostaglandin E_1, ranitidine, trimethoprim-sulfamethoxazole, and vancomycin.

Incompatibility: Pentobarbital and phenobarbital.

Selected References

♦ Bhutani VK, Abbasi S, Sivieri EM: Continuous skeletal muscle paralysis: Effect on neonatal pulmonary mechanics. *Pediatrics* 1988;81:419.

♦ Costarino AT, Polin RA: Neuromuscular relaxants in the neonate. *Clin Perinatol* 1987;14:965.

♦ Cabal LA, Siassi B, Artal R, et al: Cardiovascular and catecholamine changes after administration of pancuronium in distressed neonates. *Pediatrics* 1985;75:284.

Text updated 1/93, Compatibilities updated 3/2003

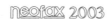

Dose and Administration
2 to 6 mg/kg IV slow push.

Uses
Sedative/hypnotic, for short-term use.

Monitoring
Monitor respiratory status and blood pressure closely.
Serum concentration for sedation: 0.5 to 3 mcg/mL.

Adverse Effects/Precautions
Respiratory depression. Tolerance, dependence, and cardiovascular depression occur with continued use. Enhances metabolism of phenytoin, sodium valproate, and corticosteroids by microsomal enzyme induction.

Pharmacology
Short-acting barbiturate. Pentobarbital has no analgesic effects. Serum half-life is dose-dependent (15 to 50 hours in adults) and unknown in neonates. Metabolized by hepatic microsomal enzyme system.

Special Considerations/Preparation
Available as a 50-mg/mL solution in 2-, 20-, and 50-mL vials. Solution contains propylene glycol 40%, and alcohol 10%. Irritating to veins—pH is 9.5.
A 5 mg/mL dilution may be made by adding 1 mL of the 50 mg/mL solution to 9 mL of preservative-free normal saline. Use immediately.

Solution compatibility: D_5W, $D_{10}W$, and NS. No data are currently available on Dex/AA.

Terminal injection site compatibility: Acyclovir, amikacin, aminophylline, atropine, calcium chloride, chloramphenicol, erythromycin lactobionate, hyaluronidase, insulin, lidocaine, linezolid, neostigmine, penicillin G, and sodium bicarbonate.

Incompatibility: Fat emulsion. Cefazolin, cimetidine, clindamycin, fentanyl, hydrocortisone succinate, midazolam, morphine, pancuronium bromide, phenytoin, propofol, ranitidine, and vancomycin. No data are currently available on heparin and potassium chloride.

Selected Reference
♦ Strain JD, Harvey LA, Foley LC, Campbell JB: Intravenously administered pentobarbital sodium for sedation in pediatric CT. *Radiology* 1986;161:105.

Text updated 3/97
Compatibilities updated 3/2002

CNS DRUGS

Phenobarbital

Dose & Administration

Loading dose: 20 mg/kg IV, given slowly over 10 to 15 minutes.
Refractory seizures: Additional 5 mg/kg doses, up to a total of 40 mg/kg.
Maintenance: 3 to 4 mg/kg **per day** beginning 12 to 24 hours after the load.
Frequency/Route: Daily (Q12 hours probably unnecessary). IV slow push (most rapid control of seizures), IM, PO, or PR.

Uses

Anticonvulsant. May improve outcomes in severely asphyxiated infants (40 mg/kg IV infusion over 1 hour, prior to onset of seizures). May enhance bile excretion in patients with cholestasis before ^{99}Tc-IDA scanning.

Monitoring

Phenobarbital monotherapy will control seizures in 43 to 85% of affected neonates - adding a second drug (phenytoin or lorazepam) is often needed. Therapeutic serum concentration is 15 to 40 mcg/mL. Drug accumulation may occur using recommended maintenance dose during the first two weeks of life. Altered (usually increased) serum concentrations may occur in patients also receiving phenytoin or valproate. Observe IV site for signs of extravasation and phlebitis.

Adverse Effects/Precautions

Sedation at serum concentrations above 40 mcg/mL. Respiratory depression at concentrations above 60 mcg/mL. Irritating to veins - pH is approximately 10 and osmolality is approximately 15,000 mOsm/kg H_2O.

Pharmacology

Phenobarbital limits the spread of seizure activity, possibly by increasing inhibitory neurotransmission. Approximately 30% protein bound. Primarily metabolized by liver, then excreted in the urine as p-hydroxyphenobarbital (no anticonvulsant activity). Serum half-life in neonates is 40 to 200 hours.

Special Considerations/Preparation

Injectable solution available in 1-mL Tubex® and vials, in concentrations of 30-, 60-, 65- and 130-mg/mL, all containing 10% (100 mg/mL) alcohol and 67.8% propylene glycol. Use within 30 minutes of opening.
Oral elixirs are available in 15 mg/5 mL and 20 mg/5 mL concentrations. All contain 13.5% alcohol (135 mg/mL).

Solution Compatibility: D_5W, $D_{10}W$, and NS. No data are currently available on neonatal Dex/AA solutions.

Terminal Injection Site Compatibility: Amikacin, aminophylline, calcium chloride, calcium gluconate, enalaprilat, fosphenytoin, heparin, linezolid, meropenem, propofol, prostaglandin E_1, and sodium bicarbonate.

Incompatibility: Fat emulsion. Cimetidine, clindamycin, hydralazine, hydrocortisone succinate, insulin, methadone, midazolam, morphine, pancuronium, ranitidine, and vancomycin. No data available on potassium chloride.

Selected References

♦ Volpe JJ: *Neurology of the Newborn,* ed 4. Philadelphia: WB Saunders Co, 2001, p 203-204.
♦ Hall RT, Hall FK, Daily SK: High-dose phenobarbital therapy in term newborn infants with severe perinatal asphyxia: A randomized, prospective study with three-year follow-up. *J Pediatr* 1998;132:345-348.

Text updated 3/2002, Compatibilities updated 3/2003

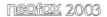

Dose & Administration

Loading dose: 15 to 20 mg/kg IV infusion over at least 30 minutes.
Maintenance dose: 4 to 8 mg/kg Q24 hours IV slow push, or PO.
(Up to 8 mg/kg per dose Q8 to 12 hours after 1 week of age).
Maximum rate of infusion 0.5 mg/kg per minute. Flush IV with saline before and after administration. **Avoid using in central lines because of the risk of precipitation. IM route not acceptable;** drug crystallizes in muscle.

Uses

Anticonvulsant often used to treat seizures refractory to phenobarbital.

Monitoring

Monitor for bradycardia, arrhythmias, and hypotension during infusion. Observe IV site for extravasation. Follow serum concentration closely: therapeutic range is 6 to 15 mcg/mL in the first weeks, then 10 to 20 mcg/mL due to changes in protein binding. Obtain initial trough level 48 hours after IV loading dose.

Adverse Effects/Precautions

Extravasation causes tissue inflammation and necrosis due to high pH and osmolality. High serum concentrations are associated with seizures. Drowsiness may be difficult to identify. Hypersensitivity reactions have been reported in infants. Toxicities with long-term therapy include cardiac arrhythmias, hypotension, gingivitis, nystagmus, rickets, hyperglycemia, and hypoinsulinemia. Phenytoin interacts with carbamazepine, cimetidine, corticosteroids, digoxin, furosemide, phenobarbital, and valproate.

Pharmacology

Hepatic metabolism capacity is limited—saturation may occur within therapeutic range. Oral absorption is erratic. Pharmacokinetics are dose-dependent. Elimination rate is increased during first weeks of life. Serum half-life is 18 to 60 hours. 85% to 90% protein bound. Bilirubin displaces phenytoin from protein-binding sites, resulting in increased free drug.

Special Considerations/Preparation

Injectable solution available in a concentration of 50 mg/mL. Contains 40% propylene glycol and 10% alcohol (100 mg/mL).
Oral suspension interacts with milk proteins in the stomach, resulting in subtherapeutic serum phenytoin concentrations.

Solution Compatibility: Phenytoin is highly unstable in any IV solution.

Solution Incompatibility: D_5W and $D_{10}W$.

Terminal Injection Site Compatibility: Esmolol, famotidine, fluconazole, sodium bicarbonate.

Incompatibility: Dex/AA, and fat emulsion. Amikacin, aminophylline, chloramphenicol, clindamycin, dobutamine, enalaprilat, fentanyl, heparin, hydrocortisone succinate, insulin, lidocaine, linezolid, methadone, morphine, pentobarbital, potassium chloride, propofol, and ranitidine.

Selected References

♦ Volpe JJ: *Neurology of the Newborn,* ed 4. Philadelphia: WB Saunders, 2001, p 204.
♦ Wheless JW: Pediatric use of intravenous and intramuscular phenytoin: lessons learned. *J Child Neurol* 1998;13(Suppl 1):S11-14.

Text updated 3/2002, Compatibilities updated 3/2003

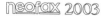

Vecuronium

Dose and Administration

0.1 mg/kg (0.03 to 0.15 mg/kg) IV push, as needed for paralysis. Usual dosing interval is 1 to 2 hours. Adjust dose as needed based on duration of paralysis.

Uses

Skeletal muscle relaxation/paralysis in infants requiring mechanical ventilation. Proposed desirable effects are improved oxygenation/ventilation, reduced barotrauma, and reduced fluctuations in cerebral blood flow.

Monitoring

Monitor vital signs frequently, blood pressure continuously. Use some form of eye lubrication.

Adverse Effects/Precautions

Hypoxemia may occur because of inadequate mechanical ventilation and deterioration in pulmonary mechanics. When used alone, cardiovascular side effects are minimal; however, decreases in heart rate and blood pressure have been observed when used concurrently with narcotics.

Pharmacology

Nondepolarizing muscle-relaxant that competitively antagonizes autonomic cholinergic receptors. Sympathetic stimulation is minimal. Vecuronium is metabolized rapidly in the liver to 3-desacetyl-vecuronium, which is 50% to 70% active, and is excreted renally. Newborns, particularly premature infants, are especially sensitive to vecuronium; this sensitivity diminishes with age. Onset of action is 1 to 2 minutes; duration of effect is prolonged with higher doses and in premature infants. Skeletal relaxation/paralysis is reversed by neostigmine and atropine.

Factors affecting duration of neuromuscular blockade:

Potentiation: Acidosis, hypothermia, neuromuscular disease, hepatic disease, cardiovascular disease, aminoglycosides, hypokalemia, hypermagnesemia, renal failure, and younger age.

Antagonism: Alkalosis, epinephrine, and hyperkalemia.

Sensation remains intact; analgesia should be used for painful procedures.

continued...

Special Considerations/Preparation

Available as powder for injection in 10-mg vials.

A 0.1-mg/mL dilution may be made by diluting 1 mL of 1-mg/mL concentration with 9 mL of preservative-free normal saline. Dilution is stable for 24 hours at room temperature.

Solution compatibility: D_5W and NS.

Terminal injection site compatibility: Dex/AA. Aminophylline, cefazolin, cefoxitin, cimetidine, dobutamine, dopamine, epinephrine, esmolol, fentanyl, fluconazole, gentamicin, heparin, hydrocortisone succinate, isoproterenol, linezolid, lorazepam, midazolam, morphine, nitroglycerin, nitroprusside, propofol, ranitidine, trimethoprim-sulfamethoxazole, and vancomycin.

Incompatibility: Diazepam, furosemide, and sodium bicarbonate.

Selected References

♦ Martin LD, Bratton SL, O'Rourke P: Clinical uses and controversies of neuromuscular blocking agents in infants and children. *Crit Care Med* 1999;27:1358-1368.

♦ Segredo V, Matthay MA, Sharma ML, et al: Prolonged neuromuscular blockage after long-term administration of vecuronium in two critically ill patients. *Anesthesiology* 1990;72:566.

♦ Bhutani VK, Abbasi S, Sivieri EM: Continuous skeletal muscle paralysis: Effect on neonatal pulmonary mechanics. *Pediatrics* 1988;81:419.

♦ Gravlee GP, Ramsey FM, Roy RC, et al: Rapid administration of a narcotic and neuromuscular blocker: A hemodynamic comparison of fentanyl, sufentanil, pancuronium, and vecuronium. *Anesth Analg* 1988;67:39.

♦ Meretoja OA, Wirtavuori K, Neuvonen PJ: Age-dependence of the dose-response curve of vecuronium in pediatric patients during balanced anesthesia. *Anesth Analg* 1988;67:21.

♦ Costarino AT, Polin RA: Neuromuscular relaxants in the neonate. *Clin Perinatol* 1987;14:965.

References updated 3/2002
Compatibilities updated 3/2002

CNS DRUGS

Sucrose

Dose & Administration

Administer orally 2 minutes prior to the painful procedure by using a pacifier dipped in the sweet solution, up to a maximum of 2 mL.

0.5 mL of 24% sucrose is equivalent to 0.12 grams of sucrose. Other solutions containing 50% sucrose and artificial sweetener have also been shown to be effective.

Uses

Mild analgesia and behavioral comforting.

Monitoring

Assess for signs of pain and discomfort.

Adverse Effects/Precautions

Sucrose 24% has an osmolarity of ~1000 mOsm/L. The adverse effects of repeated doses in premature infants are unknown.

Special Considerations/Preparation

Sweet-Ease™, a 24% sucrose and water solution, is aseptically packaged in an 11-ml cup with a peel off lid that is suitable for dipping a pacifier or for administration via a dropper.

Selected References

♦ Stevens B, Yamada J, Ohlsson A: Sucrose for analgesia in newborn infants undergoing painful procedures (Cochrane Review). In: *The Cochrane Library* , Issue 1, 2003. Oxford Update Software.

♦ Abad F, Diaz-Gomez NM, Domenech E, et al: Oral sucrose compares favorably with lidocaine-prilocaine cream for pain relief during venepuncture in neonates. *Acta Paediatr* 2001;90:160-165.

♦ Blass EM, Watt LB: Suckling and sucrose-induced analgesia in human newborns. *Pain* 1999;83:611-623.

♦ Bucher H-U, Moser T, Von Siebenthal K, et al: Sucrose reduces pain reaction to heel lancing in preterm infants: A placebo-controlled, randomized and masked study. *Pediatr Res* 1995;38:332-335.

Added 3/2003

DIURETICS

Bumetanide

Dose & Administration
0.005 to 0.05 mg/kg per dose Q6 hours IV slow push, IM, or PO.

Uses
Diuretic used in patients with renal insufficiency, congestive heart failure, or significant edema that is refractory to furosemide.

Monitoring
Serum electrolytes and urine output. Assess patients receiving digoxin concurrently for potassium depletion. Follow weight changes.

Adverse Effects/Precautions
Water and electrolyte imbalances occur frequently, especially hyponatremia, hypokalemia, and hypochloremic alkalosis. Potentially ototoxic, but less so than furosemide. May displace bilirubin from albumin binding sites when given in high doses or for prolonged periods.

Pharmacology
Bumetanide is 40 times more potent than furosemide with a similar mechanism of action. Inhibits chloride reabsorption in the ascending limb of Henle's loop and inhibits tubular sodium transport, causing major loss of sodium and chloride. Increases urinary losses of potassium, calcium, and bicarbonate. Urine sodium losses are lower with bumetanide than furosemide, but urine calcium losses are higher. Decreases CSF production by weak carbonic anhydrase inhibition. Decreases pulmonary transvascular fluid filtration. Increases renal blood flow and prostaglandin secretion. Highly protein bound (>97%). Data from adults indicate excellent oral bioavailability and significant hepatic metabolism (40%) via the cytochrome CYP pathway. Serum half-life is 2 to 6 hours in neonates.

Special Considerations/Preparation
Supplied as 2-mL ampules and 2-, 4-, and 10-mL vials (0.25-mg/mL solution). Contains 1% benzyl alcohol; pH adjusted to 6.8 to 7.8.

A 0.125 mg/mL dilution may be made by adding 3 mL of 0.25 mg/mL injectable solution to 3 mL preservative-free normal saline for injection. Refrigerated dilution is stable for 24 hours. Discolors when exposed to light.

Solution Compatibility: D_5W and NS. No data are available on Dex/AA.

Terminal Injection Site Compatibility: Fat emulsion. Aztreonam, cefepime, furosemide, lorazepam, morphine, piperacillin-tazobactam, and propofol.

Incompatibility: Dobutamine and midazolam. No other data are available.

Selected References
♦ Sullivan JE, Witte MK, Yamashita TS, Myers CM, Blumer JL: Dose-ranging evaluation of bumetanide pharmacodynamics in critically ill infants. *Clin Pharmacol Ther* 1996;60:424. (2 other related articles by same authors in same issue).

♦ Shankaran S, Liang K-C, Ilagan N, Fleischmann L: Mineral excretion following furosemide compared with bumetanide therapy in premature infants. *Pediatr Nephrol* 1995;9:159-62.

♦ Wittner M, Stefano AD, Wangemann P, Greger R: How do loop diuretics act? *Drugs* 1991;41(suppl 3):1.

♦ Brater DC: Clinical pharmacology of loop diuretics. *Drugs* 1991;41(suppl 3):14.

Test updated 3/98, Compatibilities updated 3/2003

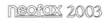

Dose and Administration
1 to 3 mg/kg per dose Q24 hours PO.

Uses
Used in combination with other diuretics in the treatment of congestive heart failure and BPD (situations of increased aldosterone secretion).

Monitoring
Follow serum potassium closely during long-term therapy. Also, measuring urinary potassium is a useful indicator of effectiveness.

Adverse Effects/Precautions
Rashes, vomiting, diarrhea, paresthesias. Dose-dependent androgenic effects in females. Gynecomastia in males. Headaches, nausea, and drowsiness. Use with caution in patients with impaired renal function. May cause false positive ELISA screening tests for congenital adrenal hyperplasia.

Pharmacology
Competitive antagonist of mineralocorticoids (e.g. aldosterone). Metabolized to canrenone and 7-α-thiomethylspironolactone, active metabolites with extended elimination half-lives. Decreases excretion of potassium. Highly protein bound. Increases excretion of calcium, magnesium, sodium, and chloride (small effect). Serum half-life with long term use is 13 to 24 hours. Addition of spironolactone to thiazide diuretic therapy in patients with BPD may yield little, if any, additional benefit.

Special Considerations/Preparation
A simple syrup suspension can be made by crushing eight 25-mg spironolactone tablets and suspending the powder in 50 mL of simple syrup. Final concentration is 4 mg/mL; solution is stable for 1 month refrigerated.

DIURETICS

Selected References
♦ Brion LP, Primhak RA, Ambrosio-Perz I: Diuretics acting on the distal renal tubule for preterm infants with (or developing) chronic lung disease (Cochrane Review). In: *The Cochrane Library* Issue 4, 2000. Oxford: Update Software.

♦ Hoffman DJ, Gerdes JS, Abbasi S: Pulmonary function and electrolyte balance following spironolactone treatment in preterm infants with chronic lung disease: a double-blind, placebo-controlled randomized trial. *J Perinatol* 2000;20:41-45.

♦ Terai I, Yamano K, Ichihara N, et al: Influence of spironolactone on neonatal screening for congenital adrenal hyperplasia. *Arch Dis Child Fetal Neonatal Ed* 1999;81:F179.

♦ Mathur LK, Wickman A: Stability of extemporaneously compounded spironolactone suspensions. *Am J Hosp Pharm* 1989;46:2040.

♦ Overdiek HW, Hermens WA, Merkus FW: New insights into the pharmacokinetics of spironolactone. *Clin Pharmacol Ther* 1985;38:469.

♦ Karim A: Spironolactone: Disposition, metabolism, pharmacodynamics, and bioavailability. *Drug Metab Rev* 1978;8:151.

♦ Loggie JMH, Kleinman LI, Van Maanen EF: Renal function and diuretic therapy in infants and children. Part II. *J Pediatr* 1975;86:657.

Text and References updated 3/2001

Chlorothiazide

Dose & Administration

Diuresis: 10 to 20 mg/kg per dose Q12 hours PO.

Adjuvant treatment of central diabetes insipidus: 5 mg/kg per dose Q12 hours PO.

Administer with food (improves absorption).

IV administration not recommended because of a lack of data.

Note: Do not confuse with hydrochlorothiazide.

Uses

Diuretic used in treating both mild to moderate edema and mild to moderate hypertension. Effects increased when used in combination with furosemide or spironolactone. May improve pulmonary function in patients with BPD. Adjuvant treatment of central diabetes insipidus.

Monitoring

Serum electrolytes, calcium, phosphorus, and glucose; urine output and blood pressure.

Adverse Effects/Precautions

Hypokalemia and other electrolyte abnormalities. Hyperglycemia. Hyperuricemia.

Do not use in patients with significant impairment of renal or hepatic function.

Pharmacology

Limited data in neonates. Variable absorption from GI tract. Onset of action within 1 hour. Elimination half-life depends on GFR, and is approximately 5 hours. Major diuretic effect results from inhibition of sodium reabsorption in the distal nephron. Increases urinary losses of sodium, potassium, magnesium, chloride, bicarbonate, and phosphorus. Decreases renal excretion of calcium. Inhibits pancreatic release of insulin. Displaces bilirubin from albumin binding sites.

Special Considerations/Preparation

Available as a 250 mg/5mL suspension for oral use.

Selected References

♦ Pogacar PR, Mahnke S, Rivkees SA: Management of central diabetes insipidus in infancy with low renal solute load formula and chlorothiazide. *Curr Opin Pediatr* 2000;12:405-411.

♦ Wells TG: The pharmacology and therapeutics of diuretics in the pediatric patient. *Pediatr Clin North Am* 1990;37:463.

♦ Albersheim SG, Solimano AJ, Sharma AK, et al: Randomized, double-blind, controlled trial of long-term diuretic therapy for bronchopulmonary dysplasia. *J Pediatr* 1989;115:615.

♦ Roberts RJ: *Drug Therapy in Infants.* Philadelphia: WB Saunders Co, 1984, p 244.

♦ Kao LC, Warburton D, Cheng MH, et al: Effect of oral diuretics on pulmonary mechanics in infants with chronic bronchopulmonary dysplasia: Results of a double-blind crossover sequential trial. *Pediatrics* 1984;74:37.

Updated 3/2003

Dose and Administration

1 to 2 mg/kg per dose Q12 hours PO.
Administer with food (improves absorption).

Note: Do not confuse with chlorothiazide.

Uses

Diuretic used in treating both mild to moderate edema and mild to moderate hypertension. Effects increased when used in combination with furosemide or spironolactone. May improve pulmonary function in patients with BPD.

Monitoring

Serum electrolytes, calcium, phosphorus, and glucose; urine output and blood pressure.

Adverse Effects/Precautions

Hypokalemia and other electrolyte abnormalities. Hyperglycemia. Hyperuricemia.

Do not use in patients with significant impairment of renal or hepatic function.

Pharmacology

Limited data in neonates. Rapidly absorbed from GI tract. Onset of action is within 1 hour. Elimination half-life depends on GFR and is longer than that of chlorothiazide. Major diuretic effect results from inhibition of sodium reabsorption in the distal nephron. Increases urinary losses of sodium, potassium, magnesium, chloride, phosphorus, and bicarbonate. Decreases renal excretion of calcium. Inhibits pancreatic release of insulin. Displaces bilirubin from albumin.

Special Considerations/Preparation

Supplied as a 50-mg/5mL oral solution.

Selected References

♦ Albersheim SG, Solimano AJ, Sharma AK, et al: Randomized, double-blind, controlled trial of long-term diuretic therapy for bronchopulmonary dysplasia. *J Pediatr* 1989;115:615.

♦ Roberts RJ: *Drug Therapy in Infants*. Philadelphia: WB Saunders Co, 1984, p 244.

Updated 1/94

DIURETICS

Furosemide

Dose & Administration

Initial dose: 1 mg/kg IV slow push, IM, or PO.
May increase to a maximum of 2 mg/kg per dose IV or
6 mg/kg per dose PO.

Initial intervals: Premature infant: Q24 hours.
Fullterm infant: Q12 hours.
Fullterm infant older than 1 month: Q6 to 8 hours.
Consider alternate-day therapy for long-term use.

Uses

Diuretic that may also improve pulmonary function.

Monitoring

Follow urine output and serum electrolytes and phosphorus. Assess closely
for potassium depletion in patients receiving digoxin concurrently. Follow
weight changes.

Adverse Effects/Precautions

Water and electrolyte imbalances occur frequently, especially hyponatremia,
hypokalemia, and hypochloremic alkalosis. Hypercalciuria and development
of renal calculi occur with long-term therapy. Potentially ototoxic, especially
in patients also receiving aminoglycosides. Cholelithiasis has been reported
in patients with BPD or congenital heart disease who received long-term
TPN and furosemide therapy.

Pharmacology

The diuretic actions of furosemide are primarily at the ascending limb of
Henle's loop, and are directly related to renal tubular drug concentration.
Furosemide causes major urinary losses of sodium, potassium, and
chloride. Urinary calcium and magnesium excretion, and urine pH are
also increased. Prostaglandin production is stimulated, with increases in
renal blood flow and renin secretion. Free water clearance is increased
and CSF production is decreased by weak carbonic anhydrase inhibition.
Nondiuretic effects include decreased pulmonary transvascular fluid
filtration and improved pulmonary function. Protein binding is extensive,
but bilirubin displacement is negligible when using normal doses. Oral
bioavailability is good. Time to peak effect when given IV is 1 to 3 hours;
duration of effect is approximately 6 hours, although half-life may be as
long as 67 hours in the most immature neonates.

continued...

DIURETICS

Special Considerations/Preparation

Furosemide oral solution is available in a 10-mg/mL concentration with only 0.02% alcohol (Roxane). The injectable solution may also be used for oral administration.

Furosemide for injection is available as a 10-mg/mL concentration in 2-, 4-, and 10-mL ampules, single use vials, and prefilled syringes.

A 2-mg/mL dilution may be made by adding 2 mL of the 10 mg/mL injectable solution to 8 mL preservative-free normal saline for injection. Dilution should be used within 24 hours. Protect from light and do not refrigerate.

Solution Compatibility: NS and sterile water for injection.

Acidic solutions (pH <5.5) such as D_5W, $D_{10}W$, and Dex/AA cause furosemide to degrade when they are mixed together for several hours.

Terminal Injection Site Compatibility: Fat emulsion. Amikacin, aminophylline, amiodarone, ampicillin, atropine, aztreonam, bumetanide, calcium gluconate, cefepime, cimetidine, dexamethasone, digoxin, epinephrine, famotidine, fentanyl, heparin, hydrocortisone succinate, indomethacin, lidocaine, lorazepam, linezolid, meropenem, morphine, nitroglycerin, penicillin G, piperacillin-tazobactam, potassium chloride, propofol, prostaglandin E_1, ranitidine, remifentanil, sodium bicarbonate, sodium nitroprusside, tobramycin, and tolazoline.

Incompatibility: Dobutamine, dopamine, erythromycin lactobionate, esmolol, fluconazole, gentamicin, hydralazine, isoproterenol, metoclopramide, midazolam, netilmicin, and vecuronium.

Selected References

◆ Stefano JL, Bhutani VK: Role of furosemide after booster-packed erythrocyte transfusions in infants with bronchopulmonary dysplasia. *J Pediatr* 1990;117:965.

◆ Rush MG, Engelhardt B, Parker RA, Hazinski TA: Double-blind, placebo-controlled trial of alternate-day furosemide therapy in infants with chronic bronchopulmonary dysplasia. *J Pediatr* 1990;117:112.

◆ Mirochnick MH, Miceli JJ, Kramer PA, et al: Furosemide pharmacokinetics in very low birth weight infants. *J Pediatr* 1988;112:653.

◆ Green TP: The pharmacologic basis of diuretic therapy in the newborn. *Clin Perinatol* 1987;14:951.

◆ Hufnagle KG, Khan SN, Penn D: Renal calcifications: A complication of longterm furosemide therapy in preterm infants. *Pediatrics* 1982;70:360.

◆ Ross BS, Pollak A, Oh W: The pharmacological effects of furosemide therapy in the low-birth-weight infant. *J Pediatr* 1978;92:149.

◆ Ghanekar AG, Das Gupta V, Gibbs CW Jr: Stability of furosemide in aqueous systems. *J Pharm Sci* 1978;67:808.

Text updated 1/94
Compatibilities updated 3/2003

DIURETICS

GI DRUGS

Cimetidine

Dose & Administration

2.5 to 5 mg/kg per dose Q6 to 12 hours PO or IV infusion over 15 to 30 minutes.

Uses

Prevention and treatment of stress ulcers and GI hemorrhage aggravated by gastric acid secretion.

Monitoring

Gastric pH may be measured to assess efficacy. Observe for impaired consciousness and reduced spontaneous movements.

Adverse Effects/Precautions

Known adverse effects of cimetidine in adults include mental confusion, seizures, renal dysfunction, hepatic dysfunction, flushing and transpiration, neutropenia, diarrhea, hypothalamic-pituitary-gonadal dysfunction, and muscular pain. Cimetidine has been reported to increase the serum level and potentiate toxicity of other drugs such as carbamazepine, diazepam, lidocaine, morphine, phenytoin, procainamide, propranolol, quinidine, theophylline, and warfarin.

Contraindicated in patients receiving cisapride due to precipitation of life-threatening arrhythmias.

Pharmacology

Inhibits gastric acid secretion by histamine H_2-receptor antagonism. Peak inhibition occurs in 15 to 60 minutes after both oral and IV administration. Metabolized in the liver via sulfation and hydroxylation to inactive compounds that are 90% renally eliminated. Half-life in neonates is 1.1 to 3.4 hours, and is prolonged in patients with renal or hepatic insufficiency. The sulfoxide metabolite may accumulate in the CNS and cause toxicity. Antacids interfere with absorption; therefore concomitant administration is not recommended.

continued...

Special Considerations/Preparation

Available as a 150-mg/mL injectable solution in 2-mL single-use vials and 8-mL multidose vials. A 15-mg/mL dilution may be made by adding 1 mL of 150 mg/mL concentration to 9 mL of preservative-free normal saline. Dilution stable for 48 hours . Manufacturer's oral solution (60 mg/mL) contains 2.8% alcohol. A 2.4 mg/mL oral dilution may be prepared by adding 1 mL (60 mg) of manufacturer's oral solution to 24 mL of sterile water. Stable for 14 days refrigerated. Also available in 300-, 400-, and 800-mg tablets.

Solution Compatibility: D_5W, $D_{10}W$, and NS.

Terminal Injection Site Compatibility: Dex/AA and fat emulsion. Acetazolamide, acyclovir, amikacin, aminophylline, ampicillin, amrinone, atropine, aztreonam, cefoxitin, ceftazidime, clindamycin, dexamethasone, diazepam, digoxin, enalaprilat, epinephrine, erythromycin lactobionate, esmolol, fentanyl, fluconazole, flumazenil, furosemide, gentamicin, glycopyrolate, heparin, insulin, isoproterenol, lidocaine, linezolid, lorazepam, meperidine, meropenem, metoclopramide, midazolam, morphine, nafcillin, nitroprusside, pancuronium, penicillin G, piperacillin-tazobactam, potassium chloride, propofol, prostaglandin E_1, protamine, remifentanil, sodium bicarbonate, tolazoline, vancomycin, vecuronium, vitamin K_1, and zidovudine.

Incompatibility: Amphotericin B (Immediate precipitation occurs), cefazolin, cefepime, indomethacin, pentobarbital, phenobarbital, and secobarbital.

Selected References

♦ Vandenplas Y, Sacre L: The use of cimetidine in newborns. *Am J Perinatol* 1987;4:131.
♦ Lloyd CW, Martin WJ, Taylor BD: The pharmacokinetics of cimetidine and metabolites in a neonate. *Drug Intell Clin Pharm* 1985;19:203.
♦ Ziemniak JA, Wynn RJ, Aranda JV, et al: The pharmacokinetics and metabolism of cimetidine in neonates. *Dev Pharmacol Ther* 1984;7:30.
♦ Aranda JV, Outerbridge EW, Shentag JJ: Pharmacodynamics and kinetics of cimetidine in a premature newborn. *Am J Dis Child* 1983;137:1207.

Text Updated 3/97
Compatibilities updated 3/2003

GI DRUGS

Cisapride

NOTE: Cisapride (Propulsid®) is no longer marketed in the United States. Janssen Pharmaceuticals has established an investigational limited access program. Call 1-877-795-4247 for information.

Dose and Administration

0.1 to 0.2 mg/kg per dose PO Q6 to 12 hours.
Administer 15 to 30 minutes before feeding.

Uses

Prokinetic agent used to increase gastric emptying and GI motility, and to decrease the severity of gastroesophageal reflux.

Monitoring

EKG, both pretreatment and after several days of therapy, to check for QTc prolongation. Assess for decreases in baseline heart rate and severity of bradycardia episodes. Monitor serum potassium, calcium, and magnesium in patients at risk. Measure gastric residuals. Observe for diarrhea.

Adverse Effects/Precautions

Cisapride is contraindicated in patients receiving : macrolide antibiotics (e.g. erythromycin) azole antifungals (e.g. fluconazole, ketoconazole, itraconazole), protease inhibitors (e.g. indinavir, ritonavir) class IA and class III antiarrhythmics (e.g. quinidine, procainamide, sotalol) and other agents. Do not use in breastfeeding infants whose mothers are receiving one of the above-referenced drugs, or in patients with hepatic or cardiac dysfunction. Asymptomatic QTc interval prolongation occurs frequently in term and preterm infants, though serious cardiac arrhythmias have only been associated with inadvertently high doses or exposure to the above-referenced drugs. Diarrhea usually resolves by reducing the dose.

Pharmacology

Cisapride stimulates acetylcholine release and acts as a 5-HT$_4$ receptor agonist. Peak plasma concentrations are increased by cimetidine and administration with food (enhanced absorption). Absorption of orally administered drugs may be altered. Highly protein bound. Extensively metabolized by the hepatic cytochrome CYP3A4 isoenzyme system, (limited in preterm infants). Elimination half-life in healthy adults is 7 to 10 hours. Approximately 40% is converted (in adults) to the active metabolite norcisapride, which has a half-life of 10 to 16 hours. No pharmacokinetic studies have been published in neonates. Cardiac toxicity is caused by high cisapride concentrations that selectively block the rapid component of the delayed rectifier potassium current (I_{Kr}) in the heart.

Selected References

♦ McClure RJ, Kristensen JH, Grauaug A: Randomized controlled trial of cisapride in preterm infants. *Arch Dis Child* 1999;80:F174-F177.

♦ Shulman RJ, Boyle JT, Colletti RB, et al: The use of cisapride in children: An updated medical position statement of the North American Society for Pediatric Gastroenterology and Nutrition. *J Pediatr Gastroenterol Nutr* 2000;31:232-233.

♦ Vandenplas Y, and the ESPGHAN Cisapride Panel: Current pediatric indications for cisapride. *J Pediatr Gastroenterol Nutr* 2000;31:480-489.

♦ Ward RM, Lemons JA, Molteni RA: Cisapride: A survey of the frequency of use and adverse events in premature newborns. *Pediatrics* 1999;103:469-472.

Updated 3/2001

GI DRUGS

Famotidine

Dose & Administration

IV: 0.5 mg/kg per dose Q24 hours IV slow push.
An oral formulation is available, but there are no data regarding bioavailability in infants.

Uses

Prevention and treatment of stress ulcers and GI hemorrhage aggravated by gastric acid secretion.

Monitoring

Gastric pH may be measured to assess efficacy (>4.0).

Adverse Effects/Precautions

No adverse events have been reported in infants and children, although data are limited to a few small studies. Thrombocytopenia, bradycardia, elevated liver enzymes, and bronchospasm have been reported in adults.

Pharmacology

Inhibits gastric acid secretion by histamine H_2-receptor antagonism. Primarily eliminated by the kidney as unchanged drug. Elimination half-life in neonates ranges from 5 to 22 hours (mean half-life 10.5 hours), and is prolonged with renal insufficiency.

Special Considerations/Preparation

Available as 10-mg/mL solution for intravenous use in 2-mL preservative-free single-dose vials, and 4-mL multidose vials containing 0.9% (9 mg/mL) benzyl alcohol as a preservative.

A 1-mg/mL dilution may be made by adding 1 mL of the 10 mg/mL concentrated solution to 9 mL of sterile water for injection. Dilution stable for 14 days refrigerated.

Solution Compatibility: D_5W, $D_{10}W$, and NS.

Terminal Injection Site Compatibility: Dex/AA and fat emulsion. Acyclovir, aminophylline, ampicillin, atropine, aztreonam, calcium gluconate, cefazolin, cefotaxime, cefoxitin, ceftazidime, ceftriaxone, dexamethasone, digoxin, dobutamine, dopamine, enalaprilat, epinephrine, erythromycin lactobionate, esmolol, fluconazole, flumazenil, furosemide, gentamicin, heparin, hydrocortisone succinate, imipenem/cilastatin, insulin, isoproterenol, lidocaine, linezolid, lorazepam, magnesium sulfate, metoclopramide, mezlocillin, midazolam, morphine, nafcillin, nitroglycerin, oxacillin, phenytoin, piperacillin, potassium chloride, propofol, remifentanil, sodium bicarbonate, sodium nitroprusside, ticarcillin/clavulanate, vancomycin, and vitamin K_1.

Incompatibility: Cefepime and piperacillin-tazobactam.

Selected References

♦ James LP, Marotti T, Stowe CD, et al: Pharmacokinetics and pharmacodynamics of famotidine in infants. *J Clin Pharmacol* 1998;38:1089-1095.
♦ James LP, Marshall JD, Heulitt MJ, et al: Pharmacokinetics and pharmacodynamics of famotidine in children. *J Clin Pharmacol* 1996;21:48-54.
♦ Echizen H, Ishizadki T: Clinical pharmacokinetics of famotidine. *Clin Pharmacokinet* 1991;21:178-194.
♦ Takabatake T Ohta H, Maekawa M, et al: Pharmacokinetics of famotidine, a new H_2-receptor antagonist, in relation to renal function. *Eur J Clin Pharmacol* 1985;28:327-331.

Added 3/99 Compatibilities updated 3/2003

GI Drugs

Lansoprazole

Dose & Administration

0.5 to 2 mg/kg per dose PO, once a day.
See below for oral preparation.

Monitoring

Observe for symptomatic improvement within 3 days.
Consider intraesophageal pH monitoring to assess for efficacy (pH >4.0).
Measure AST and ALT if duration of therapy is greater than 8 weeks.

Adverse Effects/Precautions

Hypergastrinemia and mild transaminase elevations are the only Adverse Effects reported in children who received lansoprazole for extended periods of time. Available data are limited to small studies of infants and children.

Pharmacology

Lansoprazole inhibits gastric acid secretion by inhibition of hydrogen-potassium ATPase, the enzyme responsible for the final step in the secretion of hydrochloric acid by the gastric parietal cell ("proton pump"). Extensively metabolized in the liver by CYP 2C19 and 3A4. Onset of action is within one hour of administration, maximal effect is at approximately 1.5 hours. Average elimination half-life is 1.5 hours. Inhibition of acid secretion is about 50% of maximum at 24 hours and the duration of action is approximately 72 hours.

Special Considerations/Preparation

Prevacid® is supplied in delayed-release capsules and oral suspension containing either 15, and 30-mg lansoprazole as enteric-coated granules. A 1 mg/mL oral liquid preparation can be prepared as follows: Empty the contents of one 30-mg lansoprazole capsule into the barrel of a 60-mL syringe. Replace the plunger in the syringe and draw up 30-mL of sterile water. Replace the needle on the 60-mL syringe with a fluid-dispensing connector. Connect a second 60-mL syringe to the fluid-dispensing connector and gently transfer the contents of the syringes back and forth until the granules are completely dissolved. Transfer the entire 30-mL solution into one of the 60-mL syringes removing the fluid-dispensing connector. Attach a 19-gauge needle and transfer the contents to an empty vial. Withdraw the patient specific dose. Use immediately after mixing.

Selected References

♦ Tran A, Rey E, Pons G, Pariente-Khayat A, et al: Pharmacokinetic-pharmacodynamic study of oral lansoprazole in children. *Clin Pharmacol Ther* 2002;71:359-67.

♦ Franco M, Salvia G, Terrin G, Spadaro R, et al: Lansoprazole in the treatment of gastro-oesophageal reflux disease in childhood. *Dig Liver Dis* 2000;32:660-6.

♦ Delhotal L, Petite J, Flouvat B. Clinical pharmacokinetics of lansoprazole. *Clin Pharmacokinet* 1995;28:458-70.

♦ Product information, TAP Pharmaceuticals: *Physicians' Desk Reference*, ed 57. Montvale, NJ: Thomson PDR, 2003, p 3200.

Added 3/2003

Dose & Administration

0.033 to 0.1 mg/kg per dose PO or IV slow push Q8 hours.

Uses

To facilitate gastric emptying and GI motility. May improve feeding intolerance. Use in GE reflux patients is controversial.
(Also used to enhance lactation—10 mg Q8 hours.)

Monitoring

Measure gastric residuals. Observe for increased irritability or vomiting.

Adverse Effects/Precautions

Intended for short-term use (several weeks). Dystonic reactions and extrapyramidal symptoms are seen frequently at higher doses and with prolonged use; children are more susceptible than adults.

Pharmacology

Derivative of procainamide. Exact mode of action is unknown; however, metoclopramide has both dopamine-receptor blocking activity and peripheral cholinergic effects. Well absorbed from GI tract. Variable first-pass metabolism by liver. Significant fraction excreted unchanged in urine. Lipid-soluble, large volume of distribution. Serum half-life in adults is 4 hours; prolonged in patients with renal failure.

Special Considerations/Preparation

Available as a 5-mg/mL injectable solution (osmolarity 280 mOsm/kg) in 2-, 10-, 30-, 50-, and 100-mL vials. **Protect from light.** A 0.1 mg/mL dilution may be made by adding 0.4 mL of the 5-mg/mL concentration to 19.6 mL of preservative-free NS. Dilution is stable for 24 hours refrigerated.

Oral preparation available in 1-mg/mL and 10-mg/mL concentrations. A 0.1 mg/mL oral dilution may be made by adding 1 mL of the 1 mg/mL concentration to 9 mL simple syrup. Stable for 4 weeks at room temperature.

Solution Compatibility: D_5W, and NS.

Terminal Injection Site Compatibility: Dex/AA and fat emulsion. Acyclovir, aminophylline, atropine, aztreonam, cimetidine, clindamycin, dexamethasone, famotidine, fentanyl, fluconazole, heparin, hydrocortisone, insulin, lidocaine, linezolid, meropenem, midazolam, morphine, multivitamins, piperacillin-tazobactam, potassium chloride, potassium phosphate, prostaglandin E_1, ranitidine, remifentanil, and zidovudine.

Incompatibility: Ampicillin, calcium chloride, calcium gluconate, cefepime, chloramphenicol, erythromycin lactobionate, furosemide, penicillin G, propofol, and sodium bicarbonate.

GI DRUGS

Selected References

♦ Meadow WL, Bui K, Strates E, et al: Metoclopramide promotes enteral feeding in preterm infants with feeding intolerance. *Dev Pharmacol Ther* 1989;13:38.
♦ Machida HM, Forbes DA, Gall DG, et al: Metoclopramide in gastroesophageal reflux of infancy. *J Pediatr* 1988;112:483.
♦ Ehrenkranz RA, Ackerman BA: Metoclopramide effect on faltering milk production by mothers of premature infants. *Pediatrics* 1986;78:614.
♦ Sankaran K, Yeboah E, Bingham WT, Ninan A: Use of metoclopramide in premature infants. *Dev Pharmacol Ther* 1982;5:114.

Compatibilities updated 3/2003

Omeprazole

Dose & Administration

0.5 to 1.5 mg/kg per dose PO, once a day.
See below for oral preparation.

Uses

Short-term (less than 8 weeks) treatment of documented reflux esophagitis or duodenal ulcer refractory to conventional therapy.

Monitoring

Observe for symptomatic improvement within 3 days. Consider intraesophageal pH monitoring to assess for efficacy (pH >4.0). Measure AST and ALT if duration of therapy is greater than 8 weeks.

Adverse Effects/Precautions

Hypergastrinemia and mild transaminase elevations are the only Adverse Effects reported in children who received omeprazole for extended periods of time. Available data are limited to small studies of infants and children.

Pharmacology

Omeprazole inhibits gastric acid secretion by inhibition of hydrogen-potassium ATPase, the enzyme responsible for the final step in the secretion of hydrochloric acid by the gastric parietal cell ("proton pump"). Onset of action is within one hour of administration, maximal effect is at approximately 2 hours. Inhibition of acid secretion is about 50% of maximum at 24 hours and the duration of action is approximately 72 hours.

Special Considerations/Preparation

Prilosec® is supplied in delayed-release capsules containing either 10, 20, and 40-mg omeprazole as enteric-coated granules.

A 2 mg/mL oral liquid preparation can be prepared as follows: Empty the contents of five 20-mg omeprazole capsules into the barrel of a 60-mL syringe. Replace the plunger in the syringe and draw up 50 mL of 8.4% sodium bicarbonate injection. Replace the needle on the 60-mL syringe with a fluid-dispensing connector. Connect a second 60-mL syringe to the fluid-dispensing connector and gently transfer the contents of the syringes back and forth until the granules are completely dissolved. Transfer the entire 50-mL solution into one of the 60-mL syringes removing the fluid-dispensing connector. Attach a 19-gauge needle and transfer the contents to an empty vial. Stable for 30 days refrigerated. Protect from light.

Selected References

♦ Alliet P, Raes M, Bruneel E, Gillis P: Omeprazole in infants with cimetidine-resistant peptic esophagitis. *J Pediatr* 1998;132:352-354.

♦ Quercia RA, Fan C, Liu X, et al: Stability of omeprazole in an extemporaneously prepared oral liquid. *Am J Health-Syst Pharm* 1997;54:1833-1836.

♦ Kato S, Ebina K, Fujii K, et al: Effect of omeprazole in the treatment of refractory acid-related diseases in childhood: endoscopic healing and twenty-four-hour intragastric acidity. *J Pediatr* 1996;128:415-421.

♦ Faure C, Michaud L, Shaghagi EK, Popon M, et al: Intravenous omeprazole in children: pharmacokinetics and effect on 24-hour intragastric pH. *J Pediatr Gastroenterol Nutr* 2001;33:144-8.

♦ Product information, AstraZeneca, LP: *Physicians' Desk Reference*, ed 57. Montvale, NJ: Medical Economics Data, 2003, p 627.

Updated 3/2001, References Updated 2003

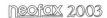
GI DRUGS

(Ursodeoxycholic acid)

Dose and Administration

10 to 15 mg/kg per dose Q 12 hours PO.

Uses

Treatment of cholestasis associated with parenteral nutrition, biliary atresia, and cystic fibrosis. Also used to dissolve cholesterol gallstones.

Monitoring

Hepatic transaminases and direct bilirubin concentration.

Adverse Effects/Precautions

Nausea/vomiting, abdominal pain, constipation, and flatulence.

Pharmacology

Ursodiol is a hydrophobic bile acid that decreases both the secretion of cholesterol from the liver and its intestinal absorption. It is well absorbed orally. After conjugation with taurine or glycine, it then enters the enterohepatic circulation where it is excreted into the bile and intestine. It is hydrolyzed back to the unconjugated form or converted to lithocholic acid which is excreted in the feces. Serum half-life is 3 to 4 days in adults. Dissolution of gallstones may take several months. Aluminum-containing antacids bind ursodiol and inhibit absorption.

Special Considerations/Preparation

Available in 300-mg capsules. A liquid suspension may be made by opening ten (10) 300-mg capsules into a glass mortar. Mix this powder with 10 mL of glycerin and stir until smooth. Add 60 mL of Ora-Plus® to the mixture and stir. Transfer the contents of the mortar to a glass amber bottle and shake well. Add a small amount of Orange Syrup to the mortar and rinse. Pour the remaining contents into the amber glass bottle, then add enough simple syrup to make the final volume 120 mL, with a final concentration of 25-mg/mL. Shake vigorously. Mixture is stable for 60 days stored at room temperature or refrigerated.

Selected References

♦ Levine A, Maayan A, Shamir R, et al: Parenteral nutrition-associated cholestasis in preterm neonates: Evaluation of ursodeoxycholic acid treatment. *J Pediatr Endocrinol Metab* 1999;12:549-553.

♦ Balisteri WF: Bile acid therapy in pediatric hepatobiliary disease: the role of ursodeoxycholic acid. *J Pediatr Gastroenterol Nutr* 1997;24:573-89.

♦ Teitelbaum DH: Parenteral nutrition-associated cholestasis. *Curr Opin Pediatr* 1997;9:270-75.

♦ Mallett MS Hagan RL, Peters DA: Stability of ursodiol 25mg/mL in an extemporaneously prepared oral liquid. *Am J Health-Syst Pharm* 1997;54:1401.

♦ Spagnuolo MI, Iorio R, Vegnente A, Guarino A: Ursodeoxycholic acid for treatment of cholestasis in children. *Gastroenterol* 1996;111:716-719.

♦ Ward A, Brodgen RN, Heel RC, et al: Ursodeoxycholic acid: A review of its pharmacological properties and therapeutic efficacy. *Drugs* 1984;27:95.

Updated 3/2000

GI DRUGS

Ranitidine

Dose & Administration

PO: 2 mg/kg per dose Q8 hours.
IV: Term: 1.5 mg/kg per dose Q8 hours slow push.
Preterm: 0.5 mg/kg per dose Q12 hours slow push.
Continuous IV infusion: 0.0625 mg/kg per hour.

Uses

Prevention and treatment of stress ulcers and GI hemorrhage aggravated by gastric acid secretion.

Monitoring

Gastric pH may be measured to assess efficacy.

Adverse Effects/Precautions

One case report of thrombocytopenia. No other adverse effects have been reported in infants or children. Elevations in hepatic enzymes, leukopenia, and bradycardia have been reported in adults.

Pharmacology

Inhibits gastric acid secretion by histamine H_2-receptor antagonism. Peak serum concentration occurs 1 to 3 hours after oral administration and is not influenced by food. Bioavailability is quite variable. Hepatic biotransformation predominates after oral absorption, with 30% excreted unchanged in the urine. In contrast, 70% of an IV dose is excreted unchanged in the urine. Elimination half-life in neonates is 3 to 7 hours, and is prolonged in preterm infants and patients with renal or hepatic insufficiency.

Special Considerations/Preparation

Available as a 1 mg/mL preservative-free solution for injection in 50 mL single-dose plastic containers, and a 25 mg/mL injectable solution in 2-, and 6-mL vials. A 1 mg/mL dilution may be made by adding 0.4 mL of the 25 mg/mL concentration to 9.6 mL preservative-free sterile water or normal saline for injection. Stable for 7 days refrigerated. May be given orally; absorption is equivalent to that of the oral solution.

Manufacturer's oral solution (15 mg/mL) contains 7.5% alcohol.

Also available as 150- and 300-mg tablets. May prepare oral solution by crushing a 150-mg tablet and dissolving in 60 mL of sterile water to yield a final concentration of 2.5 mg/mL. Stable for 28 days refrigerated.

continued...

Solution Compatibility: D_5W, $D_{10}W$, and NS.

Terminal Injection Site Compatibility: Dex/AA and fat emulsion. Acyclovir, acetazolamide, amikacin, aminophylline, ampicillin, atropine, aztreonam, cefazolin, cefepime, cefoxitin, ceftazidime, chloramphenicol, clindamycin, dexamethasone, digoxin, dobutamine, dopamine, enalaprilat, epinephrine, erythromycin lactobionate, fentanyl, fluconazole, flumazenil, furosemide, gentamicin, glycopyrrolate, heparin, insulin, isoproterenol, lidocaine, linezolid, lorazepam, meropenem, metoclopramide, midazolam, morphine, nitroprusside, pancuronium bromide, penicillin G, piperacillin, piperacillin-tazobactam, potassium chloride, propofol, prostaglandin E_1, protamine, remifentanil, tobramycin, vancomycin, vecuronium, vitamin K_1, and zidovudine.

Incompatibility: Amphotericin B, pentobarbital, phenobarbital, and phenytoin.

Selected References

♦ Kuusela A-L: Long term gastric pH monitoring for determining optimal dose of ranitidine for critically ill preterm and term neonates. *Arch Dis Child Fetal Neonatal Ed* 1998;78:F151-F153.

♦ Kelly EJ, Chatfield SL, Brownlee kg, et al: The effect of intravenous ranitidine on the intragastric pH of preterm infants receiving dexamethasone. *Arch Dis Child* 1993;69:37.

♦ Fontana M, Massironi E, Rossi A, et al: Ranitidine pharmacokinetics in newborn infants. *Arch Dis Child* 1993;68:602.

♦ Sutphen JL, Dillard VL: Effect of ranitidine on twenty-four-hour gastric acidity in infants. *J Pediatr* 1989;114:472.

♦ Grant SM, Langtry HD, Brogden RN: Ranitidine: An updated review of its pharmacodynamic and pharmacokinetic properties and therapeutic use in peptic ulcer disease and other allied diseases. *Drugs* 1989;37:801.

Text updated 3/2002
Compatibilities updated 3/2003

GI DRUGS

RESPIRATORY DRUGS

Albuterol

Dose & Administration

Bronchodilation: 0.1 to 0.5 mg/kg per dose Q2 to 6 hours as nebulized solution.

1 MDI actuation per dose (approx. 0.1 mg or 100 mcg) Q2 to 6 hours.

Studies in vitro indicate that approximately 5% of a MDI dose administered using an in-line holding chamber/spacer device, versus less than 1% of a nebulizer dose, is delivered to the lung. Optimal aerosol dose in neonates is uncertain due to differences in aerosol drug delivery techniques. The therapeutic margin appears to be wide.

Treatment of hyperkalemia: 0.4 mg/kg per dose Q2 hours as nebulized solution.

Oral: 0.1 to 0.3 mg/kg per dose Q6 to 8 hours PO.

Uses

Bronchodilator. Treatment of hyperkalemia.

Monitoring

Assess degree of bronchospasm. Continuous EKG monitoring. **Consider not administering when heart rate is greater than 180 beats per minute.** Serum potassium.

Adverse Effects/Precautions

Tachycardia, arrhythmias, tremor, hypokalemia, and irritable behavior.

Pharmacology

Specific β_2-adrenergic agonist. Minimal cardiovascular effects unless used concurrently with aminophylline. Stimulates production of intracellular cyclic AMP, enhancing the binding of intracellular calcium to the cell membrane and endoplasmic reticulum, resulting in bronchodilation. Enhances mucociliary clearance. Drives potassium intracellular. Well absorbed when administered PO. Onset of action is 30 minutes; duration is 4 to 8 hours. Serum half-life is approximately 6 hours (adults). Time to peak serum concentration is 3 to 4 hours. Tolerance may develop.

RESPIRATORY

continued...

Albuterol

Special Considerations/Preparation

Oral dosage form: Syrup, 2 mg/5 mL.

Inhalation solution: Available as either 5 mg/mL or 0.83 mg/mL.
A 0.1 mg/mL dilution for inhalation maybe made by adding 3 mL of
0.83 mg/mL albuterol concentration to 22 mL of preservative-free normal
saline. Label for inhalation use only. Stable for 7 days refrigerated.

MDI: Available in a hydrofluroalkane pressurized metered dose inhaler
(contains no chlorofluorocarbons (CFC)). Proventil® HFA 100 mcg albuterol
per actuation.

Selected References

♦ Singh BS, Sadiq HF, Noguchi A, Keenan WJ: Efficacy of albuterol inhalation in
  treatment of hyperkalemia in premature neonates. *J Pediatr* 2002;141:16-20.

♦ Lugo RA, Kenney JK, Keenan J: Albuterol delivery in a neonatal ventilated lung
  model: nebulization versus chlorofluorocarbon- and, hydrofluoroalkane- pressurized
  metered dose inhalers. *Pediatr Pulmonol* 2001;31:247-254.

♦ Stefano JL, Bhutani VK, Fox WW: A randomized placebo-controlled study to evaluate
  the effects of oral albuterol on pulmonary mechanics in ventilator-dependent infants
  at risk of developing BPD. *Pediatr Pulmonol* 1991;10:183-90.

♦ Wong CS, Pavord ID, Williams J, et al: Bronchodilator, cardiovascular, and hypokalemic
  effects of fenoterol, salbutamol, and terbutaline in asthma. *Lancet* 1990;336:1396.

♦ Bolte RG: Nebulized β-adrenergic agents in the treatment of acute pediatric asthma.
  Pediatr Emerg Care 1986;2:250.

♦ Morgan DJ, Paull JD, Richmond BH, et al: Pharmacokinetics of intravenous and
  oral salbutamol and its sulphate conjugate. *Br J Clin Pharmacol* 1986;22:587.

♦ Beck R, Robertson C, Galdes-Sebaldt M, Levison H: Combined salbutamol and
  ipratropium bromide by inhalation in the treatment of severe acute asthma.
  J Pediatr 1985;107:605.

Text and references updated 3/2003

RESPIRATORY

Aminophylline

Dose & Administration

Loading dose: 8 mg/kg IV infusion over 30 minutes, or PO.

Maintenance: 1.5 to 3 mg/kg per dose PO, or IV slow push Q8 to 12 hours (start maintenance dose 8 to 12 hours after the loading dose). In older infants (greater than 55 weeks PMA), dosage may need to be increased to 25 to 30 mg/kg per day in divided doses Q4 to 8 hours.

If changing from IV to PO aminophylline: increase dose 20%.

If changing from IV aminophylline to PO theophylline: no adjustment.

Uses

Treatment of neonatal apnea, including post-extubation and post-anesthesia. Bronchodilator. May improve respiratory function.

Monitoring

Monitor heart rate and check blood glucose periodically with reagent strips. Assess for agitation and feeding intolerance.

Consider withholding next dose if heart rate is greater than 180 beats per minute.

When indicated by lack of efficacy or clinical signs of toxicity, serum trough concentration should be obtained. Therapeutic ranges are:

1) Apnea of prematurity: 7 to 12 mcg/mL.
2) Bronchospasm: 10 to 20 mcg/mL (older infants with bronchospasm may need these higher levels because of increased protein binding).

Adverse Effects/Precautions

GI irritation. Hyperglycemia. CNS irritability and sleeplessness. May be associated with renal calcifications when used concurrently with furosemide and/or dexamethasone.

Signs of toxicity: Sinus tachycardia, failure to gain weight, vomiting, jitteriness, hyperreflexia, and seizures.

Treatment of Serious Theophylline Toxicity:

Activated charcoal, 1 g/kg as a slurry by gavage tube Q2 to 4 hours. Avoid sorbitol-containing preparations: They may cause osmotic diarrhea.

Pharmacology

Stimulates central respiratory drive and peripheral chemoreceptor activity. May increase diaphragmatic contractility. Cerebral blood flow is acutely decreased following IV bolus dose. Renal effects include diuresis and increased urinary calcium excretion. Stimulates gastric acid secretion and may cause GE reflux. Cardiac output is increased due to higher sensitivity to catecholamines. Elimination in preterm infants is primarily as unchanged drug, although significant interconversion to caffeine occurs. In the very immature neonate, the serum half-life of theophylline is prolonged (20 to 30 hours). Theophylline metabolism and clearance mature to adult values by 55 weeks postmenstrual age. Aminophylline salt is 78.9% theophylline. Theophylline administered orally is approximately 80% bioavailable; therefore, no dosage adjustment is necessary when changing from IV aminophylline to PO theophylline.

continued...

Special Considerations/Preparation

Available as aminophylline for IV use (25 mg/mL) in 10- and 20-mL vials. Dilute 1 mL (25 mg) with 4 mL NS or D_5W to yield a final concentration of 5 mg/mL. Stable for 4 days refrigerated.

Aminophylline oral solution is available in a concentration of 21 mg/mL. Use a sugar-, preservative-, and alcohol-free preparation. Dilute with sterile water to a final concentration of 2 to 4 mg/mL for oral use.

Theophylline oral solution is available as an alcohol- and dye-free preparation in a concentration of 5.33 mg/mL.

Solution Compatibility: D_5W, $D_{10}W$, and NS.

Terminal Injection Site Compatibility: Dex/AA (white precipitate forms within 2 hours) and fat emulsion. Acyclovir, ampicillin, amikacin, aztreonam, calcium gluconate, ceftazidime, chloramphenicol, cimetidine, dexamethasone, dopamine, enalaprilat, erythromycin lactobionate, esmolol, famotidine, fluconazole, flumazenil, furosemide, heparin, hydrocortisone succinate, isoproterenol, lidocaine, linezolid, methicillin, meropenem, metoclopramide, metronidazole, midazolam, morphine, nafcillin, netilmicin, nitroglycerin, nitroprusside, pancuronium bromide, pentobarbital, phenobarbital, piperacillin, piperacillin-tazobactam, potassium chloride, propofol, prostaglandin E_1, ranitidine, remifentanil, sodium bicarbonate, ticarcillin/clavulanate, tobramycin, tolazoline, vancomycin, and vecuronium.

Incompatibility: Amiodarone, cefepime, cefotaxime, ceftriaxone, ciprofloxacin, clindamycin, dobutamine, epinephrine, hydralazine, insulin, methadone, methylprednisolone, penicillin G, and phenytoin.

Selected References

♦ Hochwald C, Kennedy K, Chang J, Moya F: A randomized, controlled, double-blind trial comparing two loading doses of aminophylline. *J Perinatol* 2002;22:275-278.

♦ Carnielli VP, Verlato G, Benini F, et al: Metabolic and respiratory effects of theophylline in the preterm infant. *Arch Dis Child Fetal Neonatal Ed* 2000;83:F-39-F43.

♦ Zanardo V, Dani C, Trevisanuto D: Methylxanthines increase renal calcium excretion in preterm infants. *Biol Neonate* 1995;68:169-74.

♦ Reese J, Prentice G, Yu VYH: Dose conversion from aminophylline to theophylline in preterm infants. *Arch Dis Child* 1994;71:F51-F52.

♦ Kraus DM, Fischer JH, Reitz SJ, et al: Alterations in theophylline metabolism during the first year of life. *Clin Pharmacol Ther* 1993;54:351-59.

♦ Shannon M, Amitai Y, Lovejoy FH: Multiple dose activated charcoal for theophylline poisoning in young infants. *Pediatrics* 1987;80:368.

♦ Gal P, Boer HR, Toback J, et al: Effect of asphyxia on theophylline clearance in newborns. *South Med J* 1982;75:836.

♦ Srinivasan G, Pildes RS, Jaspan JB, et al: Metabolic effects of theophylline in preterm infants. *J Pediatr* 1981;98:815.

♦ Aranda JV, Sitar DS, Parsons WD, et al: Pharmacokinetic aspects of theophylline in premature newborns. *N Engl J Med* 1976;295:413.

Updated 3/2003
Compatibilities updated 3/2003

RESPIRATORY

Caffeine Citrate

Dose & Administration

Loading dose: 20 to 40 mg/kg of caffeine citrate
IV over 30 minutes or PO.
(Equivalent to 10 to 20 mg/kg caffeine base).

Maintenance dose: 5 to 8 mg/kg per dose of caffeine citrate
IV slow push or PO Q24 hours.
(Equivalent to 2.5 to 4 mg/kg caffeine base).

Maintenance dose should be started 24 hours after the loading dose.
(Please note that emphasis has changed to caffeine citrate due to
commercially available product. This product (Cafcit®) may be administered
both intravenously and orally).

Uses

Treatment of neonatal apnea, including post-extubation and post-anesthesia.
(More favorable therapeutic index than aminophylline).

Monitoring

Therapeutic trough serum concentration is 5 to 25 mcg/mL. Concentrations
greater than 40 to 50 mcg/mL are toxic. Monitoring of serum drug concentration
should be based on a trough level determined on approximately day 5 of
therapy. Assess for agitation. Monitor heart rate;
consider withholding dose if greater than 180 beats per minute.

Adverse Effects/Precautions

Adverse effects are usually mild, and include restlessness, vomiting, and
functional cardiac symptoms. There has been a suggested association with
NEC, but causality has never been proven. Loading doses of 25 mg/kg
caffeine (50 mg/kg caffeine citrate) have been reported to decrease cerebral
and intestinal blood flow velocity.

Pharmacology

The pharmacological effects of caffeine are mediated by its antagonism of
the actions of adenosine at cell surface receptors. It is rapidly distributed in
the brain, with CNS levels approximating plasma levels. Caffeine increases
the respiratory center output, chemoreceptor sensitivity to CO_2, smooth
muscle relaxation, and cardiac output. Oxygen consumption may be
increased and weight gain may be reduced. Renal effects include diuresis
and increased urinary calcium excretion. Orally administered caffeine
citrate is rapidly and completely absorbed. There is almost no first-pass
metabolism. In neonates, approximately 86% is excreted unchanged in the
urine, with the remainder metabolized via the CYP1A2 enzyme system. The
serum half-life of caffeine ranges from 40 to 230 hours, decreasing with
advancing postmenstrual age until 60 weeks PMA. Half-life is prolonged
in infants with cholestatic hepatitis.

continued...

RESPIRATORY

Special Considerations/Preparation

Both Cafcit® Oral Solution and Cafcit® Injection for intravenous administration (Roxane) are preservative free and available in 3-mL single use vials. Each mL of Cafcit® contains 20 mg of caffeine citrate (equivalent to 10 mg caffeine base). The osmolality is 160 mOsm/kg. Store at room temperature.

Alternatively, an oral solution may be prepared by dissolving 2.5 g of caffeine anhydrous powder in 250 mL of water, yielding a final concentration of 10 mg/mL. Solution is stable for 4 weeks refrigerated. Crystals form when stored at low temperature but dissolve at room temperature without loss of potency. **Do not freeze.**

Solution Compatibility: D_5W, $D_{50}W$, and NS.

Terminal Injection Site Compatibility: Dex/AA and fat emulsion. Calcium gluconate, dopamine, fentanyl, and heparin (concentration < 1 Unit/mL).

Selected References

♦ Comer AM, Perry CM, Figgitt DP: Caffeine citrate: A review of its use in apnoea of prematurity. *Paediatr Drugs* 2001;3:61-70.

♦ Bauer J, Maier K, Linderkamp O, Hentschel R: Effect of caffeine on oxygen consumption and metabolic rate in very low birth weight infants with idiopathic apnea. *Pediatrics* 2001;107:660-663.

♦ Erenberg A, Leff RD, Haack DG, et al: Caffeine citrate for the treatment of apnea of prematurity: A double-blind, placebo-controlled study. *Pharmacotherapy* 2000;20:644-652.

♦ Anderson BJ, Gunn TR, Holford NHG, et al: Caffeine overdose in a premature infant: Clinical course and pharmacokinetics. *Anaesth Intensive Care* 1999;27:307-311.

♦ Lane AJP, Coombs RC, Evans DH, et al: Effect of caffeine on neonatal splanchnic blood flow. *Arch Dis Child Fetal Neonatal Ed* 1999;80:F-128-F129.

♦ Lee TC, Charles B, Steer P: Population pharmacokinetics of intravenous caffeine in neonates with apnea of prematurity. *Clin Pharmacol Ther* 1997;61:628-640.

♦ Falcao AC, Fernandez de Gatta MM, Delgado Iribarnegaray MF, et al: Population pharmacokinetics of caffeine in premature neonates. *Eur J Clin Pharmacol* 1997; 52:211-217.

♦ Zanardo V, Dani C, Trevisanuto D: Methylxanthines increase renal calcium excretion in preterm infants. *Biol Neonate* 1995;68:169-74.

♦ Product information, Boehringer Ingelheim: *Physicians' Desk Reference*, ed 57. Montvale, NJ: Thomson PDR, 2003, p 1032.

Updated 3/2000
Compatibilities updated 3/2001
References updated 3/2003

RESPIRATORY

Dexamethasone

Dose & Administration

Physiologic replacement dose: 0.022 to 0.045 mg/kg per day, IV push or PO.

Stress dose: 0.07 to 0.15 mg/kg per day.

The February 2002 AAP and CPS statement strongly discourages routine use of dexamethasone.

If dexamethasone is used for CLD risk reduction, 1) Treat only those infants at highest risk; 2) Use lower than traditional pharmacologic doses; 3) Begin treatment after Day 7 but before Day 14 of life; 4) Do not give concurrently with indomethacin; 5) Use preservative-free drug wherever possible.

Uses

Anti-inflammatory glucocorticoid used to facilitate extubation and improve lung function in infants at high risk for developing chronic lung disease.

Monitoring

Assess for hyperglycemia and hyperlipidemia. Monitor blood pressure. Guaiac gastric aspirates. Echocardiogram if treating longer than 7 days.

Adverse Effects/Precautions

Data regarding neurodevelopmental outcome are increasingly worrisome, with 3 studies and a meta-analysis reporting an increased risk of cerebral palsy. Most evidence suggests no increase in the incidence of ROP or the need for cryotherapy. Gastrointestinal perforation and GI hemorrhage occur more frequently in patients treated beginning on Day 1 and in those also being treated concurrently with indomethacin. Hyperglycemia and glycosuria occur frequently after the first few doses, and one case of diabetic ketoacidosis has been reported. Blood pressure increases are common, and hypertension occurs occasionally. Cardiac effects noted by Day 14 of therapy include increased left ventricular wall thickness with outflow tract obstruction and transient impairment of left ventricular filling, systolic anterior motion of the mitral valve, and ST-segment depression. Other potential short-term adverse effects include sodium and water retention, hypokalemia, hypocalcemia, hypertriglyceridemia, increased risk of sepsis, renal stones (in patients receiving furosemide), osteopenia, and inhibition of growth. Adrenal insufficiency may occur secondary to pituitary suppression.

Special Considerations/Preparation

Dexamethasone phosphate for injection has been available in limited supply, especially preservative-free preparations. Sulfite preservative concentrations are approximately 1 mg/mL and are potentially toxic.
A 0.2 mg/mL dilution may be made by adding 1 mL of the 4 mg/mL concentration to 19 mL preservative-free sterile water for injection. Dilution is stable for 4 days refrigerated and may be used for PO administration.

Solution Compatibility: D_5W, $D_{10}W$, and NS.

Terminal Injection Site Compatibility: Dex/AA and fat emulsion. Acyclovir, amikacin, aminophylline, aztreonam, cefepime, cimetidine, famotidine, fentanyl, fluconazole, furosemide, heparin, hydrocortisone succinate, lidocaine, linezolid, lorazepam, meropenem, metoclopramide, morphine, nafcillin, netilmicin, piperacillin-tazobactam, potassium chloride, propofol, prostaglandin E_1, ranitidine, remifentanil, sodium bicarbonate, and zidovudine.

Incompatibility: Ciprofloxacin, glycopyrolate, midazolam and vancomycin.

continued...

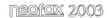

Pharmacology

Stabilizes lysosomal and cell membranes, inhibits complement-induced granulocyte aggregation, improves integrity of alveolar-capillary barrier, inhibits prostaglandin and leukotriene production, rightward shifts oxygen-hemoglobin dissociation curve, increases surfactant production, decreases pulmonary edema, relaxes bronchospasm. Hyperglycemia is caused by inhibition of glucose uptake into cells and decreased glucokinase activity. Increased triglyceride synthesis is due to hyperinsulinemia and increased acetyl-CoA carboxylase activity. Blood pressure is increased due to increased responsiveness to endogenous catechoamines. Increases protein catabolism with potential loss of muscle tissue, increases urinary calcium excretion because of bone resorption, and suppresses pituitary ACTH secretion. Biologic half-life is 36 to 54 hours.

Selected References

Reviews

♦ American Academy of Pediatrics, Canadian Paediatric Society: Postnatal corticosteroids to treat or prevent chronic lung disease in preterm infants. *Pediatrics* 2002;109:330.

♦ Kennedy KA: Controversies in the use of postnatal steroids. *Semin Perinatol* 2001;25:397-405.

♦ Halliday HL, Ehrenkranz RA: Moderately early (7-14 days) postnatal corticosteriods for preventing chronic lung disease in preterm infants. (Cochrane Review). In: *The Cochrane Library*, Issue 4, 1999. Oxford: Update Software.

♦ Arias-Camison JM, Lau J, Cole CH, Frantz ID: Meta-analysis of dexamethasone therapy started in the first 15 days of life for prevention of chronic lung disease in premature infants. *Pediatr Pulmonol* 1999;28:167-174.

Adverse Effects

♦ Stark AR, Carlo W, Tyson JE, et al: Adverse effects of early dexamethasone treatment extremely low birth weight infants. *N Engl J Med* 2001;344:95-101.

♦ Stoll BJ, Temprosa MS, Tyson JE, et al: Dexamethasone therapy increases infection in very low birth weight infants. *Pediatrics* 1999;104(5). URL:http://www.pediatrics.org/cgi/content/full/104(5)/e63.

♦ Amin SB Sinkin RA, McDermott MP, Kendig JW: Lipid intolerance in neonates receiving dexamethasone for bronchopulmonary dysplasia. *Arch Pediatr Adolesc Med* 1999;153:795-800.

♦ Bensky AS, Kothadia JM, Covitz, W: Cardiac effects of dexamethasone In very low birth weight infants. *Pediatrics* 1996;97:818.

♦ Wright K, Wright SP: Lack of association of glucocorticoid therapy and retinopathy of prematurity. *Arch Pediatr Adolesc Med* 1994;148:848.

♦ Ng PC: The effectiveness and side effects of dexamethasone in preterm infants with bronchopulmonary dysplasia. *Arch Dis Child* 1993;68:330.

Developmental Followup

♦ O'Shea TM, Kothadia JM, Klinepeter KL, et al: Randomized placebo-controlled trial of a 42-day tapering course of dexamethasone to reduce the duration of ventilator dependency in very low birth weight infants: Outcome of study participants at 1 year adjusted age. *Pediatrics* 1999;104:15-21.

♦ Shinwell ES, Karplus M, Reich D, et al: Early postnatal dexamethasone therapy and increased incidence of cerebral palsy. *Arch Dis Child Fetal Neonatal Ed* 2000; 83:F177-181.

♦ Yeh TF, Lin YJ, Huang CC et al. Early postnatal(<12 hrs) dexamethasone therapy for prevention of BPD in preterm infants with RDS: a two-year follow-up study. *Pediatrics* 1998; 101(5). URL: http://www.pediatrics.org/cgi/content/full/101/5/e7.

Text updated 3/2002, Compatibilities updated 3/2003

RESPIRATORY

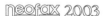

Dose & Administration

Indications:

Prophylaxis of infants at high risk for RDS (those < 29 weeks gestation)

Rescue treatment of infants with moderate to severe RDS.

Treatment of mature infants with respiratory failure due to meconium aspiration syndrome, pneumonia, or persistent pulmonary hypertension.

Monitoring

Assess ET tube patency and position. Oxygen saturation, EKG, and blood pressure should be monitored continuously during dosing. Assess for impairment of gas exchange caused by blockage of the airway. After dosing, frequent assessments of oxygenation and ventilation should be performed to prevent postdose hyperoxia, hypocarbia, and overventilation.

Adverse Effects/Precautions

Administration of exogenous surfactants should be restricted to highly supervised clinical settings, with immediate availability of clinicians experienced with intubation, ventilator management, and general care of premature infants. Reflux of exogenous surfactant up the ET tube and falls in oxygenation occur frequently. If the infant becomes dusky or agitated, heart rate slows, oxygen saturation falls more than 15%, or surfactant backs up in the ET tube, dosing should be slowed or halted. If necessary, ventilator settings and/or FiO_2 should be turned up. Pulmonary hemorrhage occurs in 2% to 4% of treated infants, primarily the smallest patients with untreated PDA. This may be due to hemorrhagic pulmonary edema caused by the rapid fall in pulmonary vascular resistance and resulting increased pulmonary blood flow.

Pharmacology

In infants with RDS, exogenous surfactant therapy reverses atelectasis and increases FRC, with rapid improvements in oxygenation. All preparations reduce mortality from RDS. Natural surfactants are more effective than synthetics in reducing pulmonary air leak. There are no significant differences between preparations in chronic lung disease or other long term outcomes. All commercially available preparations contain surfactant apoprotein C (SP-C), none contain SP-A. The lung-mince extracts Survanta® and Curosurf® contain less than 10% of the SP-B contained in the lung-wash extract Infasurf®.

Selected References

Review Articles

♦ Suresh GK, Soll RF: Current surfactant use in premature infants. *Clin Perinatol* 2001;28:671-694.

♦ Rodriguez RJ, Martin RJ: Exogenous surfactant therapy in newborns. *Resp Care Clin North Am* 1999;5:595-616.

♦ Kattwinkel J: Surfactant: Evolving issues. *Clin Perinatol* 1998; 25:17-32.

♦ Morley CJ: Systematic review of prophylactic vs rescue surfactant. *Arch Dis Child* 1997;77:F70-F74.

♦ Halliday HL: Natural vs synthetic surfactants in neonatal respiratory distress syndrome. *Drugs* 1996;51:226-237.

Selected References for Non-RDS Indications

♦ Lotze A, Mitchell BR, Bulas DI, et al: Multicenter study of surfactant (Beractant) use in the treatment of term infants with severe respiratory failure. *J Pediatr* 1998;132:40.

♦ Findlay RD, Taeusch HW, Walther FJ: Surfactant replacement therapy for meconium aspiration syndrome. *Pediatrics* 1996;97:48

References updated 3/2003

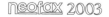

(Beractant) Intratracheal Suspension

Dose and Administration

4 mL/kg per dose intratracheally, divided into 4 aliquots.

Prophylaxis: First dose is given as soon as possible after birth, with up to three additional doses in the first 48 hours of life, if indicated.

Rescue treatment of RDS: Up to four doses in first 48 hours of life, no more frequently than Q6 hours.

Before administration, allow to stand at room temperature for 20 minutes, or warm in the hand for at least 8 minutes. **Artificial warming methods should not be used.** Shorten a 5F end-hole catheter so tip of catheter will protrude just beyond end of ET tube above infant's carina. Slowly withdraw entire contents of vial into a plastic syringe through a large (greater than 20 gauge) needle. **Do not filter or shake.** Attach shortened catheter to syringe. Fill catheter with Survanta. Discard excess Survanta through catheter so only total dose to be given remains in syringe.

Administer four quarter-doses with the infant in different positions to enhance distribution. The catheter can be inserted into the infant's endotracheal tube through a neonatal suction valve without interrupting ventilation. Alternatively, Survanta can be instilled through the catheter by briefly disconnecting the endotracheal tube from the ventilator. After administration of each quarter-dose, the dosing catheter is removed from the ET tube and the infant is ventilated for at least 30 seconds until stable.

Pharmacology

Survanta is a modified natural bovine lung extract containing phospholipids, neutral lipids, fatty acids, and surfactant-associated proteins B and C, to which colfosceril palmitate (DPPC), palmitic acid, and tripalmitin are added. Resulting drug provides 25 mg/mL phospholipids (including 11 to 15.5 mg/mL DPPC), 0.5 to 1.75 mg/mL triglycerides, 1.4 to 3.5 mg/mL fatty acids, and less than 1 mg/mL protein. Survanta is suspended in NS and heat sterilized. Animal metabolism studies show that most of a dose becomes lung-associated within hours of administration, and lipids enter endogenous surfactant pathways of reuse and recycling.

Special Considerations/Preparation

Available in 4- and 8-mL single-use vials. Refrigerate (2°C to 8°C [36°F to 46°F]) and protect from light. Inspect Survanta for discoloration; normal color is off-white to light-brown. If settling occurs during storage, **swirl** vial gently. **Do not shake.** Vials should be entered only once. Used vials with residual drug should be discarded. Unopened vials that have been warmed to room temperature one time may be refrigerated within 24 hours and stored for future use.

Selected References

♦ Zola EM, Overbach AM, Gunkel JH, et al: Treatment investigational new drug experience with Survanta (beractant). *Pediatrics* 1993;91:546.

♦ Hoekstra RE, Jackson JC, Myers TF, et al: Improved neonatal survival following multiple doses of bovine surfactant in very premature neonates at risk for respiratory distress syndrome. *Pediatrics* 1991;88:10.

♦ Liechty EA, Donovan E, Purohit D, et al: Reduction of neonatal mortality after multiple doses of bovine surfactant in low birth weight neonates with respiratory distress syndrome. *Pediatrics* 1991;88:19.

Updated 3/2001

RESPIRATORY

Curosurf®

(Poractant alfa) Intratracheal Suspension

Dose and Administration

Initial dose is 2.5 mL/kg per dose intratracheally, divided into 2 aliquots followed by up to two subsequent doses of 1.25 mL/kg per dose administered at 12-hour intervals if needed.

Clear the trachea of secretions. Shorten a 5F end-hole catheter so the tip of the catheter will protrude just beyond end of ET tube above infant's carina. Slowly withdraw entire contents of vial into a plastic syringe through a large (greater than 20 gauge) needle. **Do not filter or shake.** Attach shortened catheter to syringe. Fill catheter with surfactant. Discard excess through catheter so only total dose to be given remains in syringe. Administer in two to four aliquots with the infant in different positions to enhance distribution in the lungs. The catheter can be inserted into the infant's endotracheal tube without interrupting ventilation by passing the catheter through a neonatal suction valve attached to the endotracheal tube. Alternatively, surfactant can be instilled through the catheter by briefly disconnecting the endotracheal tube from the ventilator. After administration of each aliquot, the dosing catheter is removed from the ET tube and the infant is ventilated for at least 30 seconds until stable.

Pharmacology

Pulmonary lung surfactants are essential for effective ventilation by modifying alveolar surface tension thereby stabilizing the alveoli. Curosurf® is a modified porcine-derived minced lung extract containing phospholipids, neutral lipids, fatty acids, and surfactant-associated proteins B and C. Each mL of surfactant contains 80 mg of total phospholipids (54 mg of phosphatidylcholine of which 30.5 mg dipalmitoyl phosphatidylcholine) and 1 mg of protein including 0.3 mg of SP-B.

Special Considerations/Preparation

Available in 1.5 mL (120 mg phospholipid) and 3 mL (240 mg phospholipid) vials. Refrigerate (2°C to 8°C [36°F to 46°F]) and protect from light. Inspect Curosurf® for discoloration; normal color is creamy white. If settling occurs during storage, gently turn vial upside-down in order to uniformly suspend. **Do not shake.** Used vials with residual drug should be discarded. Unopened vials that have been warmed to room temperature one time may be refrigerated within 24 hours and stored for future use.

Selected References

♦ Collaborative European Multicenter Study Group: Surfactant replacement therapy for severe neonatal respiratory distress syndrome: A international randomized clinical trial. *Pediatrics* 1988;82:683-691.

♦ Bevilacqua G, Parmigiani S, Robertson B: Prophylaxis of respiratory distress syndrome by treatment with modified porcine surfactant at birth: a multicentre prospective randomized trial. *J Perinat Med* 1996;24:609-620.

♦ Egberts J, de Winter JP, Sedin G, et al: Comparison of prophylaxis and rescue treatment with Curosurf® in neonates less than 30 weeks' gestation: A randomized trial. *Pediatrics* 1993;92:768-774.

♦ Halliday HL, Tarnow-Mordi WO, Corcoran JD, et al: Multicentre randomised trial comparing high and low dose surfactant regimens for the treatment of respiratory distress syndrome (the Curosurf® 4 trials). *Arch Dis Child* 1993;69:276-280.

Added 3/2000

(Calfactant) Intratracheal Suspension

Dose and Administration

Initial dose is 3 mL/kg per dose intratracheally, divided into 2 aliquots followed by up to three subsequent doses of 3 mL/kg per dose administered at 12-hour intervals if needed.

Clear the trachea of secretions. Shorten a 5F end-hole catheter so the tip of the catheter will protrude just beyond end of ET tube above infant's carina. Slowly withdraw entire contents of vial into a plastic syringe through a large (greater than 20 gauge) needle. **Do not filter or shake.** Attach shortened catheter to syringe. Fill catheter with surfactant. Discard excess through catheter so only total dose to be given remains in syringe. Administer in two to four aliquots with the infant in different positions to enhance distribution in the lungs. The catheter can be inserted into the infant's endotracheal tube without interrupting ventilation by passing the catheter through a neonatal suction valve attached to the endotracheal tube. Alternatively, surfactant can be instilled through the catheter by briefly disconnecting the endotracheal tube from the ventilator. After administration of each aliquot, the dosing catheter is removed from the ET tube and the infant is ventilated for at least 30 seconds until stable.

Pharmacology

Pulmonary lung surfactants are essential for effective ventilation by modifying alveolar surface tension thereby stabilizing the alveoli. Infasurf® is a sterile, non-pyrogenic natural surfactant extracted from calf lungs containing phospholipids, neutral lipids, fatty acids, and surfactant-associated proteins B and C. Preservative free. Each mL of Infasurf® contains 35 mg of total phospholipids (26 mg of phosphatidylcholine of which 16 mg is disaturated phosphatidylcholine) and 0.65 mg of proteins including 0.26 mg of SP-B.

Special Considerations/Preparation

Available in 6 mL single-use vials. Refrigerate (2°C to 8°C [36°F to 46°F]) and protect from light. Inspect Infasurf® for discoloration; normal color is off-white. If settling occurs during storage, gently turn vial upside-down in order to uniformly suspend. **Do not shake.** Used vials with residual drug should be discarded. Unopened vials that have been warmed to room temperature one time may be refrigerated within 24 hours and stored for future use.

Selected References

♦ Bloom BT, Kattwinkel J, Hall RT, et al: Comparison of Infasurf® (calf lung surfactant extract) to Survanta (beractant) in the treatment and prevention of respiratory distress syndrome. *Pediatrics* 1997;100:31-38.

♦ Hudak ML, Farrell EE, Rosenberg AA, et al: A multicenter randomized, masked comparison trial of natural versus synthetic surfactant for the treatment of respiratory distress syndrome. *J Pediatr* 1996;128:396-406.

♦ Kendig JW, Ryan RM, Sinkin RA, et al: Comparison of two strategies for surfactant prophylaxis in very premature infants: A multicenter randomized trial. *Pediatrics* 1998;101:1006-1012.

Added 3/2000

RESPIRATORY

Exosurf®

(Synthetic Surfactant)

Dose and Administration

5 mL/kg per dose ET.

Prophylaxis (for neonates less than 29 weeks gestation):
The first dose is given as soon as possible after birth. Two additional doses are given at 12 and 24 hours if indicated.

Rescue treatment of RDS: Two doses 12 hours apart; the first dose given as soon as possible after intubation for respiratory deterioration.

After ET suctioning, administer in two 2.5-mL/kg aliquots using the sideport on the supplied ET tube adapter without interrupting mechanical ventilation. Each half-dose is instilled over 1 to 2 minutes in small bursts timed with inspiration, with the infant's head in the midline position. After each half dose, the head and torso are turned 45° to the side for 30 seconds to improve distribution. After dosing, frequent assessments of oxygenation and ventilation should be performed to prevent postdose hyperoxia and hypocarbia. Suctioning should not be performed for 2 hours following administration, except when dictated by clinical necessity.

Adverse Effects/Precautions

Reflux of Exosurf® up the ET tube and falls in oxygenation occur frequently. If the infant becomes dusky or agitated, heart rate slows, oxygen saturation falls more than 15%, or Exosurf® backs up in the ET tube, dosing should be slowed or halted. If necessary, ventilator settings and/or FiO$_2$ should be turned up. Pulmonary hemorrhage occurs in 2% to 4% of treated infants, primarily the smallest patients with untreated PDA possibly the result of hemorrhagic pulmonary edema caused by the rapid fall in pulmonary vascular resistance and resulting increased pulmonary blood flow.

Pharmacology

Synthetic, protein-free surfactant, supplied as a sterile lyophilized powder. After reconstitution, each mL of Exosurf® suspension contains 13.5 mg colfosceril palmitate (DPPC, the major lipid component of natural surfactant), 1.5 mg cetyl alcohol (a spreading agent), and 1 mg tyloxapol (a nonionic surfactant that disperses the DPPC and cetyl alcohol).

Special Considerations/Preparation

Reconstitute immediately before administration using only preservative-free sterile water for injection (supplied) .1) Fill a 10-mL or 12-mL syringe with 8 mL of sterile water .2) Allow vacuum in the Exosurf® vial to draw sterile water into vial .3) Aspirate as much as possible out of vial back into syringe (while maintaining vacuum), then suddenly release syringe plunger .4) Step 3 should be repeated 3 or 4 times to assure adequate mixing .5) Draw appropriate dosage volume into syringe **from below froth** in vial.

Each vial yields 7.5 to 8 mL of Exosurf® suspension (enough to treat an infant weighing up to ~1600 g. The suspension appears milky white, has a pH of 5 to 7, and an osmolality of 185 mOsm/L. The reconstituted suspension is stable for 12 hours when stored at 2°C to 30°C (36°F to 86°F).

Selected References

♦ Corbet A: Clinical trials of synthetic surfactant in the respiratory distress syndrome of premature infants. *Clin Perinatol* 1993;20:737.
♦ The OSIRIS Collaborative Group: Early versus delayed neonatal administration of a synthetic surfactant: The judgment of OSIRIS. *Lancet* 1992;2(340):1363.

Updated 3/2000

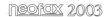

Dose and Administration

Administer Q6 to 8 hours as nebulized solution.

Doses studied in intubated neonates range from 36 to 72 mcg via metered dose inhaler (MDI) with spacer, and 75 to 175 mcg via jet nebulizer. Studies in adults indicate that approximately 10% of an MDI dose, versus 1 to 2% of a nebulizer dose, is delivered to the lung. MDI devices are not recommended for use in infants with tidal volumes less than 100 mL because of safety concerns: Potentially hypoxic mixture of ventilator gas and propellant, and unknown hazards of exposure to chlorofluorocarbons.

Optimal dose in neonates has yet to be determined due to differences in aerosol drug delivery techniques, although the therapeutic margin appears to be wide.

Uses

Anticholinergic bronchodilator for primary treatment of chronic obstructive pulmonary diseases and adjunctive treatment of acute bronchospasm. Ipratropium is not useful in the treatment of bronchiolitis.

Monitoring

Assess degree of bronchospasm.

Adverse Effects/Precautions

Temporary blurring of vision, precipitation of narrow-angle glaucoma, or eye pain may occur if solution comes into direct contact with the eyes.

Pharmacology

Ipratropium bromide is a quaternary ammonium derivative of atropine. It produces primarily large airway bronchodilation by antagonizing the action of acetylcholine at its receptor site. It is relatively bronchospecific when administered by inhalation because of limited absorption through lung tissue. Peak effect occurs 1 to 2 hours after administration. Duration of effect is 4 to 6 hours in children. The combination of ipratropium with a beta-agonist produces more bronchodilation than either drug individually.

Special Considerations/Preparation

Inhalation solution is supplied in 2.5-mL vials, containing ipratropium bromide 0.02% (200 mcg/mL) in a sterile, preservative-free, isotonic saline solution that is pH-adjusted to 3.4 with hydrochloric acid. It may be mixed with albuterol if used within 1 hour. Compatibility data are not currently available with other drugs.
Store at room temperature in foil pouch provided. Protect from light.

Selected References

♦ Lee H, Arnon S, Silverman M: Bronchodilator aerosol administered by metered dose inhaler and spacer in subacute neonatal respiratory distress syndrome. *Arch Dis Child* 1994;70:F218.

♦ Consensus Conference in Aerosol Delivery: Aerosol Consensus Statement. *Respir Care* 1991;36:916.

♦ Brundage KL, Mohsini Kj Froese AB, Fisher JT: Bronchodilator response to ipratropium bromide in infants with bronchopulmonary dysplasia. *Am Rev Respir Dis* 1990;142:1137.

♦ Gross NJ: Ipratropium bromide. *N Engl J Med* 1988;319:486.

Added 1/95

RESPIRATORY

MISCELLANEOUS

Diazoxide

Dose and Administration

2 to 5 mg/kg per dose PO given Q8 hours. Begin therapy at the higher dosage and taper by response.

Uses

Treatment of persistent (more than a few days) or severe hypoglycemia due to hyperinsulinism.

Positive responses are usually seen within 48 to 72 hours, and occur in less than 50% of neonates.

Monitoring

Periodic CBC and serum uric acid concentrations if treating long term.

Adverse Effects/Precautions

Sodium and fluid retention is common—consider concurrent treatment with chlorothiazide (which may also potentiate the hyperglycemic action of diazoxide). Hyperuricemia, leukopenia, and neutropenia are rare complications. Excessive hair growth and coarse facial features develop with long term use. Ketoacidosis may occur during times of intercurrent illness.

Pharmacology

Diazoxide inhibits insulin release by acting as a specific ATP-sensitive potassium channel agonist in normal pancreatic beta cells. It also reduces insulin release and counters the peripheral actions of insulin via catecholamine stimulation. The serum half-life is 10 to 24 hours in infants. Diazoxide is more than 90% protein-bound in adults, and is excreted entirely by the kidneys.

Special Considerations/Preparation

Proglycem® is available as an oral suspension, 50 mg/mL concentration. Alcohol content is 7.25%. Shake well before use. Protect from light. Store at 2 to 36°C (36 to 80°F).

Selected References

♦ Schwitzgebel VM, Gitelman SE: Neonatal hyperinsulinism. *Clin Perinatol* 1998;25:1015-1038.

♦ Kane C, Lindley KJ, Johnson PRV, et al: Therapy for persistent hyperinsulinemic hypoglycemia of infancy: understanding the responsiveness of beta cells to diazoxide and somatostatin. *J Clin Investig* 1997;100:1888-1893.

♦ Stanley CA: Hyperinsulinism in infants and children. *Pediatr Clin North Am* 1997;44:363-374.

Added 3/99

(Eutectic Mixture of Local Anesthetics)

Dose & Administration

Apply 1 to 2 gm to distal half of the penis, then wrap with occlusive dressing. Allow dressing to remain intact for 60 to 90 minutes, remove and clean treated area completely prior to circumcision to avoid systemic absorption.

Uses

Topical analgesia for circumcision. Not effective for heel lancing.

Monitoring

Blood methemoglobin concentration if concerned about toxicity.

Adverse Effects/Precautions

Blanching and redness resolve without treatment. When measured, blood levels of methemoglobin in neonates after the application of 1 g of EMLA cream have been well below toxic levels. Two cases of methemoglobinemia in infants occurred after >3 g of EMLA cream was applied; in 1 of these cases, the infant also was receiving sulfamethoxazole. EMLA cream should not be used in neonates who are receiving other drugs known to induce methemoglobinemia: sulfonamides, acetaminophen, nitrates, nitroglycerin, nitroprusside, phenobarbital, and phenytoin.

Pharmacology

EMLA cream, containing 2.5% lidocaine and 2.5% prilocaine, attenuates the pain response to circumcision when applied 60 to 90 minutes before the procedure. The analgesic effect is limited during the phases associated with extensive tissue trauma such as during lysis of adhesions and tightening of the clamp. Stabilizes the neuronal membranes by inhibiting the ionic fluxes required for conduction and initiation of nerve impulses. There is a theoretic concern about the potential for neonates to develop methemoglobinemia after the application of EMLA cream, because a metabolite of prilocaine can oxidize hemoglobin to methemoglobin. Neonates are deficient in methemoglobin NADH cytochrome b_5 reductase. Lidocaine is metabolized rapidly by the liver to a number of active metabolites and then excreted renally.

Special Considerations/Preparation

Available in 5-gm and 30-gm tubes with Tegaderm dressing and in a 1-gm Anesthetic Disc, boxes of 2 and 10. Each gram of EMLA contains lidocaine 25 mg and prilocaine 25 mg in a eutectic mixture. pH of the product is 9. Contains no preservatives.

Selected References

♦ American Academy of Pediatrics, Task Force on Circumcision. Circumcision policy statement. *Pediatrics* 1999;103:686-693.

♦ Taddio A, Ohlsson A, Einarson TR, et al: A systematic review of lidocaine-prilocaine cream (EMLA) in the treatment of acute pain in neonates. *Pediatrics* 1998;101:1-9.

♦ Lander J, Brady-Fryer B, Metcalfe JB, et al: Comparison of ringblock, dorsal penile nerve block, and topical anesthesia for neonatal circumcision: A randomized controlled trial. *JAMA* 1997;278:2157-2162.

♦ Taddio A, Stevens B, Craig K, et al: Efficacy and safety of lidocaine-prilocaine cream for pain during circumcision. *N Engl J Med* 1997;336:1197-1201.

♦ Product information, AstraZeneca: *Physicians' Desk Reference*, ed 57. Montvale, NJ: Medical Economics Data, 2003, p 599.

References updated 2003

MISCELLANEOUS

Glucagon

Dose & Administration

200 mcg/kg per dose (0.2 mg/kg per dose) IV push, IM, or SC.
Maximum dose: 1 mg.
Continuous infusion: Begin with 10 to 20 mcg/kg per hour (0.5 to 1 mg per day) using reconstituted solution. Rise in blood glucose should occur with one hour of starting infusion.

Uses

Treatment of hypoglycemia refractory to intravenous dextrose infusions, or when dextrose infusion is unavailable, or in cases of documented glucagon deficiency.

Monitoring

Follow blood glucose concentration closely. Watch for rebound hypoglycemia. Rise in blood glucose will last approximately 2 hours.

Adverse Effects/Precautions

Nausea and vomiting, tachycardia, and ? ileus.

Pharmacology

Glucagon stimulates synthesis of cyclic AMP, especially in liver and adipose tissue. Stimulates gluconeogenesis. In high doses, glucagon has a cardiac inotropic effect. Inhibits small-bowel motility and gastric-acid secretion.

Special Considerations/Preparation

Supplied in 1-mg single-dose vials and 10-mg multiple-use vials. Dissolve the lyophilized product in the supplied diluent. Precipitates in chloride solutions. One unit (1 U) of glucagon and 1 mg of glucagon are equivalent. Use immediately after reconstitution.

Solution Compatibility: No data are currently available on Dex/AA and other intravenous solutions.

Terminal Injection Site Compatibility: No data are currently available.

Selected References

♦ Miralles RE, Lodha A, Perlman M, Moore AM: Experience with intravenous glucagon infusions as a treatment for resistant neonatal hypoglycemia. *Arch Pediatr Adolesc Med* 2002;156:99-1004.

♦ Hawdon JM, Aynsley-Green A, Ward Platt MP: Neonatal blood glucose concentrations: metabolic effect of intravenous glucagon and intragastric medium chain triglyceride. *Arch Dis Child* 1993;68:255.

♦ Mehta A, Wootton R, Cheng KN, et al: Effect of diazoxide or glucagon on hepatic production rate during extreme neonatal hypoglycemia. *Arch Dis Child* 1987;62:924.

♦ Davis SN, Granner DK: Insulin and oral hypoglycemic agents and the pharmacology of the endocrine pancreas, in Hardman JG, Limbird LE, Gilman AG (eds): *The Pharmacological Basis of Therapeutics*, ed 10. New York: Macmillan Co, 2001, p 1707-08.

Dose and References Updated 3/2003

Dose & Administration

Subcutaneous or intradermal: Inject 1 mL (150 U) as 5 separate 0.2-mL injections around periphery of extravasation site. Use 25- or 26-gauge needle and change after each injection.

Use within 1 hour of extravasation for best results.

Uses

Prevention of tissue injury caused by IV extravasation. Suggested indications (some anecdotal) are for extravasations involving drugs that are irritating to veins because of hyperosmolarity or extreme pH (e.g. aminophylline, amphotericin B, calcium, diazepam, erythromycin, gentamicin, methicillin, nafcillin, oxacillin, phenytoin, potassium chloride, rifampin, sodium bicarbonate, tromethamine, vancomycin, and TPN, and concentrated IV solutions). Hyaluronidase is **not** indicated for treatment of extravasations of vasoconstrictive agents (e.g. dopamine, epinephrine, and norepinephrine).

Monitoring

No specific monitoring required.

Adverse Effects/Precautions

Not recommended for IV use.

Pharmacology

Hyaluronidase is a mucolytic enzyme that disrupts the normal intercellular barrier and allows rapid dispersion of extravasated fluids through tissues.

Special Considerations/Preparation

Supplied as both a stabilized solution and lyophilized powder.

The solution is available in 1-mL and 10-mL vials (150 U/mL).

The powder is also available in 1-mL and 10-mL vials that are reconstituted to a concentration of 150 U/mL. **Dilute only with NS.** Reconstituted powder is stable at room temperature for 2 weeks; stabilized solution is potent for up to 2 years refrigerated. Do not use if solution is discolored or contains a precipitate.

Terminal Injection Site Compatibility: Amikacin, pentobarbital, and sodium bicarbonate.

Incompatibility: Epinephrine and heparin.

Selected References

♦ Raszka WV, Kueser TK, Smith FR, Bass JW: The use of hyaluronidase in the treatment of intravenous extravasation injuries. *J Perinatol* 1990;10:146.

♦ Zenk KE, Dungy CI, Greene GR: Nafcillin extravasation injury. *Am J Dis Child* 1981;135:1113.

♦ Tilden SJ, Craft C, Cano R, Daum RS: Cutaneous necrosis associated with intravenous nafcillin therapy. *Am J Dis Child* 1980;134:1046.

♦ Britton RC, Habif DV: Clinical use of hyaluronidase. *Surgery* 1953;33:917.

Updated 3/98
Compatibilities Updated 3/2001

Note: Hyaluronidase is no longer manufactured or marketed in the USA.

MISCELLANEOUS

Hydrocortisone

Dose & Administration

Physiologic replacement: 6 to 8 mg/m^2 per day IV or PO, in 2 or 3 doses.
Treatment of pressor- and volume-resistant hypotension (Stress doses):
20 to 40 mg/m^2 per day IV or PO, in 2 or 3 doses.

Body Surface Area

Weight (kg)	Surface Area* (sq meters)
0.6	0.08
1	0.1
1.4	0.12
2	0.15
3	0.2
4	0.25
* BSA (m^2) = (0.05 x kg) + 0.05	

Treatment of cortisol-deficient ELBW infants to decrease risk of CLD:
Initial dose: 0.5 mg/kg/dose IV Q12 hours for 9 days, followed by
0.25 mg/kg IV Q 12 hours for 3 days.

Uses

Treatment of cortisol deficiency. Blood pressure support. Adjunctive
therapy for persistent hypoglycemia.

Monitoring

Measure blood pressure and blood glucose frequently during acute illness.

Adverse Effects/Precautions

Hyperglycemia, hypertension, salt and water retention. Two studies have
also reported an increased risk of disseminated *Candida* infections. Adverse
effects of long-term treatment with pharmacologic doses are probably
similar to those due to dexamethasone.

Pharmacology

Hydrocortisone is the main adrenal corticosteroid, with primarily
glucocorticoid effects. It increases the expression of adrenergic receptors
in the vascular wall, thereby enhancing vascular reactivity to other
vasoactive substances, such as norepinephrine and angiotensin II. It
stimulates the liver to form glucose from amino acids and glycerol, and
also stimulates the deposition of glucose as glycogen. Peripheral glucose
utilization is diminished, protein breakdown is increased, and lipolysis
is activated. The net result is an increase in blood glucose levels. Renal
effects include increased calcium excretion.

continued...

MISCELLANEOUS

Special Considerations/Preparation

Available as hydrocortisone sodium phosphate injection 50 mg/mL in 2- and 10-mL vials and hydrocortisone sodium succinate 125 mg/mL in 2-, 4-, and 8-mL vials (contains 9 mg/mL benzyl alcohol). Make a 1 mg/mL dilution by adding 0.5 mL of the 50 mg/mL concentration to 24.5 mL of preservative-free normal saline. Dilution stable for 3 days refrigerated. Also available as hydrocortisone cypionate oral suspension in a 2 mg/mL concentration.

Hydrocortisone acetate is not suitable for IV or IM administration.

Hydrocortisone phosphate

Solution compatibility: D_5W and NS.

Terminal Injection Site Compatibility: Fat emulsion. Amikacin, amphotericin B, aztreonam, fluconazole, metoclopramide, and sodium bicarbonate.

Hydrocortisone succinate

Solution compatibility: D_5W, $D_{10}W$, and NS.

Terminal Injection Site Compatibility: Dex/AA and fat emulsion. Acyclovir, amikacin, aminophylline, amphotericin B, ampicillin, atropine, aztreonam, calcium chloride, calcium gluconate, chloramphenicol, clindamycin, dexamethasone, digoxin, dopamine, enalaprilat, epinephrine, erythromycin lactobionate, esmolol, famotidine, fentanyl, furosemide, heparin, hydralazine, insulin, isoproterenol, lidocaine, lorazepam, magnesium, methicillin, metoclopramide, metronidazole, morphine, neostigamine, netilmicin, oxacillin, pancuronium, penicillin G, piperacillin, piperacillin-tazobactam, potassium chloride, propofol, propranolol, prostaglandin E_1, remifentanil, sodium bicarbonate, vecuronium and vitamin K_1.

Incompatibility: Midazolam, nafcillin, pentobarbital, phenobarbital, and phenytoin.

Selected References

♦ Seri I, Tan R, Evans J: Cardiovascular effects of hydrocortisone in preterm infants with pressor-resistant hypotension. *Pediatrics* 2001;107:1070-1074.

♦ Watterberg KL, Gerdes JS, Gifford KL, Lin H-M: Prophylaxis against early adrenal insufficiency to prevent chronic lung disease in premature infants. *Pediatrics* 1999;104: 1258-1263.

♦ Botas CM, Kurlat I, Young SM, Sola A: Disseminated candidal infections and intravenous hydrocortisone in preterm infants. *Pediatrics* 1995;95:883.

♦ Schimmer BP, Parker KL: ACTH: Adrenocortical steroids and their synthetic analogs, in Hardman JG, Gilman AG, Limbird LE (eds): *The Pharmacological Basis of Therapeutics*, ed 9. New York: Macmillan Co, 1995, p 1465.

♦ Helbock HJ, Insoft RM, Conte FA: Glucocorticoid-responsive hypotension in extremely low birth weight newborns. *Pediatrics* 1993;92:715.

♦ Briars GL, Bailey BJ: Surface area estimation: pocket calculator versus nomogram. *Arch Dis Child* 1994;70:246-247.

♦ Ramanathan R, Siassi B, Sardesai S, deLemos R: Dexamethasone versus hydrocortisone for hypotension refractory to high dose inotropic agents and incidence of Candida infections in extremely low birth weight infants. *Pediatr Res* 1996; 39:240A.

Updated 3/2002, Compatibilities updated 3/2003

MISCELLANEOUS

Insulin

Dose & Administration

Continuous IV infusion: 0.01 to 0.1 U/kg per hour.

Only regular insulin for injection may be administered intravenously.
To saturate plastic tubing binding sites, fill IV tubing with insulin solution
and wait for at least 20 minutes before infusing . The use of higher insulin
concentrations and longer wait times will shorten the time to steady-state.
Titrate using blood glucose concentration/reagent strips.

Intermittent dose: 0.1 to 0.2 U/kg Q6 to 12 hours SC.

Uses

Treatment of VLBW hyperglycemic infants with persistent glucose
intolerance. Adjuvant therapy for hyperkalemia.

Monitoring

Follow blood glucose concentration frequently (Q15 to 30 minutes) after
starting insulin infusion and after changes in infusion rate.

Adverse Effects/Precautions

May rapidly induce hypoglycemia. Insulin resistance may develop, causing
a larger dose requirement. Euglycemic hyperinsulinemia due to exogenous
insulin administration may cause metabolic acidosis.

Pharmacology

Degraded in liver and kidney. Enhances cellular uptake of glucose,
conversion of glucose to glycogen, amino acid uptake by muscle tissue,
synthesis of fat, and cellular uptake of potassium. Inhibits lipolysis and
conversion of protein to glucose. Plasma half-life in adults is 9 minutes.

Special Considerations/Preparation

Available as 100 Unit/mL concentration in 10-mL vials. Dilute with sterile
water or NS to a concentration of 1 U/mL. **Keep refrigerated.**

Solution Compatibility: D_5W, and $D_{10}W$.

Terminal Injection Site Compatibility: Dex/AA and fat emulsion. Amiodarone,
ampicillin, aztreonam, cefazolin, cefoxitin, cimetidine, digoxin, dobutamine,
esmolol, famotidine, gentamicin, heparin, hydrocortisone succinate,
imipenem, indomethacin, lidocaine, meropenem, metoclopramide,
midazolam, morphine, nitroglycerin, pentobarbital, potassium chloride,
propofol, ranitidine, sodium bicarbonate, sodium nitroprusside, ticarcillin/
clavulanate, tobramycin, and vancomycin.

Incompatibility: Aminophylline, dopamine, nafcillin, phenobarbital,
and phenytoin.

Selected References

♦ Mena P, Llanos A, Uauy R: Insulin homeostasis in the extremely low birth weight
  infant. *Semin Perinatol* 2001;25:436-446.

♦ Fuloria M, Friedberg MA, DuRant RH, Aschner JL: Effect of flow rate and insulin
  priming on the recovery of insulin from microbore infusion tubing. *Pediatrics*
  1998;102:1401-1406.

♦ Poindexter BB, Karn CA, Denne SC: Exogenous insulin reduces proteolysis and protein
  synthesis in extremely low birth weight infants. *J Pediatr* 1998;132:948-953.

♦ Ostertag SG, Jovanovic L, Lewis B, Auld PAM: Insulin pump therapy in the very low
  birth weight infant. *Pediatrics* 1986;78:625.

References updated 3/2003, Compatibilities updated 3/2001

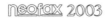
neofax 2003

Dose and Administration

Initial oral dose: 10 to 14 mcg/kg per dose PO Q24 hours.
(37.5 to 50 mcg/dose for an average term infant).
Dosage is adjusted in 12.5mcg increments. Always round upward.
Initial IV dose: 5 to 8 mcg/kg per dose Q24 hours.

Uses

Treatment of hypothyroidism.

Monitoring

After 4 weeks of treatment, serum T$_4$ should be high normal—10 to 16 mcg/dL. Maintain in this range for the first year. Free T$_4$ should also be high normal—values are assay-dependent, direct dialysis method is preferred. Serum T$_3$ should be normal (70 to 220 ng/dL), and TSH should have declined from initial value. After 12 weeks, serum TSH should be in the normal range, less than 15 mU/L. Serum T$_4$, free T$_4$, and TSH concentrations should be measured every 1 to 2 months, or 2 weeks after any dosage change. Assess for signs of hypothyroidism: Lethargy, poor feeding, constipation, intermittent cyanosis, and prolonged neonatal jaundice. Assess for signs of thyrotoxicosis: hyperreactivity, altered sleep pattern, tachycardia, tachypnea, fever, exophthalmos, and goiter. Periodically assess growth, development, and bone-age advancement.

Adverse Effects/Precautions

Prolonged over-treatment can produce premature craniosynostosis and acceleration of bone age.

Pharmacology

Tissue deiodination converts T$_4$ to T$_3$, the active metabolite. Elimination of both T$_4$ and T$_3$ is equally in the urine and feces. Clinical effects will persist for 1 week after discontinuation of the drug. Levothyroxine prepared as an oral suspension is 50% to 80% bioavailable. Oral dosing produces effects within 3 to 5 days, while IV dosing produces effects in 6 to 8 hours.

Special Considerations/Preparation

Available only as scored tablets ranging from 25 to 300 mcg per tablet. Prepare oral dosage form by crushing tablet(s) and suspending in a small amount of sterile water, breast milk, or non-soy formula. **Use immediately**. Monitor patients closely when switching brand of drug, due to differences in bioavailability. **The injectable form should not be given orally,** as it crystallizes when exposed to acid. Injectable form is available as lyophilized powder in vials containing 200 or 500 mcg. **Use only NS for reconstitution.** Manufacturer's suggested final concentrations are 40 or 100 mcg/mL; however, we suggest diluting to a final concentration of 20 mcg/mL. **Use immediately. Do not add to any other IV solution.**

Selected References

♦ AAP Section on Endocrinology and Committee on Genetics, and Committee on Public Health, American Thyroid Association: Newborn screening for congenital hypothyroidism: Recommended guidelines. *Pediatrics* 1993;91:1203-1209.

♦ Selva KA, Mandel SH, Rien L, et al: Initial treatment dose of L-thyroxine in congenital hypothyroidism. *J Pediatr* 2002;141:786-92.

♦ Germak JA, Foley TP: Longitudinal assessment of L-thyroxine therapy for congenital hypothyroidism. *J Pediatr* 1990;117:211.

Updated 3/2003

MISCELLANEOUS

Sodium Bicarbonate

Dose & Administration
Resuscitation: 1 to 2 mEq/kg IV slow push over at least 2 minutes.

Correction of metabolic acidosis:
HCO_3 needed (mEq) = HCO_3 deficit (mEq/L) x (0.3 x body wt [kg])
Administer half of calculated dose, then assess need for remainder.

Maximum concentration used: 0.5 mEq/mL dilute if desired. Can also be administered by continuous IV infusion or PO.

Uses
Treatment of documented metabolic acidosis during prolonged resuscitation after establishment of effective ventilation. Treatment of bicarbonate deficit caused by renal or GI losses.

Monitoring
Follow acid/base status, ABGs.

Adverse Effects/Precautions
Rationale against use in resuscitation:
1) Rapid infusion of hypertonic solution is linked to IVH.
2) When administered during inadequate ventilation, PCO_2 increases, thereby decreasing pH.
3) Carbon dioxide diffuses more readily across cell membranes than bicarbonate, thereby decreasing intracellular pH.

Other adverse effects: Local tissue necrosis, hypocalcemia, and hypernatremia.

Pharmacology
Rationale for use in prolonged resuscitation:
1) Decreases pulmonary vasculature resistance.
2) Improves myocardial function.
3) Increases response of myocardium to sympathomimetics.

continued...

Special Considerations/Preparation

Will precipitate with calcium or phosphate. Dilute with sterile water for injection. Maximum concentration used is 0.5 mEq/mL.

Osmolarity

Concentration by		Approximate Osmolarity
(%)	(mEq/mL)	(mOsm/L)
8.4	1	1800
4.2	0.5	900
2.8	0.33	600
2.1	0.25	450

Solution Compatibility: D_5W, $D_{10}W$, and NS.

Terminal Injection Site Compatibility: Fat emulsion. Acyclovir, amikacin, aminophylline, amphotericin B, ampicillin, atropine, aztreonam, cefepime, cefoxitin, ceftazidime, ceftriaxone, chloramphenicol, cimetidine, clindamycin, dexamethasone, erythromycin lactobionate, esmolol, famotidine, fentanyl, furosemide, heparin, hyaluronidase, hydrocortisone succinate, indomethacin, insulin, lidocaine, linezolid, meropenem, morphine, nafcillin, netilmicin, oxacillin, penicillin G, pentobarbital, phenobarbital, phenytoin, piperacillin-tazobactam, potassium chloride, propofol, remifentanil, tolazoline, vancomycin, and vitamin K_1.

Incompatibility: Dex/AA (note change from previous editions). Amiodarone, calcium chloride, calcium gluconate, cefotaxime, dobutamine, dopamine, epinephrine, glycopyrolate, imipenem/cilastatin, isoproterenol, magnesium sulfate, methadone, methicillin, metoclopramide, midazolam, norepinephrine, ticarcillin/clavulanate, and vecuronium.

Selected References

♦ Ammari AN, Schulze KF: Uses and abuses of sodium bicarbonate in the neonatal intensive care unit. *Curr Opin Pediatr* 2002;14:151-156.

♦ Wyckoff MH, Perlman J, Niermeyer S: Medications during resuscitation - what is the evidence? *Semin Neonatol* 2001;6:251-259.

♦ International Guidelines for Neonatal Resuscitation: An Excerpt from the Guidelines 2000 for Cardiopulmonary Resuscitation and Emergency Cardiovascular Care: International Consensus on Science. *Pediatrics* 2000;106(3) URL:http://www.pediatrics.org/cgi/content/full/106/3/e29.

♦ Howell JH: Sodium bicarbonate in the perinatal setting—revisited. *Clin Perinatol* 1987;14:807.

References updated 3/2003
Compatibilities updated 3/2003

THAM acetate

(Tromethamine)

Dose and Administration

1 to 2 mMol/kg (3.3 to 6.6 mL/kg) per dose IV.

Infuse in a large vein over at least 30 minutes.

Dose (of the 0.3 M solution) may be calculated from the following formula:

Dose (mL) = Weight (kg) x Base deficit (mEq/L)

Maximum dose in neonates with normal renal function is approximately 5 to 7 mMol/kg per 24 hours. Clinical studies support only short term use.

Uses

Treatment of metabolic acidosis, primarily in mechanically ventilated patients with significant hypercarbia or hypernatremia. **Do not use in patients who are anuric or uremic.** THAM is not indicated for treatment of metabolic acidosis caused by bicarbonate deficiency.

Monitoring

Observe IV site closely for signs of extravasation. Follow blood-gas results to assess therapeutic efficacy. Follow urine output. Monitor for respiratory depression, hypoglycemia, and hyperkalemia when using several doses.

Adverse Effects/Precautions

Most reports of toxicity in neonates (hypoglycemia, hyperkalemia, liver necrosis) were related to rapid umbilical venous infusion of high doses of THAM base solutions that were more alkaline and hypertonic than the THAM acetate solution currently available from Abbott (pH 8.6; osmolarity 380 mOsm/L). **Irritating to veins.**

Pharmacology

THAM (Tris-Hydroxymethyl Aminomethane) is a proton acceptor that generates NH_3^+ and HCO_3^- without generating CO_2. The protonated $R-NH_3^+$ is eliminated by the kidneys. Unlike bicarbonate, THAM does not require an open system for CO_2 elimination in order to exert its buffering effect.

Special Considerations/Preparation

Supplied as a 0.3-M solution (1 mMol = 3.3 mL) in a 500-mL single-dose container with no bacteriostatic agent. Use within 24 hours of opening. **Compatibilities:** No data are currently available on solutions and additives.

Selected References

♦ Holmdahl MH, Wiklund L, Wetterberg T, et al: The place of THAM in the management of acidemia in clinical practice. *Acta Anaethesiol Scand* 2000;44:524-527.

♦ Nahas GG, Sutin KM, Fermon C, et al: Guidelines for the treatment of acidemia with THAM. *Drugs* 1998;55:191-224. (Errata published 1998;55:517).

♦ Baum JD, Robertson NRC: Immediate effects of alkaline infusion in infants with respiratory distress syndrome. *J Pediatr* 1975;87:255.

♦ Strauss J: Tris (hydroxymethyl amino-methane [THAM]): A pediatric evaluation. *Pediatrics* 1968;41:667.

♦ Gupta JM, Dahlenburg GW, Davis JW: Changes in blood gas tensions following administration of amine buffer THAM to infants with respiratory distress syndrome. *Arch Dis Child* 1967;42:416-427.

Text and references updated 3/2001

Dose and Administration

1 or 2 drops instilled in the eye 10 to 30 minutes prior to funduscopy. Use solutions containing concentrations of 0.5% or less in neonates. May be used in conjunction with 1 drop of Phenylephrine 2.5% ophthalmic solution.

Apply pressure to the lacrimal sac during and for 2 minutes after instillation to minimize systemic absorption.

Uses

Induction of mydriasis and cycloplegia for diagnostic and therapeutic ophthalmic procedures.

Monitoring

Monitor heart rate and assess for signs of ileus prior to feeding.

Adverse Effects/Precautions

Feedings should be withheld for 4 hours following procedure. Systemic effects are those of anticholinergic drugs: Fever, tachycardia, vasodilatation, dry mouth, restlessness, delayed gastric emptying and decreased gastrointestinal motility, and urinary retention. The use of solutions with concentrations of 1% or greater have caused systemic toxicity in infants.

Pharmacology

Anticholinergic drug that produces pupillary dilation by inhibiting the sphincter pupillae muscle, and paralysis of accommodation. Maximal mydriasis occurs 30 to 60 minutes following administration. Recovery of accommodation occurs in 6 to 24 hours. Without lacrimal sac occlusion, approximately 80% of each drop may pass through the nasolacrimal system and be available for rapid systemic absorption by the nasal mucosa.

Special Considerations/Preparation

Supplied as ophthalmic solution in 0.5%, 1% and 2% concentrations in 2- and 15-mL bottles. Store away from heat. **Do not refrigerate.**

A preparation containing cyclopentolate 0.2% and phenylephrine 1% (Cyclomydril®) is commercially available in 2- and 8-mL Drop-tainers.

A combination eye drop solution ("Caputo drops") may be prepared in a 15-mL bottle with 3.75 mL of cyclopentolate 2%, 7.5 mL of tropicamide 1%, and 3.75 mL of phenylephrine 10%. The final solution contains cyclopentolate 0.5%, tropicamide 0.5%, and phenylephrine 2.5%.

MISCELLANEOUS

Selected References

♦ Bonthala S, Sparks JW, Musgrove KH, Berseth CL: Mydriatics slow gastric emptying in preterm infants. *J Pediatr* 2000;137:327-30.

♦ Wallace DK, Steinkuller PG: Ocular medications in children. *Clin Pediatr* 1998;37:645.

♦ Laws DE, Morton C, Weindling M, Clark D: Systemic effects of screening for retinopathy of prematurity. *Br J Ophthalmol* 1996;80:425-428.

♦ McGregor MLK: Anticholinergic agents, in Mauger TF, Craig EL (eds): *Havener's Ocular Pharmacology,* ed 6. St. Louis: Mosby-YearBook, 1994, pp 148-155.

♦ Caputo AR, Schnitzer RE, Lindquist TD, Sun S: Dilation in neonates: a protocol. *Pediatrics* 1982;69:77-80.

♦ Isenberg S, Everett S: Cardiovascular effects of mydriatics in low-birth-weight infants. *J Pediatr* 1984;105:111-112.

References updated 3/2001

Phenylephrine (Ophthalmic)

Dose and Administration

1 drop instilled in the eye at least 10 minutes prior to funduscopic procedures. Use **only** the 2.5% ophthalmic solution in neonates.

Apply pressure to the lacrimal sac during and for 2 minutes after instillation to minimize systemic absorption.

Uses

Induction of mydriasis and cycloplegia for diagnostic and therapeutic ophthalmic procedures.

Monitoring

Monitor heart rate and oxygen saturation in babies with BPD.

Adverse Effects/Precautions

May cause decreased pulmonary compliance, tidal volume, and peak airflow in babies with BPD. Do not use in patients receiving beta-blocker medications (e.g. propranolol). The use of 10% solutions has caused systemic hypertension and tachycardia in infants.

Pharmacology

Alpha-adrenergic. Mydriasis begins within 5 minutes of instillation and lasts for 60 minutes. Without lacrimal sac occlusion, approximately 80% of each drop may pass through the nasolacrimal system and be available for rapid systemic absorption by the nasal mucosa.

Special Considerations/Preparation

Supplied as ophthalmic solution in 0.12%, 2.5%, and 10% concentrations in 2 to 15 mL quantities. Do not use solution that becomes discolored or contains precipitate. **Do not refrigerate.**

A preparation containing cyclopentolate 0.2% and phenylephrine 1% (Cyclomydril®) is commercially available in 2- and 8-mL Drop-tainers.

Supplied as a combination eye drop solution ("Caputo drops") with final concentrations of cyclopentolate 0.5%, tropicamide 0.5%, and phenylephrine 2.5%, may be prepared in a 15-mL bottle with 3.75 mL of cyclopentolate 2%, 7.5 mL of tropicamide 1%, and 3.75 mL of phenylephrine 10%.

Selected References

♦ Wallace DK, Steinkuller PG: Ocular medications in children. *Clin Pediatr* 1998;37:645-652.

♦ Laws DE, Morton C, Weindling M, Clark D: Systemic effects of screening for retinopathy of prematurity. *Br J Ophthalmol* 1996;80:425-428.

♦ McGregor MLK: Adrenergic agonists, in Mauger TF, Craig EL (eds): *Havener's Ocular Pharmacology,* ed 6. St. Louis: Mosby-YearBook, 1994, pp 70-72.

♦ Mirmanesh SJ, Abbasi S, Bhutani VK: Alpha-adrenergic bronchoprovocation in neonates with bronchopulmonary dysplasia. *J Pediatr* 1992;121:622-625.

♦ Isenberg S, Everett S: Cardiovascular effects of mydriatics in low-birth-weight infants. *J Pediatr* 1984;105:111-112

♦ Caputo AR, Schnitzer RE, Lindquist TD, Sun S: Dilation in neonates: a protocol. *Pediatrics* 1982;69:77-80.

♦ Borromeo-McGrall V, Bordiuk JM, Keitel H: Systemic hypertension following ocular administration of 10% phenylephrine in the neonate. *Pediatrics* 1973;51:1032-1036.

Added 3/99

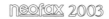

Dose and Administration

1 drop instilled in the eye at least 10 minutes prior funduscopic procedures.
Use **only** the 0.5% ophthalmic solution in neonates.

Apply pressure to the lacrimal sac during and for 2 minutes after instillation to minimize systemic absorption.

Uses

Induction of mydriasis and cycloplegia for diagnostic and therapeutic ophthalmic procedures.

Monitoring

Monitor heart rate and assess for signs of ileus prior to feeding.

Adverse Effects/Precautions

Feedings should be withheld for 4 hours following procedure. Systemic effects are those of anticholinergic drugs: Fever, tachycardia, vasodilatation, dry mouth, restlessness, decreased gastrointestinal motility, and urinary retention. The use of solutions with concentrations of 1% or greater have caused systemic toxicity in infants

Pharmacology

Anticholinergic drug that produces pupillary dilation by inhibiting the sphincter pupillae muscle, and paralysis of accommodation. Mydriasis begins within 5 minutes of instillation, cycloplegia occurs in 20 to 40 minutes. Recovery of accommodation occurs in 6 hours. Without lacrimal sac occlusion, approximately 80% of each drop may pass through the nasolacrimal system and be available for rapid systemic absorption by the nasal mucosa.

Special Considerations/Preparation

Supplied as ophthalmic solution in 0.5%, and 1% concentrations in 2- and 15-mL dropper bottles. Store away from heat. **Do not refrigerate.**

A combination eye drop solution ("Caputo drops") may be prepared in a 15-mL bottle with 3.75 mL of cyclopentolate 2%, 7.5 mL of tropicamide 1%, and 3.75 mL of phenylephrine 10%. The final solution contains cyclopentolate 0.5%, tropicamide 0.5%, and phenylephrine 2.5%. Use within 24 hours, as the solution contains no preservatives.

Selected References

♦ Wallace DK, Steinkuller PG: Ocular medications in children. *Clin Pediatr* 1998;37:645-652.

♦ Laws DE, Morton C, Weindling M, Clark D: Systemic effects of screening for retinopathy of prematurity. *Br J Ophthalmol* 1996;80:425-428.

♦ McGregor MLK: Anticholinergic agents, in Mauger TF, Craig EL (eds): *Havener's Ocular Pharmacology,* ed 6. St. Louis: Mosby-YearBook, 1994, pp 148-155.

♦ Caputo AR, Schnitzer RE, Lindquist TD, Sun S: Dilation in neonates: a protocol. *Pediatrics* 1982;69:77-80.

Added 3/99

MISCELLANEOUS

VITAMINS/MINERALS

Calcium

Dose and Administration

Symptomatic hypocalcemia—acute treatment:

Drug	mg/kg/dose	mL/kg/dose
Elemental calcium	10 to 20	—
10% Calcium gluconate	100 to 200	1 to 2
10% Calcium chloride	35 to 70	0.35 to 0.7

Infuse IV over 10 to 30 minutes while monitoring for bradycardia (stop infusion if heart rate is less than 100 beats per minute). Dilute Calcium chloride at least 1:1 with water.
Do not give intra-arterially.

Maintenance treatment:

Drug	mg/kg/day	mL/kg/day
Elemental calcium	20 to 80	—
10% Calcium gluconate (IV or PO)	200 to 800	2 to 8
10% Calcium chloride (IV)	75 to 300	0.75 to 3
6.5% Calcium glubionate (PO)	360 to 1260	1 to 3.5

Administer PO in 4 divided doses after diluting in feeding, or by continuous IV infusion. Treat for 3 to 5 days, and follow serum concentrations closely.

Exchange transfusion:

Drug	mg/dose*	mL/dose*
Elemental calcium	9	—
10% Calcium gluconate	100	1
10% Calcium chloride	33	0.33
* Dose per 100 mL citrated blood exchanged		

Uses

Treatment and prevention of hypocalcemia, usually defined as a serum ionized calcium concentration less than approximately 4 mg/dL (or total serum calcium less than approximately 8 mg/dL).
Treatment of asymptomatic infants is controversial.

continued...

VITAMINS & MINERALS

Calcium

Monitoring

If possible, measure ionized calcium directly. Avoid hypercalcemia during treatment. Correct hypomagnesemia if present. Observe IV infusion site closely for extravasation. Observe IV tubing for precipitates. Monitor continuously for bradycardia. Assess for GI intolerance when treating PO.

Adverse Effects/Precautions

Rapid administration is associated with bradycardia or cardiac standstill. Cutaneous necrosis or calcium deposition occurs with extravasation. Bolus infusions by UAC have been associated with intestinal bleeding and lower-extremity tissue necrosis. Gastric irritation and diarrhea may occur during oral therapy; NEC has been related to oral administration of hyperosmolar preparations (e.g. Calcium glubionate). Calcium gluconate may be given orally if infant can tolerate the drug volume.

Pharmacology

Ionized calcium is the physiologically active fraction, accounting for approximately 50% of total blood calcium. The remainder is bound to albumin (40%) or complexed (10%) with citrate, phosphate, and bicarbonate. Early hypocalcemia is common in asphyxiated infants, premature infants, and infants of diabetic mothers. Significant decreases in ionized calcium may occur during acute alkalosis and following exchange transfusions with citrated blood. Clinical signs suggestive of hypocalcemia in neonates include muscle twitching, jitteriness, generalized seizures, and QT_c above 0.40 second. Calcium chloride may be more bioavailable than calcium gluconate, but it also is more likely to cause metabolic acidosis. Administration by continuous infusion is more efficacious than intermittent bolus dosing due to less renal calcium loss.

Special Considerations/Preparation

| Salt | Formulation | Elemental Calcium | | Osmolarity |
		(mg/mL)	*(mEq/mL)*	*(mOsm/L)*
Calcium glubionate	6.5% syrup	23	1.16	2500
Calcium chloride	10% injection	27	1.36	2040
Calcium gluconate	10% injection	9.3	0.46	700

Injectable calcium salts should be stored at room temperature and are stable indefinitely.

continued...

VITAMINS & MINERALS

Calcium gluconate

Solution Compatibility: D_5W, $D_{10}W$, and NS.

Terminal Injection Site Compatibility: Dex/AA and fat emulsion. Amikacin, aminophylline, ampicillin, aztreonam, caffeine citrate, cefazolin, chloramphenicol, dobutamine, enalaprilat, epinephrine, famotidine, furosemide, heparin, hydrocortisone, isoproterenol, lidocaine, meropenem, methicillin, midazolam, netilmicin, penicillin G, phenobarbital, piperacillin-tazobactam, potassium chloride, propofol, remifentanil, tobramycin, tolazoline, and vancomycin.

Incompatibility: Amphotericin B, clindamycin, esmolol, fluconazole, indomethacin, methylprednisolone, metoclopramide, sodium bicarbonate, and phosphate and magnesium salts when mixed directly.

Calcium chloride

Solution compatibility: D_5W, $D_{10}W$, and NS.

Terminal Injection Site Compatibility: Dex/AA and fat emulsion. Amikacin, chloramphenicol, dobutamine, dopamine, epinephrine, esmolol, hydrocortisone, isoproterenol, lidocaine, methicillin, morphine, penicillin G, pentobarbital, phenobarbital, potassium chloride, and prostaglandin E_1.

Incompatibility: Amphotericin B, methylprednisolone, metoclopramide, sodium bicarbonate, and phosphate and magnesium salts when mixed directly.

Selected References

♦ Koo WWK, Tsang RC: Calcium and magnesium homeostasis. In: Avery GB, Fletcher MA, MacDonald MG (eds): *Neonatology: Pathophysiology and Management of the Newborn*, ed 5. Philadelphia: Lippincott Williams & Wilkins, 1999, pp 725-726.

♦ Porcelli PJ, Oh W: Effects of single dose calcium gluconate infusion in hypocalcemic preterm infants. *Am J Perinatol* 1995;12:18-21.

♦ Mimouni F, Tsang RC: Neonatal hypocalcemia: to treat or not to treat? (A review). *J Am Coll Nutr* 1994;13:408-15.

♦ Broner CW, Stidham GL, Westernkirchner DF, Watson DC: A prospective, randomized, double-blind comparison of calcium chloride and calcium gluconate therapies for hypocalcemia in critically ill children. *J Pediatr* 1990;117:986.

♦ Roberts RJ: *Drug Therapy in Infants*. Philadelphia: WB Saunders Co, 1984, p 294.

♦ Scott SM, Ladenson JH, Aguanna JJ, et al: Effect of calcium therapy in the sick premature infant with early neonatal hypocalcemia. *J Pediatr* 1984;104:747.

Compatibilities updated 3/2003

VITAMINS & MINERALS

Ferrous sulfate

Dose & Administration

2 mg/kg per day of elemental iron for growing premature infants.
(Maximum of 15 mg/day). Begin therapy after 2 weeks of age.
Infants with birthweights less than 1000 grams may need 4 mg/kg per day.
6 mg/kg per day of elemental iron for patients receiving erythropoietin.
Administer PO in 1 or 2 divided doses, preferably diluted in formula.

Uses

Iron supplementation for prevention and treatment of anemia.

Monitoring

Monitor hemoglobin and reticulocyte counts during therapy.
Observe stools, check for constipation.

Adverse Effects/Precautions

In growing premature infants, iron supplementation should not be started
until adequate vitamin E is supplied in the diet; otherwise, iron may increase
hemolysis. Nausea, constipation, black stools, lethargy, hypotension, and
erosion of gastric mucosa.

Pharmacology

Well absorbed from stomach.

Special Considerations/Preparation

Drops: Contain 15 mg elemental iron per 0.6 mL (0.02% alcohol).
Syrup: Contains 18 mg elemental iron per 5 mL (5% alcohol).
Elixir: Contains 44 mg elemental iron per 5 mL (some with 5% alcohol).

Selected References

♦ Rao R, Georgieff MK: Neonatal iron nutrition. *Semin Neonatol* 2001;6:425-435.

♦ Ehrenkranz RA: Iron, folic acid, and vitamin B$_{12}$. In: Tsang RC, Lucas A, Uauy R, Zlotkin S (eds): *Nutritional Needs of the Preterm Infant: Scientific Basis and Practical Guidelines*. Pauling, New York: Caduceus Medical Publishers, 1993, pp 177-187.

♦ Siimes MA, Järvenpää A-L: Prevention of anemia and iron deficiency in very low-birth-weight infants. *J Pediatr* 1982;101:277-280.

♦ Oski FA: Iron requirements of the premature infant, in Tsang R (ed): *Vitamin and Mineral Requirements in Preterm Infants*. New York: Marcel Dekker, 1985, p 18.

References updated 3/2003

VITAMINS & MINERALS

Dose and Administration

0.4 to 1 mg/kg (400 to 1000 mcg/kg) per day IV continuous infusion in Dex/AA solutions containing at least 2% amino acids.

Uses

Iron supplementation in patients unable to tolerate oral iron, especially those also being treated with erythropoietin.

Monitoring

Periodic CBC and reticulocyte count. Observe Dex/AA solution for rust-colored precipitates.

Adverse Effects/Precautions

No adverse effects have been observed in patients who have received low doses infused continuously. Large (50 mg) intramuscular doses administered to infants were associated with increased risk of infection. Retrospective reviews of adult patients who received larger doses injected over a few minutes report a 0.7% risk of immediate serious allergic reactions, and a 5% risk of delayed such as myalgia, arthralgia, phlebitis, and lymphadenopathy.

Pharmacology

Iron dextran for intravenous use is a complex of ferric hydroxide and low molecular mass dextran. The dextran serves as a protective lipophilic colloid. Radiolabeled iron dextran injected into adult subjects localized to the liver and spleen before being incorporated into RBC hemoglobin. Complete clearance occurred by 3 days. Approximately 40% of the labeled iron was bound to transferrin within 11 hours. The addition of iron dextran to Dex/AA solutions inhibits the spontaneous generation of peroxides.

Special Considerations/Preparation

Available as a 50 mg/mL concentration in 2-mL and 10-mL vials. Store at room temperature.

***Mix only in Dex/AA solutions containing at least 2% amino acids.**

Selected References

♦ Mayhew SL, Quick MW: Compatibility of iron dextran with neonatal parenteral nutrition solutions. *Am J Health-Syst Pharm* 1997;54:570-1.

♦ Lavoie J-C, Chessex P: Bound iron admixture prevents the spontaneous generation of peroxides in total parenteral nutrition solutions. *J Pediatr Gastroenterol Nutr* 1997;25:307-11.

♦ Friel JK, Andrews WL, Hall MS, et al: Intravenous iron administration to very-low-birth-weight newborns receiving total and partial parenteral nutrition. *JPEN* 1995;19:114-18.

♦ Burns DL, Mascioli EA, Bistrian BR: Parenteral iron dextran therapy: a review. *Nutrition* 1995;11:163-68.

♦ Kanakakorn K, Cavill I, Jacobs A: The metabolism of intravenously administered iron-dextran. *Br J Haematol* 1973;25:637-43.

Added 3/98

VITAMINS & MINERALS

Potassium chloride

Dose and Administration

Initial oral replacement therapy: 0.5 to 1 mEq/kg per day divided and administered with feedings (small, more frequent aliquots preferred). Adjust dosage based on monitoring of serum potassium concentrations.

$$1 \text{ g KCl} = 13.4 \text{ mEq K}^+ \qquad 1 \text{ mEq K}^+ = 74.6 \text{ mg KCl}$$

Acute treatment of symptomatic hypokalemia: Begin with 0.5 to 1 mEq/kg IV over 1 hour, then reassess. Maximum concentration: 40 mEq/L for peripheral, 80 mEq/L for central venous infusions.

Monitoring

Continuous EKG monitoring is mandatory if administering by the IV route, especially for central infusions. Observe IV site closely for signs of extravasation when using concentrated solutions. Monitor serum potassium concentration. Assess for GI intolerance.

Adverse Effects/Precautions

Rapid IV infusions, especially those through central lines, may cause arrhythmias including heart block and cardiac arrest. Peripheral IV administration of concentrated potassium solutions is associated with thrombophlebitis and pain at the injection site. GI irritation is common—most commonly diarrhea, vomiting, and bleeding— minimized by dividing oral doses and administering with feedings. Use with caution (if at all) in patients receiving potassium-sparing diuretics, e.g. spironolactone.

Pharmacology

Potassium is the major intracellular cation. Hypokalemia in critically ill neonates is usually the result of diuretic (furosemide, thiazides) therapy or diarrhea. Other causes include congenital adrenal hyperplasia and renal disorders. Alkalosis, as well as insulin infusions, will lower serum potassium concentrations by driving the ion intracellularly. Symptoms of hypokalemia include neuromuscular weakness and paralysis, ileus, urine retention, and EKG changes (ST segment depression, low-voltage T wave, and appearance of U wave). Hypokalemia increases digitalis toxicity. Oral potassium preparations are completely absorbed.

Special Considerations/Preparation

Potassium chloride for injection is supplied as 2-mEq/mL solution (equals 2000 mEq/L). **Always dilute before administration.** Hyperosmolar - 4355 mOsm/kg determined by freezing-point depression. pH ranges from 4 to 8 depending on buffering. Various oral solutions are available, with concentrations ranging from 10 to 40 mEq per 15 mL. Other oral forms available include powder packets, tablets, and sustained-release capsules.

Terminal injection site compatibility: Most drugs.

Incompatibility: Amphotericin B, diazepam, and phenytoin.

Selected References

♦ Satlin LM, Schwartz GJ: Disorders of potassium metabolism, in Ichikawa I (ed): *Pediatric Textbook of Fluids and Electrolytes.* Baltimore: Williams & Wilkins, 1990, p 227.
♦ Morgan BC: Rapidly infused potassium chloride therapy in a child. *JAMA* 1981;245:2446.
♦ DeFronzo RA, Bia M: Intravenous potassium chloride therapy. *JAMA* 1981;245:2446.

Updated 3/97

VITAMINS & MINERALS

Dose and Administration

Initial diagnostic dose: 50 to 100 mg IV push, or IM.

Maintenance dose: 50 to 100 mg PO Q24 hours. High doses may be required during periods of intercurrent illness.

Uses

Diagnosis and treatment of pyridoxine-dependent seizures.

Monitoring

When possible, initial administration of pyridoxine should be accompanied by EEG monitoring.

Adverse Effects/Precautions

Risk of profound sedation. Ventilator support may be necessary.

Pharmacology

Pyridoxine-dependent seizures are a result of defective binding of pyridoxine in the formation of GABA (an inhibitory neurotransmitter). Administration of pharmacologic doses of pyridoxine will correct this GABA deficiency.

Special Considerations/Preparation

Injectable form available in concentration of 100 mg/mL in 10- and 30-mL vials. May use injectable form orally; mix in simple syrup if desired. **Protect from light.**

Solution incompatibility: Alkaline solutions. No data are currently available on Dex/AA.

Terminal injection site compatibilities: Fat emulsion.

Incompatibility: Iron salts and oxidizing agents. No data are currently available on heparin and potassium chloride.

Selected References

♦ Gospe SM: Current perspectives on pyridoxine-dependent seizures. *J Pediatr* 1998;132:919-923.

♦ Gordon N: Pyridoxine dependency: An update. *Dev Med Child Neurol* 1997;39:63.

♦ Mikati MA, Trevathan E, Krishnamoorthy KS, Lombroso CT: Pyridoxine-dependent epilepsy: Investigations and long-term followup. *Electroencephalogr Clin Neurophysiol* 1991;78:215

♦ Kroll JS: Pyridoxine for neonatal seizures: An unexpected danger. *Dev Med Child Neurol* 1985;27:369.

♦ Bankier A, Turner M, Hopkins IJ: Pyridoxine-dependent seizures: A wider clinical spectrum. *Arch Dis Child* 1983;58:415.

Updated 3/99
Compatibilities updated 3/99

VITAMINS & MINERALS

Vitamin A

(Retinyl Palmitate)

Dose and Administration

Parenteral treatment of Vitamin A deficiency: 5000 IU IM 3 times weekly for 4 weeks.

Administer using 29-g needle and insulin syringe.

DO NOT ADMINISTER IV.

Uses

To reduce the risk of Chronic Lung Disease in high risk premature neonates with Vitamin A deficiency. In the NICHD-sponsored trial, 14 infants needed to be treated to prevent 1 case of Chronic Lung Disease.

Monitoring

Assess regularly for signs of toxicity: full fontanel, lethargy, irritability, hepatomegaly, edema, mucocutaneous lesions, and bony tenderness. Consider measuring plasma retinol concentrations if available, especially if patient is also receiving glucocorticoid therapy. Desired concentrations are approximately 30 to 60 mcg/dL.

Concentrations < 20 mcg/dL indicate deficiency, while those > 100 mcg/dL are potentially toxic.

Adverse Effects/Precautions

See monitoring section. Coincident treatment with glucocorticoids should be avoided, as it significantly raises plasma vitamin A concentrations.

Pharmacology

The pulmonary histopathologic changes of BPD and Vitamin A deficiency are remarkably similar. Vitamin A is the generic name for a group of fat soluble compounds which have the biological activity of the primary alcohol, retinol. Retinol metabolites exhibit potent and site-specific effects on gene expression and on lung growth and development. Retinol is supplied in the diet as retinyl esters.

Special Considerations/Preparation

Available as Aquasol A® Parenteral (water-miscible vitamin A palmitate) (AstraZeneca), 50,000 IU per mL, equivalent to 15 mg retinol per mL, in 2 mL vials.

Protect from light. Store refrigerated at 36 to 46°F (2 to 8°C). Do not freeze.

Selected References

♦ Tyson JE, Wright LL, Oh W, Kennedy K, et al: Vitamin A supplementation for extremely-low-birth-weight infants. *New Engl J Med* 1999;340:1962-68.

♦ Darlow BA, Graham PJ: Vitamin A supplementation for preventing morbidity and mortality in very low birthweight infants (Cochrane Review). In: *The Cochrane Library* 4, 1999. Oxford: Update Software.

♦ Shenai JP: Vitamin A supplementation in very low birthweight neonates: rationale and evidence. *Pediatrics* 1999;104:1369-74.

♦ Product information, AstraZeneca, 2002.

Added 3/2000
References updated: 3/2002

(dl-alpha-tocopherol acetate)

Dose and Administration

5 to 25 IU per day PO. Dilute with feedings. Do not administer simultaneously with iron—iron absorption is impaired.

Uses

Prevention of vitamin E deficiency. May be indicated in babies receiving erythropoietin and high iron dosages. Higher doses used to reduce oxidant-induced injury (ROP, BPD, IVH) remain controversial.

Monitoring

Assess feeding tolerance. Signs of vitamin E deficiency include hemolytic anemia and thrombocytosis. Physiologic serum vitamin E concentrations are between 0.8 and 3.5 mg/dL.

Adverse Effects/Precautions

Feeding intolerance may occur due to hyperosmolarity of preparation. Pharmacologic doses of alpha tocopherol have been associated with increased rates of sepsis (antioxidant effect of drug) and NEC (? osmolarity of oral formulation).

Pharmacology

Alpha-tocopherol is the most active antioxidant of the group of tocopherols known as Vitamin E. The amount required by the body is primarily dependent upon the dietary intake of fat, especially polyunsaturated fatty acids (PUFA). Human milk and currently available infant formulas contain adequate Vitamin E and have appropriate E:PUFA ratios to prevent hemolytic anemia. Infants receiving supplemental iron amounts above 2 mg/kg/day may also require additional Vitamin E. Oral absorption of vitamin E is dependent upon hydrolysis that requires bile salts and pancreatic esterases. This can be quite variable in very immature infants and those with fat malabsorption. Free tocopherol is absorbed in the small intestine, taken via chylomicrons into the gastrointestinal lymphatics, then carried via low-density lipoproteins to be incorporated into cell membranes. Significant tissue accumulation may occur with pharmacologic doses.

Special Considerations/Preparation

Available as liquid drops: Aquasol E® (AstraZeneca) and Aquavit E® (Cypress Pharmaceutical), 15 IU (=15 mg) per 0.3 mL. Water solubilized with polysorbate 80. Also contains propylene glycol. Hyperosmolar (3620 mOsm/kg H2O). Store at controlled room temperature.

Selected References

♦ Gross SJ: Vitamin E. In Tsang RC, Lucas A, Uauy R, Zlotkin S (eds): *Nutritional Needs of the Preterm Infant: Scientific Basis and Practical Guidelines.* Pauling, New York: Caduceus Medical Publishers, 1993, pp 101-109.

♦ Roberts RJ, Knight ME: Pharmacology of vitamin E in the newborn. *Clin Perinatol* 1987;14:843-855.

♦ Raju TNK, Langenberg P, Bhutani V, Quinn GE: Vitamin E prophylaxis to reduce retinopathy of prematurity: A reappraisal of published trials. *J Pediatr* 1997;131:844-850.

Added 3/2001

Dose and Administration

Recommended Prophylaxis: 0.5 to 1 mg IM at birth.

Preterm infants with BW < 1000 grams: 0.3 mg IM.

Alternate strategy for healthy, term, exclusively breast-fed infants:
2 mg PO with the first feed, at 1 week, 4 weeks, and 8 weeks of age.
***Note:** there is no approved oral formulation in the United States.

Oral prophylaxis is contraindicated in infants who are premature, ill, on antibiotics, have cholestasis, or have diarrhea. There has been an increased number of cases of hemorrhagic disease of the newborn in countries that have changed to oral prophylaxis, primarily in patients who received only a single oral dose.

Also: Maternal daily intake of 5 mg/day of phylloquinone significantly increases Vitamin K concentrations in breastmilk and infant plasma.

Treatment of severe hemorrhagic disease: 1 to 10 mg IV slow push. (See Adverse Effects/Precautions for rate of administration.)

Uses

Prophylaxis and therapy of hemorrhagic disease of the newborn. Treatment of hypoprothrombinemia secondary to factors limiting absorption or synthesis of vitamin K$_1$.

Monitoring

Check prothrombin time when treating clotting abnormalities. (A minimum of 2 to 4 hours is needed for measurable improvement.)

Adverse Effects/Precautions

Severe reactions, including death, have been reported with IV administration in adults. These reactions have resembled anaphylaxis and included shock and cardiac/respiratory arrest.
With IV administration, give very slowly, not exceeding 1 mg per minute, with physician present.
Pain and swelling may occur at IM injection site. Efficacy of treatment with vitamin K$_1$ is decreased in patients with liver disease. The risk of childhood cancer is not increased by IM administration of vitamin K$_1$.

Note: A new (May 2001) box warning statement in the AquaMEPHYTON® product information states that intramuscular administration "should be restricted to those situations where the subcutaneous route is not feasible and the serious risk is considered justified". However, this does not apply to newborns, and the American Academy of Pediatrics recommends the single intramuscular dose at birth as above. The product information labeling will likely be modified again in the near future to better reflect recommended newborn dosing.

Pharmacology

Vitamin K$_1$ (phytonadione) promotes formation of the following clotting factors in the liver: active prothrombin (factor II), proconvertin (factor VII), plasma thromboplastin component (factor IX), and Stuart factor (factor X). Vitamin K$_1$ does **not** counteract the anticoagulant action of heparin.

continued...

Special Considerations/Preparation

Available as a 2 mg/mL aqueous dispersion in 0.5-mL ampules and 10 mg/mL aqueous dispersion in 1-mL ampules and 2.5- and 5-mL vials. Contains 0.9% (9 mg/mL) benzyl alcohol as a preservative.

*** Efficacy with giving this preparation orally is uncertain. ***

Protect from light.

Solution compatibility: D_5W, $D_{10}W$, and NS.

Terminal injection site compatibility: Dex/AA. Amikacin, ampicillin, dobutamine, chloramphenicol, cimetidine, epinephrine, famotidine, heparin, hydrocortisone succinate, netilmicin, potassium chloride, ranitidine, sodium bicarbonate, and tolazoline.

Incompatibility: Phenytoin.

Selected References

♦ Product information, Merck & Co, Inc: *Physicians' Desk Reference,* ed 56. Montvale, NJ: Thomson PDR, 2003, p1944.

♦ Kumar D, Greer FR, Super DM, et al: Vitamin K status of premature infants: implications for current recommendations. *Pediatrics* 2001;108:1117-1122.

♦ Zipursky AL: Prevention of vitamin K deficiency bleeding in newborns. *Br J Haematol* 1999;104:430-437.

♦ American Academy of Pediatrics Committee on Nutrition: Nutritional needs of preterm infants. In: *Pediatric Nutrition Handbook.* 4th ed. Elk Grove Village, Il: American Academy of Pediatrics 1998: pp 55-87.

♦ Brousson MA, Klein MC: Controversies surrounding the administration of vitamin K to newborns: a review. *Can Med Assoc J* 1996;154:307.

♦ Greer FR: Vitamin K deficiency and hemorrhage in infancy. *Clin Perinatol* 1995;22:759.

♦ Thorp JA, Gaston L, Caspers DR, Pal ML: Current concepts and controversies in the use of vitamin K. *Drugs* 1995;49:376.

♦ Huysman MWA, Sauer PJJ: The vitamin K controversy. *Curr Opin Pediatr* 1994;6:129.

♦ American Academy of Pediatrics, Vitamin K Ad Hoc Task Force: Controversies concerning vitamin K and the newborn. *Pediatrics* 1993;91:1001.

♦ Greer FR, Marshall SP, Foley AL, Suttie JW: Improving the vitamin K status of breast-feeding infants with maternal vitamin K supplements. *Pediatrics* 1997;99:88.

Compatibilities updated 3/2001
Updated 3/2002

Dose and Administration

1 dropperful (1 mL) Q24 hours, or as directed by physician. Percentages of the Reference Daily Intakes (%RDIs) listed in the table below are for infants.

	Vi-Daylin® ADC Vitamin Drops		Vi-Daylin® ADC Vitamins + Iron Drops		Vi-Daylin® Multivitamin Drops		Vi-Daylin® Multivitamin + Iron Drops	
	Amt	%RDI	Amt	%RDI	Amt	%RDI	Amt	%RDI
Vitamins								
A (IU)	1350	90	1350	90	1350	90	1350	90
D (IU)	400	100	400	100	360	90	360	90
C (mg)	32	90	32	90	32	90	32	90
E (IU)					5	90	5	90
Thiamine (B_1) (mg)					0.4	80	0.5	89
Riboflavin (B_2) (mg)					0.5	90	0.5	90
Niacin (mg)					7	90	7	90
B_6 (mg)					0.4	90	0.4	90
B_{12} (mcg)					1.4	68		
Minerals								
Iron (mg)			9	60			9	60

Dose and Administration

1 dropperful (1 mL) Q24 hours, or as directed by physician. Percentages of the Reference Daily Intakes (%RDIs) listed in the table below are for infants.

	Tri-Vi-Sol® Multivitamin Drops		Tri-Vi-Sol® Multivitamin with Iron Drops		Poly-Vi-Sol® Multivitamin Drops		Poly-Vi-Sol® Multivitamin with Iron Drops	
	Amt	%RDI	Amt	%RDI	Amt	%RDI	Amt	%RDI
Vitamins								
A (IU)	1500	100	1500	100	1500	100	1500	100
D (IU)	400	100	400	100	400	100	400	100
C (mg)	35	100	35	100	35	100	35	100
E (IU)					5	100	5	100
Thiamine (B_1) (mg)					0.5	100	0.5	100
Riboflavin (B_2) (mg)					0.6	100	0.6	100
Niacin (mg)					8	100	8	100
B_6 (mg)					0.4	100	0.4	100
B_{12} (mcg)					2	100		
Minerals								
Iron (mg)			10	67			10	67

INFUVITE™ *Pediatric*, Multiple Vitamins for Infusion.
Dose and Administration

IV administration: Infuvite™ *Pediatric* is a sterile product consisting of two vials: a 4 mL vial labeled **Vial 1** and a 1 mL vial labeled **Vial 2**. The daily dose is a function of infant weight as indicated in the following table. **Do not exceed this daily dose.**

Weight of Infant

	<1 kg	≥ 1 kg and < 3 kg	≥ 3 kg
Vial 1	1.2 mL	2.6 mL	4 mL
Vial 2	0.3 mL	0.65 mL	1 mL

INFUVITE™ *Pediatric*

Vial 1 (4 mL)	Amt*	
Vitamin A** (as palmitate)	2300	(equals 0.7 mg)
Vitamin D** (IU) (cholecalciferol)	400	IU (equals 10 mcg)
Ascorbic Acid (vitamin C)	80	mg
Vitamin E** (dl-alpha tocopheryl acetate)	7	IU (equals 7 mg)
Thiamine (as hydrochloride) B_1	1.2	mg
Riboflavin (as phosphate) B_2	1.4	mg
Niacinamide B_3	17	mg
Pyridoxine hydrochloride B_6	1	mg
d-Panthenol	5	mg
Vitamin K_1**	0.2	mg

Vial 2 (1 mL)		
Biotin	20	mcg
Folic Acid	140	mcg
Vitamin B_{12} (cyanocobalamin)	1	mcg

* Amounts based upon guidelines published by the American Medical Association Department of Foods and Nutrition, *JPEN* 3(4);258-62:1979.

Vial 1 (4 mL) Inactive ingredients: 50 mg polysorbate 80, sodium hydroxide and/or hydrochloric acid for pH adjustment and water for injection.

** Polysorbate 80 is used to water solubilize the oil-soluble vitamins A, D, E, and K.

Vial 2 (1 mL) Inactive ingredients: 75 mg mannitol, citric acid and/or sodium citrate for pH adjustment and water for injection.

continued...

Adverse Effects/Precautions

Warnings: INFUVITE™ *Pediatric* is administered in intravenous solutions, which may contain aluminum that may be toxic. Aluminum may reach toxic levels with prolonged parenteral administration if kidney function is impaired. Premature neonates are particularly at risk because their kidneys are immature, and they require large amounts of calcium and phosphate solution, which contain aluminum.

Research indicates that patients with impaired kidney function, including premature neonates who receive parenteral levels of aluminum at greater than 4 to 5 mcg/kg per day accumulate aluminum at levels associated with central nervous system and bone toxicity. Tissue loading may occur at even lower rates of administration.

Special Considerations/Preparation

After INFUVITE™ *Pediatric* is diluted in an intravenous infusion, the resulting solution is ready for immediate use. Inspect visually for particulate matter and discoloration prior to administration, whenever solution and container permit. Exposure to light should be minimized. Discard any unused portion. **Store between 2-8°C (36-46°F).**

Incompatibility: Alkaline solutions or moderately alkaline drugs: acetazolamide, aminophylline, ampicillin, and chlorothiazide.

Direct addition to intravenous fat emulsions is not recommended.

Selected References

Product Information, Baxter Clinitec 2001

Added 3/2002

NUTRITIONALS

The following information, although accurate at the time of publication, is subject to change. The most current information may be obtained by referring to product packaging.

Potential renal solute load is estimated as follows:

$$[\text{Protein (g)} \times 5.714] + [\text{Na(mOsm)} + \text{K(mOsm)} + \text{Cl(mOsm)} + \text{P(mOsm)}]$$

Dilution Tables

To reconstitute standard infant formulas (Similac®, Similac® Advance®, Similac® Lactose Free, Similac® PM 60/40, Alimentum® Powder, Enfamil®, Enfamil® Lipil®, LactoFree®, Isomil® Advance®, ProSobee®, Nutramigen®, and Pregestimil®) from Powder:

Dilution	Water (fl oz)	Level Unpacked Scoopful	Approximate Yield (fl oz)
13 Cal/fl oz	6.5	2	7
20 Cal/fl oz (Standard mixture)	2	1	2
24 Cal/fl oz	5	3	6
27 Cal/fl oz	4.25	3	5

To reconstitute Similac NeoSure® Advance® Powder and Enfamil® EnfaCare® Lipil®:

Dilution	Water (fl oz)	Level Unpacked Scoopful	Approximate Yield (fl oz)
20 Cal/fl oz	4.5	2	5
22 Cal/fl oz (Standard mixture)	2	1	2
24 Cal/fl oz	5.5	3	6.5
27 Cal/fl oz	8	5	9

To reconstitute Similac®, Similac® Lactose Free, Enfamil®, Isomil®, Isomil® Advance®, LactoFree®, ProSobee®, and Nutramigen® Concentrated Liquid:

Dilution	Water (fl oz)	Concentrated Liquid (fl oz)	Approximate Yield (fl oz)
13 Cal/fl oz	2	1	3
20 Cal/fl oz (Standard mixture)	1	1	2
24 Cal/fl oz	2	3	5
27 Cal/fl oz	1	2	3

Nutrient per Liter	Term*	Preterm
Energy, Cal	699	671
Protein, g	9.09	14.09
% of total calories [†]	5	8
Fat, g	41.96	38.93
% of total calories [††]	54	52
Linoleic acid, mg	3021	3691
Carbohydrate, g	72.7	66.4
% of total calories [§]	42	40
Water, g	881	879
Minerals		
Calcium, mg (mEq)	280 (14.0)	248 (12.4)
Phosphorus, mg	147	128
Magnesium, mg	30.1	30.9
Iron, mg	0.42	1.21
Zinc, mg	1.19	3.42
Manganese, mcg	6	6
Copper, mcg	252	644
Iodine, mcg	112	107
Selenium, mcg	20.3	20.1
Sodium, mg (mEq)	182 (7.9)	248 (10.8)
Potassium, mg (mEq)	580 (14.8)	570 (14.6)
Chloride, mg (mEq)	420 (11.8)	550 (15.5)
Vitamins		
Vitamin A, IU	2231	3899
Vitamin D, IU	21	20
Vitamin E, IU	2.8	10.7
Vitamin K, mcg	2.1	2.0
Thiamine (B_1), mcg	210	208
Riboflavin (B_2), mcg	350	483
Vitamin B_6, mcg	930	148
Vitamin B_{12}, mcg	0.28	0.47
Niacin, mcg	1497	1503
Folic acid (Folacin), mcg	85	33
Pantothenic acid, mcg	1797	1805
Biotin, mcg	6.3	6.0
Vitamin C (Ascorbic acid), mg	40	110
Choline, mg	92	92
Inositol, mg	149	149
Renal Solute Load, mOsm	91.3	125.6
Osmolality, mOsm/kg water	286	290

* American Academy of Pediatrics Committee on Nutrition: *Pediatric Nutrition Handbook*, 4th ed. Elk Grove Village: American Academy of Pediatrics, 1998:655-658, 258, 217.

[†] Protein Source: Mother's milk

[††] Fat Source: Mother's milk

[§] Carbohydrate Source: Lactose

NUTRITIONALS

Preterm Human Milk + Similac® Human Milk Fortifier

Nutrient per Liter	1 pk/50 mL	1 pk/25 mL
Energy, Cal	731	789
Volume, mL	1000	1000
Protein, g	18.8	23.5
% of total calories [†]	10	12
Fat, g	40.2	41.4
% of total calories [††]	49	47
Linoleic acid, mg	3642	3594
Carbohydrate, g	74.4	82.2
% of total calories [§]	41	42
Water, g	867	856
Minerals		
Calcium, mg (mEq)	822 (41.0)	1381 (68.9)
Phosphorus, mg	456	777
Magnesium, mg	65.0	98.2
Iron, mg	2.92	4.58
Zinc, mg	8.31	13.07
Manganese, mcg	41	76
Copper, mcg	1474	2283
Iodine, mcg	106	105
Selenium, mcg	17	19.2
Sodium, mg (mEq)	319 (13.9)	388 (16.9)
Potassium, mg (mEq)	874 (22.3)	1169 (29.9)
Chloride, mg (mEq)	730 (20.6)	906 (25.5)
Vitamins		
Vitamin A, IU	6906	9834
Vitamin D, IU	612	1188
Vitamin E, IU	26.4	41.6
Vitamin K, mcg	42.9	82.8
Thiamine (B_1), mcg	1355	2471
Riboflavin (B_2), mcg	2534	4531
Vitamin B_6, mcg	1187	2198
Vitamin B_{12}, mcg	3.62	6.69
Niacin, mcg	19096	36225
Folic acid (Folacin), mcg	146	256
Pantothenic acid, mcg	9181	16354
Biotin, mcg	132.2	257.1
Vitamin C (Ascorbic acid), mg	229	348
Choline, mg	102	109
Inositol, mg	165	181
Renal Solute Load, mOsm	179.1	231.3
Osmolality, mOsm/kg water	343	385

[†] Protein Source: Preterm human milk/whey protein concentrate, nonfat milk

[††] Fat Source: Preterm human milk and MCT oil

[§] Carbohydrate Source: Lactose and corn syrup solids

Preterm Human Milk + Enfamil® Human Milk Fortifier

Nutrient per Liter	1 pk/50 mL	1 pk/25 mL
Energy, Cal	730	788
Volume, mL	1000	1000
Protein, g	22	27
% of total calories †	11.4	13.2
Fat, g	38	42
% of total calories ††	48	50
Linoleic acid, mg	2980	2939
Carbohydrate, g	78	84
% of total calories §	43	42.5
Water, g	867	855
Minerals		
Calcium, mg (mEq)	710 (35.4)	1150 (57.4)
Phosphorus, mg	370	600
Magnesium, mg	38	43
Iron, mg	8.1	15.3
Zinc, mg	7.3	10.9
Manganese, mcg	53.6	104
Copper, mcg	600	820
Iodine, mcg	190	200
Selenium, mcg	25	26
Sodium, mg (mEq)	340 (14.8)	390 (16.9)
Potassium, mg (mEq)	600 (15.3)	700 (17.9)
Chloride, mg (mEq)	630 (17.8)	670 (18.9)
Vitamins		
Vitamin A, IU	5280	10000
Vitamin D, IU	840	1580
Vitamin E, IU	30	50
Vitamin K, mcg	42	64
Thiamine (B$_1$), mcg	850	1600
Riboflavin (B$_2$), mcg	1400	2500
Vitamin B$_6$, mcg	640	1210
Vitamin B$_{12}$, mcg	1	2
Niacin, mcg	17100	32000
Folic acid (Folacin), mcg	150	280
Pantothenic acid, mcg	5960	9600
Biotin, mcg	19	32
Vitamin C (Ascorbic acid), mg	104	164
Carnitine, mg	114	156
Renal Solute Load, mOsm	182	230
Osmolality, mOsm/kg water	350	350
Osmolarity, mOsm/L	303	350

† Protein Source: Mature preterm human milk/whey protein concentrate/sodium caseinate

†† Fat Source: Lactose and corn syrup solids

§ Carbohydrate Source: Lactose

Similac® Human Milk Fortifier

Nutrient	per 1 packet	per 4 packets
Energy, Cal	3.5	14
Protein, g	0.25	1.0
Fat, g	0.09	0.36
Carbohydrate, g	0.45	1.8
Minerals		
Calcium, mg	29.25	117
Phosphorus, mg	16.8	67
Magnesium, mg	1.75	7.0
Iron, mg	0.08*	0.35*
Zinc, mg	0.26	1.0
Manganese, mcg	1.8	7.2
Copper, mcg	42.5	170
Iodine, mcg		
Selenium, mcg	0.12	0.48
Sodium, mg (mEq)	3.75 (0.2)	15 (0.68)
Potassium, mg (mEq)	15.75 (0.41)	63 (1.6)
Chloride, mg (mEq)	9.5 (0.26)	38 (1.07)
Vitamins		
Vitamin A, IU	155	620
Vitamin D, IU	30	120
Vitamin E, IU	0.8	3.2
Vitamin K, mcg	2.07	8.3
Thiamine (B_1), mcg	58.3	233
Riboflavin (B_2), mcg	104	417
Vitamin B_6, mcg	53	211
Vitamin B_{12}, mcg	0.16	0.64
Niacin, mcg	893	3570
Folic acid (Folacin), mcg	5.75	23
Pantothenic acid, mcg	375	1500
Biotin, mcg	6.6	26
Vitamin C (Ascorbic acid), mg	6.3	25
Choline, mg	0.45	1.8
Inositol, mg	0.96	3.84
Renal Solute Load, mOsm	1.8	7.3

* Additional iron should be supplied from other sources.

Enfamil® Human Milk Fortifier

Nutrient	per 1 pk	per 4 pks
Energy, Cal	3.5	14
Protein, g	0.28	1.1
Fat, g	0.26	1
Carbohydrate, g	0.06	<0.4
Minerals		
Calcium, mg	23	90
Phosphorus, mg	12.5	50
Magnesium, mg	0.25	1
Iron, mg	0.36*	1.44*
Zinc, mg	0.18	0.72
Manganese, mcg	2.5	10
Copper, mcg	11	44
Iodine, mcg	0	0
Selenium, mcg	0	0
Sodium, mg (mEq)	4 (0.17)	16 (0.7)
Potassium, mg (mEq)	7.3 (0.19)	29 (0.74)
Chloride, mg (mEq)	3.3 (0.09)	13 (0.37)
Vitamins		
Vitamin A, IU	240	950
Vitamin D, IU	38	150
Vitamin E, IU	1.15	4.6
Vitamin K, mcg	1.1	4.4
Thiamine (B_1), mcg	38	150
Riboflavin (B_2), mcg	55	220
Vitamin B_6, mcg	29	115
Vitamin B_{12}, mcg	0.05	0.18
Niacin, mcg	750	3000
Folic acid (Folacin), mcg	6.3	25
Pantothenic acid, mcg	183	730
Biotin, mcg	0.68	2.7
Vitamin C (Ascorbic acid), mg	3	12
Carnitine, mg	0	0

* Additional iron should be supplied from other sources.

Term Human Milk + Similac NeoSure® Advance® Powder

Term Milk + Similac NeoSure® Advance® Powder*

Nutrient per 100 mL	22 Cal/fl oz	24 Cal/fl oz	27 Cal/fl oz
Energy, Cal	76	83	93
Protein, g	1.27	1.45	1.73
% of total calories [†]	6.7	7	7.4
Fat, g	4.33	4.7	5.27
% of total calories [††]	51.4	51.2	51
Linoleic acid, mg	120	175	567
Carbohydrate, g	8.01	8.69	9.77
% of total calories [§]	42.2	42.1	42
Water, g	87	86	87
Minerals			
Calcium, mg	37	44	56
Phosphorus, mg	19	24	31
Magnesium, mg	4.2	4.9	5.9
Iron, mg	0.19	0.32	0.53
Zinc, mg	0.22	0.31	0.45
Manganese, mcg	1	2	3
Copper, mcg	35	44	57
Iodine, mcg	12	13	15
Selenium, mcg	1.7	1.8	2.1
Sodium, mg	21	23	26
Potassium, mg	65	74	90
Chloride, mg	48	53	61
Vitamins			
Vitamin A, IU	263	294	344
Vitamin D, IU	8	13	21
Vitamin E, IU	0.7	1	1.4
Vitamin K, mcg	1.2	2	3.3
Thiamine (B_1), mcg	40	56	81
Riboflavin (B_2), mcg	48	58	75
Vitamin B_6, mcg	29	36	47
Vitamin B_{12}, mcg	0.08	0.11	0.16
Niacin, mcg	320	461	685
Folic acid (Folacin), mcg	7.1	8.9	11.7
Pantothenic acid, mcg	248	305	395
Biotin, mcg	1.2	1.8	2.9
Vitamin C (Ascorbic acid), mg	5	6	8
Choline, mg	10	12	13
Inositol, mg	15	16	16
Renal Solute Load, mOsm	9	10.2	12.1
Osmolality, mOsm/kg water	-	-	-

* Nutrient needs of small premature infants may not be met by this fortification strategy. Compare nutrient profile to fortification with Similac Human Milk Fortifier.

† Protein Source: Term human milk, nonfat milk and whey protein concentrate

†† Fat Source: High-oleic sunflower, soy, MCT, coconut, and C.cohnii[1] and M. alpina[2] oils

[1] A source of docosahexaenoic acid (DHA).

[2] A source of arachidonic acid (ARA).

§ Carbohydrate Source: Lactose, maltodextrin

Preparation

22 Calorie = 1 tsp level powder + 130 mL Term Human Milk

24 Calorie = 1 tsp level powder + 70 mL Term Human Milk

27 Calorie = 1 tsp level powder + 40 mL Term Human Milk

Term Human Milk + EnfaCare® Powder

Nutrient	22 Cal/fl oz	24 Cal/fl oz	27 Cal/fl oz
Energy, Cal	74	81	91
Volume, mL	100	100	100
Protein, g	1.22	1.41	1.69
% of total calories [†]	7	7	7
Fat, g	4.2	4.6	5.1
% of total calories [††]	-	-	-
Linoleic acid, mg			
Carbohydrate, g	7.8	8.6	9.7
% of total calories [§]	-	-	-
Water, g	-	-	-
Minerals			
Calcium, mg (mEq)	35	44	56
Phosphorus, mg	18	23	29
Magnesium, mg	4	4.5	5.3
Iron, mg	0.14	0.26	0.44
Zinc, mg	0.2	0.28	0.41
Manganese, mcg	1.5	2.6	4.1
Copper, mcg	32	41	53
Iodine, mcg	11.9	13	14.5
Selenium, mcg	0	0	26
Sodium, mg (mEq)	20	23	77
Potassium, mg (mEq)	59	66	60
Chloride, mg (mEq)	47	52	
Vitamins			
Vitamin A, IU	250	280	330
Vitamin D, IU	7	12.6	21
Vitamin E, IU	0.55	0.83	1.23
Vitamin K, mcg	0.69	1.25	2.1
Thiamine (B$_1$), mcg	33	47	67
Riboflavin (B$_2$), mcg	47	61	81
Vitamin B$_6$, mcg	27	34	44
Vitamin B$_{12}$, mcg	0.07	0.09	0.12
Niacin, mcg	270	410	610
Folic acid (Folacin), mcg	6.6	8.4	11
Pantothenic acid, mcg	230	290	380
Biotin, mcg	0.76	1.18	1.78
Vitamin C (Ascorbic acid), mg	5	6.1	7.7
Choline, mg	-	-	-
Inositol, mg	-	-	-
Renal Solute Load, mOsm	-	-	-
Osmolality, mOsm/kg water	-	-	-
Osmolarity, mOsm/L	-	-	-

† Protein Source: Mature preterm human milk, nonfat milk and whey protein concentrate

†† Fat Source: High-oleic sunflower, soy, MCT, and coconut oils

§ Carbohydrate Source: Lactose, corn syrup solids

Preparation

22 Calorie = 1/4 tsp packed powder + 45 mL Human Milk
24 Calorie = 1/2 tsp packed powder + 45 mL Human Milk
27 Calorie = 1 tsp packed powder + 45 mL Human Milk

NUTRITIONALS

Preterm Human Milk +
Similac Natural Care® Advance®

Nutrient per Liter	75:25 ratio	50:50 ratio
Energy, Cal	706	741
Volume, mL	1000	1000
Protein, g	16.07	18.04
% of total calories [†]	9	10
Fat, g	40.21	41.5
% of total calories [††]	51	50
Linoleic acid, mg	4189	4686
Carbohydrate, g	71.3	76
% of total calories [§]	40	41
Water, g	881	882
Minerals		
Calcium, mg (mEq)	612 (30.4)	971 (48.4)
Phosphorus, mg	331	539
Magnesium, mg	47.5	64.1
Iron, mg	1.66*	2.11*
Zinc, mg	5.61	7.76
Manganese, mcg	29	52
Copper, mcg	990	1337
Iodine, mcg	93	78
Selenium, mcg	14.7	14.6
Sodium, mg (mEq)	273 (11.9)	299 (12.9)
Potassium, mg (mEq)	690 (17.6)	809 (20.6)
Chloride, mg (mEq)	577 (16.2)	604 (17.0)
Vitamins		
Vitamin A, IU	5461	7022
Vitamin D, IU	319	619
Vitamin E, IU	16.2	21.6
Vitamin K, mcg	26	50
Thiamine (B_1), mcg	663	1118
Riboflavin (B_2), mcg	1620	2757
Vitamin B_6, mcg	618	1088
Vitamin B_{12}, mcg	1.47	2.47
Niacin, mcg	11272	21041
Folic acid (Folacin), mcg	100	166
Pantothenic acid, mcg	5209	8612
Biotin, mcg	78.1	152.2
Vitamin C (Ascorbic acid), mg	156	204
Choline, mg	91	88
Inositol, mg	122	96
Renal Solute Load, mOsm	148	170.4
Osmolality, mOsm/kg water	288	285

* Additional iron should be supplied from other sources as necessary.

† Protein Source: Preterm human milk, nonfat milk and whey protein concentrate

†† Fat Source: Preterm human milk, medium-chain triglycerides, soy, coconut oils, and, C. cohnii[1] and M. alpina oils[2]

[1] A source of docosahexaenoic acid (DHA).

[2] A source of arachidonic acid (ARA).

§ Carbohydrate Source: Lactose, corn syrup solids

Similac Natural Care® Advance® Low Iron Human Milk Fortifier*
24 Cal/fl oz

Nutrient	per 100 Cal	per Liter
Energy, Cal	100	812
Volume, mL	124	1000
Protein, g	2.71	21.99
% of total calories [†]	11	11
Fat, g	5.43	44.07
% of total calories [††]	47	47
Linoleic acid, mg	700	5681
Carbohydrate, g	10.60	86.0
% of total calories [§]	42	42
Water, g	109	885
Minerals		
Calcium, mg (mEq)	210 (10.5)	1694 (84.5)
Phosphorus, mg	116	935
Magnesium, mg	12	96.8
Iron, mg	0.37*	3*
Zinc, mg	1.5	12.10
Manganese, mcg	12	97
Copper, mcg	250	2016
Molybdenum, mcg	0	0
Iodine, mcg	6	48
Selenium, mcg	1.8	14.5
Sodium, mg (mEq)	43 (1.9)	347 (15.1)
Potassium, mg (mEq)	129 (3.3)	1040 (26.6)
Chloride, mg (mEq)	81 (2.3)	653 (18.4)
Vitamins		
Vitamin A, IU	1250	10144
Vitamin D, IU	150	1217
Vitamin E, IU	4	32.5
Vitamin K, mcg	12	97.4
Thiamine (B_1), mcg	250	2029
Riboflavin (B_2), mcg	620	5032
Vitamin B_6, mcg	250	2029
Vitamin B_{12}, mcg	0.55	4.46
Niacin, mcg	5000	40577
Folic acid (Folacin), mcg	37	300
Pantothenic acid, mcg	1900	15419
Biotin, mcg	37	300.3
Vitamin C (Ascorbic acid), mg	37	300
Choline, mg	10	81
Inositol, mg	5.5	44.6
L-Carnitine, mg	0	0
Nucleotide fortification, mg	0	0
Renal Solute Load, mOsm	26.7	216.6
Osmolality, mOsm/kg water	280	280

---

  * Additional iron should be supplied from other sources as necessary.
  † Protein Source: Nonfat milk and whey protein concentrate
 †† Fat Source: Medium-chain triglyceride, soy, coconut, and, C. cohnii[1] and M. alpina oils[2]
  [1] A source of docosahexaenoic acid (DHA).
  [2] A source of arachidonic acid (ARA).
  § Carbohydrate Source: Corn syrup solids and lactose
  Precautions: Similac Natural Care Advance® is not intended to be fed as the sole source of nutrients. Tolerance to enteral feeding should be confirmed by offering small volumes of unfortified human milk. Once enteral feeding is well established, Similac Natural Care Advance® can be added in increasing amounts to human milk, or alternated with human milk, to assure that the infant's nutrient needs are fully met. Human milk can be fortified with Similac Natural Care Advance® until the low-birth-weight infant reaches a weight of approximately 8 lb (3629 g), or as directed by a physician.
  Shake bottle vigorously to suspend minerals before mixing with human milk and also before feeding.

NUTRITIONALS

Similac® Special Care® Advance® 20

Similac® Special Care® Advance® 20 with Iron Premature Infant Formula *
Similac® Special Care® Advance® 20 Low Iron Premature Infant Formula **
20 Cal/fl oz

Nutrient	per 100 Cal	per Liter
Energy, Cal	100	676
Volume, mL	148	1000
Protein, g	2.71	18.33
% of total calories [†]	11	11
Fat, g	5.43	36.72
% of total calories [††]	49	49
Linoleic acid, mg	700	4734
Carbohydrate, g	10.6	71.7
% of total calories [§]	42	42
Water, g	133	899
Minerals		
Calcium, mg (mEq)	180 (9.0)	1217 (60.7)
Phosphorus, mg	100	676
Magnesium, mg	12	81.2
Iron, mg	1.8* (0.4)**	12.17* (2.50)**
Zinc, mg	1.5	10.14
Manganese, mcg	12	81
Copper, mcg	250	1691
Molybdenum, mcg	0	0
Iodine, mcg	6	41
Selenium, mcg	1.8	12.2
Sodium, mg (mEq)	43 (1.9)	291 (12.6)
Potassium, mg (mEq)	129 (3.3)	872 (22.3)
Chloride, mg (mEq)	81 (2.3)	548 (15.5)
Vitamins		
Vitamin A, IU	1250	8454
Vitamin D, IU	150	1014
Vitamin E, IU	4	27.1
Vitamin K, mcg	12	81.2
Thiamine (B_1), mcg	250	1691
Riboflavin (B_2), mcg	620	4193
Vitamin B_6, mcg	250	1691
Vitamin B_{12}, mcg	0.55	3.72
Niacin, mcg	5000	33815
Folic acid (Folacin), mcg	37	250
Pantothenic acid, mcg	1900	12850
Biotin, mcg	37	250
Vitamin C (Ascorbic acid), mg	37	250
Choline, mg	10	68
Inositol, mg	5.5	37.2
L-Carnitine, mg	0	0
Nucleotide fortification, mg	0	0
Renal Solute Load, mOsm	26.2	177
Osmolality, mOsm/kg water	235	235

* The addition of iron to this formula conforms to the recommendation of the Committee on Nutrition of the American Academy of Pediatrics.
** Additional iron should be supplied from other sources.
[†] Protein Source: Nonfat milk and whey protein concentrate
[††] Fat Source: Medium-chain triglyceride, soy, coconut, and, C. cohnii[1] and M. alpina oils[2]
[1] A source of docosahexaenoic acid (DHA)
[2] A source of arachidonic acid (ARA)
[§] Carbohydrate Source: Corn syrup solids and lactose
Precautions: Tolerance to enteral feeding should be confirmed by initially offering small volumes of hypocaloric formula followed by cautious progression to higher caloric feeding. Spitting up, excessive gastric residuals, abdominal distention, abnormal stools or stool patterns, or other signs of intestinal dysfunction have been associated with enteral feeding before the intestinal tract is ready to accommodate the regimen. At the first sign of these problems, enteral feeding should be slowed or discontinued. Shake bottle vigorously to suspend minerals.

Similac® Special Care® Advance® 24 with Iron Premature Infant Formula*
Similac® Special Care® Advance® 24 Low Iron Premature Infant Formula**
24 Cal/fl oz

Nutrient	per 100 Cal	per Liter
Energy, Cal	100	812
Volume, mL	124	1000
Protein, g	2.71	21.99
% of total calories †	11	11
Fat, g	5.43	44.07
% of total calories ††	49	49
Linoleic acid, mg	700	5681
Carbohydrate, g	10.6	86.0
% of total calories §	42	42
Water, g	109	885
Minerals		
Calcium, mg (mEq)	180 (9.0)	1461 (72.9)
Phosphorus, mg	100	812
Magnesium, mg	12	97.4
Iron, mg	1.8* (0.4)**	14.61* (3.0)**
Zinc, mg	1.5	12.1
Manganese, mcg	12	97
Copper, mcg	250	2029
Molybdenum, mcg	0	0
Iodine, mcg	6	49
Selenium, mcg	1.8	14.6
Sodium, mg (mEq)	43 (1.9)	349 (15.2)
Potassium, mg (mEq)	129 (3.3)	1047 (26.8)
Chloride, mg (mEq)	81 (2.3)	657 (18.4)
Vitamins		
Vitamin A, IU	1250	10144
Vitamin D, IU	150	1217
Vitamin E, IU	4	32.5
Vitamin K, mcg	12	97.4
Thiamine (B_1), mcg	250	2029
Riboflavin (B_2), mcg	620	5032
Vitamin B_6, mcg	250	2029
Vitamin B_{12}, mcg	0.55	4.46
Niacin, mcg	5000	40577
Folic acid (Folacin), mcg	37	300
Pantothenic acid, mcg	1900	15419
Biotin, mcg	37	300.3
Vitamin C (Ascorbic acid), mg	37	300
Choline, mg	10	81
Inositol, mg	5.5	44.6
L-Carnitine, mg	0	0
Nucleotide fortification, mg	0	0
Renal Solute Load, mOsm	26.2	212.4
Osmolality, mOsm/kg water	280	280

---

* The addition of iron to this formula conforms to the recommendation of the Committee on Nutrition of the American Academy of Pediatrics.
** Low-Iron: Additional iron should be supplied from other sources.
† Protein Source: Nonfat milk and whey protein concentrate
†† Fat Source: Medium-chain triglyceride, soy, coconut, and, C. cohnii[1] and M. alpina oils[2]
[1] A source of docosahexaenoic acid (DHA)
[2] A source of arachidonic acid (ARA)
§ Carbohydrate Source: Corn syrup solids and lactose
Precautions: Tolerance to enteral feeding should be confirmed by initially offering small volumes of hypocaloric formula followed by cautious progression to higher caloric feeding. Spitting up, excessive gastric residuals, abdominal distention, abnormal stools or stool patterns, or other signs of intestinal dysfunction have been associated with enteral feeding before the intestinal tract is ready to accommodate the regimen. At the first sign of these problems, enteral feeding should be slowed or discontinued. Shake bottle vigorously to suspend minerals.

Similac® Advance®

20 Cal/fl oz

Nutrient	per 100 Cal	per Liter
Energy, Cal	100	676
Volume, mL	148	1000
Protein, g	2.07	14.00
% of total calories [†]	8	8
Fat, g	5.40	36.52
% of total calories [††]	49	49
Linoleic acid, mg	1000	6763
Carbohydrate, g	10.80	73.0
% of total calories [§]	43	43
Water, g	133	904
Minerals		
Calcium, mg (mEq)	78 (3.9)	528 (26.3)
Phosphorus, mg	42	284
Magnesium, mg	6	40.6
Iron, mg	1.8 (0.7)*	12.17 (4.7)*
Zinc, mg	0.75	5.07
Manganese, mcg	5	34
Copper, mcg	90	609
Molybdenum, mcg	0	0
Iodine, mcg	6	41
Selenium, mcg	1.8	12.2
Sodium, mg (mEq)	24 (1.0)	162 (7.1)
Potassium, mg (mEq)	105 (2.7)	710 (18.2)
Chloride, mg (mEq)	65 (1.8)	440 (12.4)
Vitamins		
Vitamin A, IU	300	2029
Vitamin D, IU	60	406
Vitamin E, IU	3	20.3
Vitamin K, mcg	8	54.1
Thiamine (B$_1$), mcg	100	676
Riboflavin (B$_2$), mcg	150	1014
Vitamin B$_6$, mcg	60	406
Vitamin B$_{12}$, mcg	0.25	1.69
Niacin, mcg	1050	7101
Folic acid (Folacin), mcg	15	101
Pantothenic acid, mcg	450	3043
Biotin, mcg	4.4	29.8
Vitamin C (Ascorbic acid), mg	9	61
Choline, mg	16	108
Inositol, mg	4.7	31.8
L-Carnitine, mg	0	0
Taurine, mg	0	0
Nucleotide fortification, mg	10.7	72
Renal Solute Load, mOsm	18.7	126.8
Osmolality, mOsm/kg water	300	300

* The addition of iron to this formula conforms to the recommendation of the Committee on Nutrition of the American Academy of Pediatrics.

† Protein Source: Nonfat milk and whey protein concentrate

†† Fat Source: High-oleic safflower, soy, coconut, and, C. cohnii[1] and M. alpina oils[2]
   [1] A source of docosahexaenoic acid (DHA)
   [2] A source of arachidonic acid (ARA)
   Similac® Advance® Powder contains 5.49 g fat and 10.56 g carbohydrate.
§ Carbohydrate Source: Lactose

Similac® 20 with Iron Infant Formula*
Similac® 20 Low Iron Infant Formula**
20 Cal/fl oz

Nutrient	per 100 Cal	per Liter
Energy, Cal	100	676
Volume, mL	148	1000
Protein, g	2.07	14.00
% of total calories [†]	8	8
Fat, g	5.40	36.52
% of total calories [††]	49	49
Linoleic acid, mg	1000	6763
Carbohydrate, g	10.8	73.0
% of total calories [§]	43	43
Water, g	133	904
Minerals		
Calcium, mg (mEq)	78 (3.9)	528 (26.3)
Phosphorus, mg	42	284
Magnesium, mg	6	40.6
Iron, mg	1.8* (0.7)**	12.17* (4.73)**
Zinc, mg	0.75	5.07
Manganese, mcg	5	34
Copper, mcg	90	609
Molybdenum, mcg	0	0
Iodine, mcg	6	41
Selenium, mcg	2.2	14.9
Sodium, mg (mEq)	24 (1.0)	162 (7.1)
Potassium, mg (mEq)	105 (2.7)	710 (18.2)
Chloride, mg (mEq)	65 (1.8)	440 (12.4)
Vitamins		
Vitamin A, IU	300	2029
Vitamin D, IU	60	406
Vitamin E, IU	1.5	10.1
Vitamin K, mcg	8	54.1
Thiamine (B_1), mcg	100	676
Riboflavin (B_2), mcg	150	1014
Vitamin B_6, mcg	60	406
Vitamin B_{12}, mcg	0.25	1.69
Niacin, mcg	1050	7101
Folic acid (Folacin), mcg	15	101
Pantothenic acid, mcg	450	3043
Biotin, mcg	4.4	29.8
Vitamin C (Ascorbic acid), mg	9	61
Choline, mg	16	108
Inositol, mg	4.7	31.8
L-Carnitine, mg	0	0
Taurine, mg	0	0
Nucleotide fortification, mg	10.7	72
Renal Solute Load, mOsm	18.7	126.8
Osmolality, mOsm/kg water	300	300

* The addition of iron to this formula conforms to the recommendation of the Committee on Nutrition of the American Academy of Pediatrics.

** Additional iron should be supplied from other sources

† Protein Source: Nonfat milk and whey protein concentrate

†† Fat Source: High-oleic safflower, coconut and soy oils

§ Carbohydrate Source: Lactose

NUTRITIONALS

Similac® PM 60/40

Similac® PM 60/40 Low Iron Infant Formula *
(Powder prepared at standard dilution, 20 Cal/fl oz)

Nutrient	per 100 Cal	per Liter
Energy, Cal	100	676
Volume, mL	148	1000
Protein, g	2.22	15.01
% of total calories [†]	9	9
Fat, g	5.59	37.80
% of total calories [††]	50	50
Linoleic acid, mg	1300	8792
Carbohydrate, g	10.2	69.0
% of total calories [§]	41	41
Water, g	134	899
Minerals		
Calcium, mg (mEq)	56 (2.8)	379 (18.9)
Phosphorus, mg	28	189
Magnesium, mg	6	40.6
Iron, mg	0.7*	4.73*
Zinc, mg	0.75	5.07
Manganese, mcg	5	34
Copper, mcg	90	609
Molybdenum, mcg	0	0
Iodine, mcg	6	41
Selenium, mcg	1.9	12.8
Sodium, mg (mEq)	24 (1.0)	162 (7.1)
Potassium, mg (mEq)	80 (2.2)	541 (14.9)
Chloride, mg (mEq)	59 (1.7)	399 (11.3)
Vitamins		
Vitamin A, IU	300	2029
Vitamin D, IU	60	406
Vitamin E, IU	2.5	16.9
Vitamin K, mcg	8	54.1
Thiamine (B_1), mcg	100	676
Riboflavin (B_2), mcg	150	1014
Vitamin B_6, mcg	60	406
Vitamin B_{12}, mcg	0.25	1.69
Niacin, mcg	1050	7101
Folic acid (Folacin), mcg	15	101
Pantothenic acid, mcg	450	3043
Biotin, mcg	4.5	30.4
Vitamin C (Ascorbic acid), mg	9	61
Choline, mg	12	81
Inositol, mg	24	162.3
L-Carnitine, mg	0	0
Taurine, mg	0	0
Nucleotide fortification, mg	0	0
Renal Solute Load, mOsm	18.5	125.1
Osmolality, mOsm/kg water	280	280

* Additional iron should be supplied from other sources.

† Protein Source: Whey protein concentrate and sodium caseinate

†† Fat Source: Corn, coconut, and soy oils

§ Carbohydrate Source: Lactose

Precautions: In conditions where the infant is losing abnormal quantities of one or more electrolytes, it may be necessary to supply electrolytes from sources other than the formula. It may be necessary to supply low-birth-weight infants (weighing less than 1500 g at birth) additional calcium, phosphorus, and sodium during periods of rapid growth.

Similac® 24 with Iron Infant Formula*
24 Cal/fl oz

Nutrient	per 100 Cal	per Liter
Energy, Cal	100	812
Volume, mL	124	1000
Protein, g	2.71	21.99
% of total calories [†]	11	11
Fat, g	5.27	42.77
% of total calories [††]	47	47
Linoleic acid, mg	1300	10550
Carbohydrate, g	10.5	85.2
% of total calories [§]	42	42
Water, g	109	885
Minerals		
Calcium, mg (mEq)	90 (4.5)	730 (36.4)
Phosphorus, mg	70	568
Magnesium, mg	7	56.8
Iron, mg	1.8*	14.61*
Zinc, mg	0.75	6.09
Manganese, mcg	5	41
Copper, mcg	90	730
Molybdenum, mcg	0	0
Iodine, mcg	9	73
Selenium, mcg	1.8	20.3
Sodium, mg (mEq)	34 (1.5)	276 (12.0)
Potassium, mg (mEq)	132 (3.4)	1071 (27.4)
Chloride, mg (mEq)	81 (2.3)	657 (18.5)
Vitamins		
Vitamin A, IU	300	2435
Vitamin D, IU	60	487
Vitamin E, IU	3	24.3
Vitamin K, mcg	8	64.9
Thiamine (B_1), mcg	100	812
Riboflavin (B_2), mcg	150	1217
Vitamin B_6, mcg	60	487
Vitamin B_{12}, mcg	0.25	2.03
Niacin, mcg	1050	8521
Folic acid (Folacin), mcg	15	122
Pantothenic acid, mcg	450	3652
Biotin, mcg	4.4	35.7
Vitamin C (Ascorbic acid), mg	9	73
Choline, mg	16	130
Inositol, mg	4.7	38.1
L-Carnitine, mg	0	0
Taurine, mg	0	0
Nucleotide fortification, mg	0	0
Renal Solute Load, mOsm	24.9	202
Osmolality, mOsm/kg water	380	380

* The addition of iron to this formula conforms to the recommendation of the Committee on Nutrition of the American Academy of Pediatrics.

† Protein Source: Nonfat milk

†† Fat Source: Soy and coconut oils

§ Carbohydrate Source: Lactose

NUTRITIONALS

Similac® Lactose Free

Similac® Lactose Free Infant Formula with Iron *
20 Cal/fl oz

Nutrient	per 100 Cal	per Liter
Energy, Cal	100	676
Volume, mL	148	1000
Protein, g	2.14	14.47
% of total calories †	9	9
Fat, g	5.40	36.52
% of total calories ††	49	49
Linoleic acid, mg	1300	8792
Carbohydrate, g	10.7	72.4
% of total calories §	43	43
Water, g	133	902
Minerals		
Calcium, mg (mEq)	84 (4.2)	568 (28.3)
Phosphorus, mg	56	379
Magnesium, mg	6	40.6
Iron, mg	1.8*	12.17*
Zinc, mg	0.75	5.07
Manganese, mcg	5	34
Copper, mcg	90	609
Molybdenum, mcg	0	0
Iodine, mcg	9	61
Selenium, mcg	1.8	12.2
Sodium, mg (mEq)	30 (1.3)	203 (8.8)
Potassium, mg (mEq)	107 (2.7)	724 (18.5)
Chloride, mg (mEq)	65 (1.8)	440 (12.4)
Vitamins		
Vitamin A, IU	300	2029
Vitamin D, IU	60	406
Vitamin E, IU	3.0	20.3
Vitamin K, mcg	8	54.1
Thiamine (B_1), mcg	100	676
Riboflavin (B_2), mcg	150	1014
Vitamin B_6, mcg	60	406
Vitamin B_{12}, mcg	0.25	1.69
Niacin, mcg	1050	7101
Folic acid (Folacin), mcg	15	101
Pantothenic acid, mcg	450	3043
Biotin, mcg	4.4	29.8
Vitamin C (Ascorbic acid), mg	9	61
Choline, mg	16	108
Inositol, mg	4.3	29.1
L-Carnitine, mg	0	0
Taurine, mg	0	0
Nucleotide fortification, mg	10.7	72
Renal Solute Load, mOsm	19.9	134.7
Osmolality, mOsm/kg water	200	200

* The addition of iron to this formula conforms to the recommendation of the Committee on Nutrition of the American Academy of Pediatrics.

† Protein Source: Milk protein isolate

†† Fat Source: Soy and coconut oils

§ Carbohydrate Source: Maltodextrin and sucrose

Familiar Nutritionals

Similac® Isomil® 20

Similac® Isomil® 20 Soy Formula with Iron*
20 Cal/fl oz

Nutrient	per 100 Cal	per Liter
Energy, Cal	100	676
Volume, mL	148	1000
Protein, g	2.45	16.57
% of total calories †	10	10
Fat, g	5.46	36.93
% of total calories ††	49	49
Linoleic acid, mg	1000	6763
Carbohydrate, g	10.3	69.7
% of total calories §	41	41
Water, g	133	901
Minerals		
Calcium, mg (mEq)	105 (5.2)	710 (35.4)
Phosphorus, mg	75	507
Magnesium, mg	7.5	50.7
Iron, mg	1.8*	12.17*
Zinc, mg	0.75	5.07
Manganese, mcg	25	169
Copper, mcg	75	507
Molybdenum, mcg	0	0
Iodine, mcg	15	101
Selenium, mcg	1.8	14.2
Sodium, mg (mEq)	44 (1.9)	298 (12.9)
Potassium, mg (mEq)	108 (2.8)	730 (18.7)
Chloride, mg (mEq)	62 (1.7)	419 (11.8)
Vitamins		
Vitamin A, IU	300	2029
Vitamin D, IU	60	406
Vitamin E, IU	1.5	10.1
Vitamin K, mcg	11	74.4
Thiamine (B_1), mcg	60	406
Riboflavin (B_2), mcg	90	609
Vitamin B_6, mcg	60	406
Vitamin B_{12}, mcg	0.45	3.04
Niacin, mcg	1350	9130
Folic acid (Folacin), mcg	15	101
Pantothenic acid, mcg	750	5072
Biotin, mcg	4.5	30.4
Vitamin C (Ascorbic acid), mg	9	61
Choline, mg	12	81
Inositol, mg	5	33.8
L-Carnitine, mg	0	0
Taurine, mg	0	0
Nucleotide fortification, mg	0	0
Renal Solute Load, mOsm	22.8	154.5
Osmolality, mOsm/kg water	200	200

* The addition of iron to this formula conforms to the recommendation of the Committee on Nutrition of the American Academy of Pediatrics.

† Protein Source: Soy protein isolate and L-methionine

†† Fat Source: High-oleic safflower, coconut, and soy oils

§ Carbohydrate Source: Corn syrup and sucrose

Precautions: This formula is not recommended for long-term feeding of very-low-birth-weight infants (less than 1500 g). If long-term feeding is necessary, an additional source of calcium and phosphorus may be indicated.

Similac® Isomil® Advance® Soy Formula with Iron*
20 Cal/fl oz

Nutrient	per 100 Cal	per Liter
Energy, Cal	100	676
Volume, mL	148	1000
Protein, g	2.45	16.57
% of total calories [†]	10	10
Fat, g	5.46	36.93
% of total calories [††]	49	49
Linoleic acid, mg	1000	6763
Carbohydrate, g	10.3	69.7
% of total calories [§]	41	41
Water, g	133	901
Minerals		
Calcium, mg (mEq)	105 (5.2)	709 (35.4)
Phosphorus, mg	75	507
Magnesium, mg	7.5	50.7
Iron, mg	1.8*	12.17*
Zinc, mg	0.75	5.07
Manganese, mcg	25	169
Copper, mcg	75	507
Molybdenum, mcg	0	0
Iodine, mcg	15	101
Selenium, mcg	1.8	12.2
Sodium, mg (mEq)	44 (1.9)	298 (12.9)
Potassium, mg (mEq)	108 (2.8)	730 (18.7)
Chloride, mg (mEq)	62 (1.7)	419 (11.8)
Vitamins		
Vitamin A, IU	300	2029
Vitamin D, IU	60	406
Vitamin E, IU	1.5	10.1
Vitamin K, mcg	11	74.4
Thiamine (B_1), mcg	60	406
Riboflavin (B_2), mcg	90	609
Vitamin B_6, mcg	60	406
Vitamin B_{12}, mcg	0.45	3.04
Niacin, mcg	1350	9130
Folic acid (Folacin), mcg	15	101
Pantothenic acid, mcg	750	5072
Biotin, mcg	4.5	30.4
Vitamin C (Ascorbic acid), mg	9	61
Choline, mg	12	81
Inositol, mg	5.0	33.8
L-Carnitine, mg	0	0
Taurine, mg	0	0
Nucleotide fortification, mg	0	0
Renal Solute Load, mOsm	22.8	154.5
Osmolality, mOsm/kg water	200	200

* The addition of iron to this formula conforms to the recommendation of the Committee on Nutrition of the American Academy of Pediatrics.

† Protein Source: Soy protein isolate and L-methionine

†† Fat Source: High-oleic safflower, soy, coconut, and, C. cohnii[1] and M. alpina oils[2]
  [1] A source of docosahexaenoic acid (DHA)
  [2] A source of arachidonic acid (ARA)

§ Carbohydrate Source: Corn syrup and sucrose

NUTRITIONALS

Similac® Alimentum®

Similac® Alimentum® Protein Hydrolysate Formula with Iron *
20 Cal/fl oz

Nutrient	per 100 Cal	per Liter
Energy, Cal	100	676
Volume, mL	148	1000
Protein, g	2.75	18.60
% of total calories [†]	11	11
Fat, g	5.54	37.47
% of total calories [††]	48	48
Linoleic acid, mg	1900	12850
Carbohydrate, g	10.2	69.0
% of total calories [§]	41	41
Water, g	133	901
Minerals		
Calcium, mg (mEq)	105 (5.2)	710 (35.4)
Phosphorus, mg	75	507
Magnesium, mg	7.5	50.7
Iron, mg	1.8*	12.17*
Zinc, mg	0.75	5.07
Manganese, mcg	8	54
Copper, mcg	75	507
Molybdenum, mcg		
Iodine, mcg	15	101
Selenium, mcg	1.8	12.2
Sodium, mg (mEq)	44 (1.9)	298 (12.9)
Potassium, mg (mEq)	118 (3.0)	798 (20.4)
Chloride, mg (mEq)	80 (2.3)	541 (15.3)
Vitamins		
Vitamin A, IU	300	2029
Vitamin D, IU	45	304
Vitamin E, IU	3.0	20.3
Vitamin K, mcg	15	101.4
Thiamine (B_1), mcg	60	406
Riboflavin (B_2), mcg	90	609
Vitamin B_6, mcg	60	406
Vitamin B_{12}, mcg	0.45	3.04
Niacin, mcg	1350	9130
Folic acid (Folacin), mcg	15	101
Pantothenic acid, mcg	750	5072
Biotin, mcg	4.5	30.4
Vitamin C (Ascorbic acid), mg	9	61
Choline, mg	8	54
Inositol, mg	5	33.8
L-Carnitine, mg	0	0
Taurine, mg	0	0
Nucleotide fortification, mg	0	0
Renal Solute Load, mOsm	25.3	171.3
Osmolality, mOsm/kg water	370	370

* The addition of iron to this formula conforms to the recommendation of the Committee on Nutrition of the American Academy of Pediatrics

† Protein Source: Casein hydrolysate, L-cystine, L-tyrosine, L-tryptophan

†† Fat Source: Safflower, medium-chain triglyceride, and soy oils

§ Carbohydrate Source: Sucrose and modified tapioca starch

Similac® Alimentum® Powder

Similac® Alimentum® Protein Hydrolysate Formula with Iron*
20 Cal/fl oz

Nutrient	Per 100 Cal	Per Liter	Per 100 g Powder
Energy, Cal	100	676	509
Volume, mL	148	1000	-
Protein, g	2.75	18.60	13.99
% of total calories †	11	11	11
Fat, g	5.54	37.7	28.19
% of total calories ††	48	48	48
Linoleic acid, mg	800	5405	4069
Carbohydrate, g	10.2	68.9	51.9
% of total calories §	41	41	41
Water, g	133	901	1.2
Minerals			
Calcium, mg (mEq)	105 (5.2)	710 (35.4)	534 (26.7)
Phosphorus, mg	75	507	382
Magnesium, mg	7.5	50.7	38.2
Iron, mg	1.8*	12.17*	9.16*
Zinc, mg	0.75	5.07	3.82
Manganese, mcg	8	54	41
Copper, mcg	75	507	382
Iodine, mcg	15	101	41
Selenium, mcg	1.8	12.2	9.2
Sodium, mg (mEq)	44 (1.9)	298 (12.9)	224 (9.7)
Potassium, mg (mEq)	118 (3.0)	798 (20.4)	600 (15.4)
Chloride, mg (mEq)	80 (2.3)	541 (15.3)	407 (11.5)
Vitamins			
Vitamin A, IU	300	2029	1527
Vitamin D, IU	45	304	229
Vitamin E, IU	3.0	20.3	15.3
Vitamin K, mcg	8	101.4	40.7
Thiamine (B$_1$), mcg	60	406	305
Riboflavin (B$_2$), mcg	90	609	458
Vitamin B$_6$, mcg	60	406	305
Vitamin B$_{12}$, mcg	0.45	3.04	2.29
Niacin, mcg	1350	9130	6870
Folic acid (Folacin), mcg	15	101	76
Pantothenic acid, mcg	750	5072	3817
Biotin, mcg	4.5	30.4	22.9
Vitamin C (Ascorbic acid), mg	9	61	46
Choline, mg	8	54	41
Inositol, mg	5	33.8	25.4
Renal Solute Load, mOsm	25.3	171.3	128.9
Osmolality, mOsm/kg water	320	370	-

* The addition of iron to this formula conforms to the recommendations of the Committee on Nutrition of the American Academy of Pediatrics.

† Protein Source: Casein Hydrolysate, L-Cystine, L-Tyrosine, and L-Tryptophan

†† Fat Source: 35% High-Oleic Safflower, 33% Medium-Chain Triglyceride & 28% Soy oils
The remaining 4% of the fat is comprised of emulsifiers, antioxidants, and fat-soluble vitamins.

§ Carbohydrate Source: 70% Maltodextrin & 30% Sucrose

	Preparation	
To Make Approx.	Water	Powder
2 fl oz bottle	2 fl oz	1 unpacked level scoop (8.7g)
4 fl oz bottle	3.5 fl oz	2 unpacked level scoops

Similac NeoSure® Advance®

Similac NeoSure® Advance® Infant Formula with Iron*
22 Cal/fl oz

Nutrient	per 100 Cal	per Liter
Energy, Cal	100	744
Volume, mL	134	1000
Protein, g	2.6	19.34
% of total calories [†]	10	10
Fat, g	5.50	40.92
% of total calories [††]	49	50
Linoleic acid, mg	750	5579
Carbohydrate, g	10.3	76.6
% of total calories [§]	41	41
Water, g	120	893
Minerals		
Calcium, mg (mEq)	105 (5.2)	781 (39.0)
Phosphorus, mg	62	461
Magnesium, mg	9	67.0
Iron, mg	1.8*	13.39*
Zinc, mg	1.2	8.93
Manganese, mcg	10	74
Copper, mcg	120	893
Molybdenum, mcg	0	0
Iodine, mcg	15	112
Selenium, mcg	2.3	17.1
Sodium, mg (mEq)	33 (1.4)	245 (10.7)
Potassium, mg (mEq)	142 (3.6)	1056 (27.0)
Chloride, mg (mEq)	75 (2.1)	558 (15.7)
Vitamins		
Vitamin A, IU	460	3422
Vitamin D, IU	70	521
Vitamin E, IU	3.6	26.8
Vitamin K, mcg	11	81.8
Thiamine (B_1), mcg	220	1637
Riboflavin (B_2), mcg	150	1116
Vitamin B_6, mcg	100	744
Vitamin B_{12}, mcg	0.4	2.98
Niacin, mcg	1950	14506
Folic acid (Folacin), mcg	25	186
Pantothenic acid, mcg	800	5951
Biotin, mcg	9	67.0
Vitamin C (Ascorbic acid), mg	15	112
Choline, mg	16	119
Inositol, mg	6	44.6
L-Carnitine, mg	0	0
Taurine, mg	0	0
Nucleotide fortification, mg	0	0
Renal Solute Load, mOsm	24	178.9
Osmolality, mOsm/kg water	250	250

* The addition of iron to this formula conforms to the recommendation of the Committee on Nutrition of the American Academy of Pediatrics.

† Protein Source: Nonfat milk and whey protein concentrate

†† Fat Source: Soy, coconut, medium-chain triglyceride, and, C. cohnii[1] and M. alpina oils[2]
  [1] A source of docosahexaenoic acid (DHA)
  [2] A source of arachidonic acid (ARA)

§ Carbohydrate Source: Maltodextrin and lactose

Enfamil® EnfaCare® LIPIL® 20
22 Cal/fl oz

Nutrient	per 100 Cal	per Liter
Energy, Cal	100	744
Volume, mL	135	1000
Protein, g	2.8	21
% of total calories [†]	11	11
Fat, g	5.3	39
% of total calories [††]	47	47
Linoleic acid, mg	950	7000
Carbohydrate, g	10.4	77
% of total calories [§]	42	42
Water, g	120	890
Minerals		
Calcium, mg (mEq)	120 (6)	890 (45)
Phosphorus, mg	66	490
Magnesium, mg	8	59
Iron, mg	1.8*	13*
Zinc, mg	1.25	9.2
Manganese, mcg	15	111
Copper, mcg	120	890
Molybdenum, mcg	0	0
Iodine, mcg	21	155
Selenium, mcg	2.8	21
Sodium, mg (mEq)	35 (1.52)	260 (11.3)
Potassium, mg (mEq)	105 (2.7)	780 (20)
Chloride, mg (mEq)	78 (2.2)	580 (16.3)
Vitamins		
Vitamin A, IU	450	3300
Vitamin D, IU	80	590
Vitamin E, IU	4	30
Vitamin K, mcg	8	59
Thiamine (B_1), mcg	200	1480
Riboflavin (B_2), mcg	200	1480
Vitamin B_6, mcg	100	740
Vitamin B_{12}, mcg	0.3	2.2
Niacin, mcg	2000	14800
Folic acid (Folacin), mcg	26	192
Pantothenic acid, mcg	850	6300
Biotin, mcg	6	44
Vitamin C (Ascorbic acid), mg	16	118
Choline, mg	24	178
Inositol, mg	30	220
L-Carnitine, mg	2	14.8
Taurine, mg	6	44
Nucleotide fortification, mg	4.2	31.1
Renal Solute Load, mOsm	24	181
Osmolality, mOsm/kg water	230	230
Osmolarity, mOsm/L	200	200

* The addition of iron to this formula conforms to the recommendation of the Committee on Nutrition of the American Academy of Pediatrics.

† Protein Source: Whey protein concentrate and nonfat milk

†† Fat Source: Soy, coconut, medium-chain triglyceride, and, C. cohnii[1] and M. alpina oils[2]
[1] A source of docosahexaenoic acid (DHA). DHA- 0.33% of fatty acids (w/w).
[2] A source of arachidonic acid (ARA). ARA- 0.67% of fatty acids (w/w).

§ Carbohydrate Source: Maltodextrin, lactose

Enfamil® Premature LIPIL® 20

Enfamil® Premature LIPIL® 20
20 Cal/fl oz

Nutrient	per 100 Cal	per Liter
Energy, Cal	100	676
Volume, mL	148	1000
Protein, g	3	20
% of total calories [†]	12	12
Fat, g	5.1	34
% of total calories [††]	44	44
Linoleic acid, mg	810	5500
Carbohydrate, g	11	74
% of total calories [§]	44	44
Water, g	133	900
Minerals		
Calcium, mg (mEq)	165 (8.3)	1120 (56)
Phosphorus, mg	83	560
Magnesium, mg	9	61
Iron, mg	1.8* (0.5)**	12.2* (3.4)**
Zinc, mg	1.5	10.1
Manganese, mcg	6.3	43
Copper, mcg	120	810
Molybdenum, mcg	0	0
Iodine, mcg	25	169
Selenium, mcg	2.8	18.9
Sodium, mg (mEq)	58 (2.5)	390 (17)
Potassium, mg (mEq)	98 (2.5)	660 (16.9)
Chloride, mg (mEq)	90 (2.5)	610 (17.2)
Vitamins		
Vitamin A, IU	1250	8500
Vitamin D, IU	240	1620
Vitamin E, IU	6.3	43
Vitamin K, mcg	8	54
Thiamine (B_1), mcg	200	1350
Riboflavin (B_2), mcg	300	2000
Vitamin B_6, mcg	150	1010
Vitamin B_{12}, mcg	0.25	1.7
Niacin, mcg	4000	27000
Folic acid (Folacin), mcg	40	270
Pantothenic acid, mcg	1200	81000
Biotin, mcg	4	27
Vitamin C (Ascorbic acid), mg	20	135
Choline, mg	20	135
Inositol, mg	44	300
L-Carnitine, mg	2.4	16.2
Taurine, mg	6	41
Nucleotide fortification, mg	4.2	28.4
Renal Solute Load, mOsm	27	181
Osmolality, mOsm/kg water	260	260
Osmolarity, mOsm/L	230	230

* The addition of iron to this formula conforms to the recommendation of the Committee on Nutrition of the American Academy of Pediatrics.

** Supplemental iron should be considered.

† Protein Source: Whey protein concentrate and nonfat milk

†† Fat Source: Medium-chain triglycerides, soy oil, high oleic, and, M. alpina[1] and C. codinium[2] oils
[1] A source of arachidonic acid (ARA). ARA- 0.67% of fatty acids (w/w).
[2] A source of docosahexaenoic acid (DHA). DHA- 0.33% of fatty acids (w/w).

§ Carbohydrate Source: Corn syrup solids and lactose

Enfamil® Premature Formula 24 and with Iron 24*
24 Cal/fl oz

Nutrient	per 100 Cal	per Liter
Energy, Cal	100	812
Volume, mL	123	1000
Protein, g	3	24
% of total calories [†]	12	12
Fat, g	5.10	41
% of total calories [††]	44	44
Linoleic acid, mg	810	6600
Carbohydrate, g	11	89
% of total calories [§]	44	44
Water, g	108	880
Minerals		
Calcium, mg (mEq)	165 (8.3)	1340 (67)
Phosphorus, mg	83	670
Magnesium, mg	9	55
Iron, mg	1.8 (0.5)*	14.6 (4.1)*
Zinc, mg	1.5	12.2
Manganese, mcg	6.3	51
Copper, mcg	120	970
Molybdenum, mcg	0	0
Iodine, mcg	25	200
Selenium, mcg	2.8	14.6
Sodium, mg (mEq)	58 (2.5)	470 (20)
Potassium, mg (mEq)	98 (2.5)	800 (20)
Chloride, mg (mEq)	90 (2.5)	730 (21)
Vitamins		
Vitamin A, IU	1250	10100
Vitamin D, IU	240	1950
Vitamin E, IU	6.3	51
Vitamin K, mcg	8	65
Thiamine (B_1), mcg	200	1620
Riboflavin (B_2), mcg	300	2400
Vitamin B_6, mcg	150	1220
Vitamin B_{12}, mcg	0.25	2
Niacin, mcg	4000	32000
Folic acid (Folacin), mcg	40	320
Pantothenic acid, mcg	1200	9700
Biotin, mcg	4	32
Vitamin C (Ascorbic acid), mg	20	162
Choline, mg	20	162
Inositol, mg	44	360
L-Carnitine, mg	2.4	19.5
Taurine, mg	6	49
Nucleotide fortification, mg	4.2	33.8
Renal Solute Load, mOsm	27	220
Osmolality, mOsm/kg water	310	310
Osmolarity, mOsm/L	270	270

  * Supplemental iron should be considered.

  † Protein Source: Whey protein concentrate and nonfat milk

  †† Fat Source: Medium-chain triglycerides, soy oil, high oleic, and, M. alpina[1] and C. codinium[2] oils
  [1] A source of arachidonic acid (ARA). ARA- 0.67% of fatty acids (w/w).
  [2] A source of docosahaxaenoic acid (DHA). DHA- 0.33% of fatty acids (w/w).

  § Carbohydrate Source: Corn syrup solids and lactose

NUTRITIONALS

Enfamil® Lipil® 20 with Iron
20 Cal/fl oz

Nutrient	per 100 Cal	per Liter
Energy, Cal	100	676
Volume, mL	148	1000
Protein, g	2.10	14.50
% of total calories [†]	8.5	8.5
Fat, g	5.30	36
% of total calories [††]	48	48
Linoleic acid, mg	860	5800
Carbohydrate, g	10.90	73
% of total calories [§]	43	43
Water, g	134	910
Minerals		
Calcium, mg (mEq)	78 (3.9)	530 (27)
Phosphorus, mg	53	360
Magnesium, mg	8	54
Iron, mg	1.8* (0.7)	12.2* (4.7)
Zinc, mg	1	6.8
Manganese, mcg	15	101
Copper, mcg	75	510
Molybdenum, mcg	0	0
Iodine, mcg	10	68
Selenium, mcg	2.8	18.9
Sodium, mg (mEq)	27 (1.2)	183 (8.0)
Potassium, mg (mEq)	108 (2.8)	730 (18.7)
Chloride, mg (mEq)	63 (1.8)	430 (12.1)
Vitamins		
Vitamin A, IU	300	2000
Vitamin D, IU	60	410
Vitamin E, IU	2	13.5
Vitamin K, mcg	8	54
Thiamine (B_1), mcg	80	540
Riboflavin (B_2), mcg	140	950
Vitamin B_6, mcg	60	410
Vitamin B_{12}, mcg	0.3	2
Niacin, mcg	1000	6800
Folic acid (Folacin), mcg	16	108
Pantothenic acid, mcg	500	3400
Biotin, mcg	3	20
Vitamin C (Ascorbic acid), mg	12	81
Choline, mg	12	81
Inositol, mg	6	41
L-Carnitine, mg	2	13.5
Taurine, mg	6	41
Nucleotide fortification, mg	4.2	28
Renal Solute Load, mOsm	19.2	132
Osmolality, mOsm/kg water	300	300
Osmolarity, mOsm/L	270	270

* The addition of iron to this formula conforms to the recommendation of the Committee on Nutrition of the American Academy of Pediatrics.

† Protein Source: Reduced minerals whey and nonfat milk

†† Fat Source: Palm olein, soy, coconut and high-oleic sunflower oils, M. alpina[1] and C. codinium[2] oils.
  [1] A source of arachidonic acid (ARA). ARA- 0.64% of fatty acids (w/w).
  [2] A source of docosahexaenoic acid (DHA). DHA- 0.32% of fatty acids (w/w).

§ Carbohydrate Source: Lactose

Enfamil® 20** and Enfamil® 20 with Iron*
20 Cal/fl oz

Nutrient	per 100 Cal	per Liter
Energy, Cal	100	676
Volume, mL	148	1000
Protein, g	2.1	14.5
% of total calories †	8.5	8.5
Fat, g	5.3	36
% of total calories ††	48	48
Linoleic acid, mg	860	5800
Carbohydrate, g	10.9	73
% of total calories §	43.5	43.5
Water, g	134	910
Minerals		
Calcium, mg (mEq)	78 (3.9)	530 (27)
Phosphorus, mg	53	360
Magnesium, mg	8	54
Iron, mg	1.8* (0.7)**	12.2* (4.7)**
Zinc, mg	1	6.8
Manganese, mcg	15	101
Copper, mcg	75	510
Molybdenum, mcg	0	0
Iodine, mcg	10	68
Selenium, mcg	2.8	18.9
Sodium, mg (mEq)	27 (1.17)	183 (8)
Potassium, mg (mEq)	108 (2.8)	730 (18.7)
Chloride, mg (mEq)	63 (1.77)	430 (12.1)
Vitamins		
Vitamin A, IU	300	2000
Vitamin D, IU	60	410
Vitamin E, IU	2	13.5
Vitamin K, mcg	8	54
Thiamine (B_1), mcg	80	540
Riboflavin (B_2), mcg	140	950
Vitamin B_6, mcg	60	410
Vitamin B_{12}, mcg	0.3	2
Niacin, mcg	1000	6800
Folic acid (Folacin), mcg	16	108
Pantothenic acid, mcg	500	3400
Biotin, mcg	3	20
Vitamin C (Ascorbic acid), mg	12	81
Choline, mg	12	81
Inositol, mg	6	41
L-Carnitine, mg	2	13.5
Taurine, mg	6	41
Nucleotide fortification, mg	4.2	28.4
Renal Solute Load, mOsm	19.2	132
Osmolality, mOsm/kg water	300	300
Osmolarity, mOsm/L	270	270

* The addition of iron to this formula conforms to the recommendation of the Committee on Nutrition of the American Academy of Pediatrics.

** Supplemental iron should be considered.

† Protein Source: Reduced minerals whey and nonfat milk

†† Fat Source: Palm olein, soy, coconut and high-oleic sunflower oils

§ Carbohydrate Source: Lactose

NUTRITIONALS

Enfamil® 24

Enfamil® 24** and Enfamil® 24 with Iron*
24 Cal/fl oz

Nutrient	per 100 Cal	per Liter
Energy, Cal	100	812
Volume, mL	123	1000
Protein, g	2.1	17.4
% of total calories †	8.5	8.5
Fat, g	5.3	43
% of total calories ††	48	48
Linoleic acid, mg	860	7000
Carbohydrate, g	10.9	88
% of total calories §	43.5	43.5
Water, g	109	880
Minerals		
Calcium, mg (mEq)	78.7 (3.9)	630 (32)
Phosphorus, mg	53	430
Magnesium, mg	8	65
Iron, mg	1.8* (0.7)**	14.6* (5.7)**
Zinc, mg	1	8.1
Manganese, mcg	15	122
Copper, mcg	75	610
Molybdenum, mcg	0	0
Iodine, mcg	10	81
Selenium, mcg	2.8	23
Sodium, mg (mEq)	27 (1.2)	220 (9.6)
Potassium, mg (mEq)	108 (2.8)	880 (23)
Chloride, mg (mEq)	63 (1.8)	510 (14.4)
Vitamins		
Vitamin A, IU	300	2400
Vitamin D, IU	60	490
Vitamin E, IU	2	16.2
Vitamin K, mcg	8	65
Thiamine (B_1), mcg	80	650
Riboflavin (B_2), mcg	140	1140
Vitamin B_6, mcg	60	490
Vitamin B_{12}, mcg	0.3	2.4
Niacin, mcg	1000	8100
Folic acid (Folacin), mcg	16	130
Pantothenic acid, mcg	500	4100
Biotin, mcg	3	24
Vitamin C (Ascorbic acid), mg	12	97
Choline, mg	12	97
Inositol, mg	6	49
L-Carnitine, mg	2	16.2
Taurine, mg	0	0
Nucleotide fortification, mg	4.2	33.8
Renal Solute Load, mOsm	19.2	158
Osmolality, mOsm/kg water	360	360
Osmolarity, mOsm/L	320	320

* The addition of iron to this formula conforms to the recommendation of the Committee on Nutrition of the American Academy of Pediatrics.

** Supplemental iron should be considered.

† Protein Source: Reduced minerals whey and nonfat milk

†† Fat Source: Palm olein, soy, coconut and high-oleic sunflower oils

§ Carbohydrate Source: Lactose

Enfamil® AR® 20

Enfamil® AR® 20
20 Cal/fl oz

Nutrient	per 100 Cal	per Liter
Energy, Cal	100	812
Volume, mL	148	1000
Protein, g	2.5	16.9
% of total calories †	10	10
Fat, g	5.1	35
% of total calories ††	46	46
Linoleic acid, mg	860	5800
Carbohydrate, g	11	74
% of total calories §	44	44
Water, g	133	900
Minerals		
Calcium, mg (mEq)	78 (3.9)	530 (27)
Phosphorus, mg	53	360
Magnesium, mg	8	54
Iron, mg	1.8* (0.7)**	12.2* (5.7)**
Zinc, mg	1.0	6.8
Manganese, mcg	15	101
Copper, mcg	75	510
Molybdenum, mcg	0	0
Iodine, mcg	10	68
Selenium, mcg	2.8	18.9
Sodium, mg (mEq)	40 (1.7)	270 (11.7)
Potassium, mg (mEq)	108 (2.8)	730 (18.9)
Chloride, mg (mEq)	75 (2.1)	510 (14.4)
Vitamins		
Vitamin A, IU	300	2000
Vitamin D, IU	60	410
Vitamin E, IU	2	13.5
Vitamin K, mcg	8	54
Thiamine (B_1), mcg	80	540
Riboflavin (B_2), mcg	140	950
Vitamin B_6, mcg	60	410
Vitamin B_{12}, mcg	0.3	2
Niacin, mcg	1000	6800
Folic acid (Folacin), mcg	16	108
Pantothenic acid, mcg	500	3400
Biotin, mcg	3	20
Vitamin C (Ascorbic acid), mg	12	81
Choline, mg	12	81
Inositol, mg	6	41
L-Carnitine, mg	2	13.5
Taurine, mg	6	41
Nucleotide fortification, mg	0	0
Renal Solute Load, mOsm	22	151
Osmolality, mOsm/kg water	240	240
Osmolarity, mOsm/L	220	220

* The addition of iron to this formula conforms to the recommendation of the Committee on Nutrition of the American Academy of Pediatrics.

** Low-Iron: Additional iron should be supplied from other sources.

† Protein Source: Nonfat milk

†† Fat Source: Palm olein, soy, coconut and high-oleic sunflower oils

§ Carbohydrate Source: Lactose, rice starch, maltodextrin

NUTRITIONALS

Enfamil® LactoFree® Lipil® 20

20 Cal/fl oz

Nutrient	per 100 Cal	per Liter
Energy, Cal	100	676
Volume, mL	148	1000
Protein, g	2.10	14.30
% of total calories [†]	8.5	8.5
Fat, g	5.30	36
% of total calories [††]	48	48
Linoleic acid, mg	860	5800
Carbohydrate, g	10.90	74
% of total calories [§]	43	43
Water, g	134	910
Minerals		
Calcium, mg (mEq)	82 (4.1)	550 (28)
Phosphorus, mg	55	370
Magnesium, mg	8	54
Iron, mg	1.8*	12.2*
Zinc, mg	1	6.8
Manganese, mcg	15	101
Copper, mcg	75	510
Molybdenum, mcg	0	0
Iodine, mcg	15	101
Selenium, mcg	2.8	18.9
Sodium, mg (mEq)	30 (1.3)	200 (8.7)
Potassium, mg (mEq)	110 (2.8)	740 (18.9)
Chloride, mg (mEq)	67 (1.9)	450 (12.7)
Vitamins		
Vitamin A, IU	300	2000
Vitamin D, IU	60	410
Vitamin E, IU	2	13.5
Vitamin K, mcg	8	54
Thiamine (B_1), mcg	80	540
Riboflavin (B_2), mcg	140	950
Vitamin B_6, mcg	60	410
Vitamin B_{12}, mcg	0.3	2
Niacin, mcg	1000	6800
Folic acid (Folacin), mcg	16	108
Pantothenic acid, mcg	500	3400
Biotin, mcg	3	20
Vitamin C (Ascorbic acid), mg	12	81
Choline, mg	12	81
Inositol, mg	6	115
L-Carnitine, mg	2	13.5
Taurine, mg	6	41
Nucleotide fortification, mg	4.2	28
Renal Solute Load, mOsm	20	132
Osmolality, mOsm/kg water	200	200
Osmolarity, mOsm/L	182	182

* The addition of iron to this formula conforms to the recommendation of the Committee on Nutrition of the American Academy of Pediatrics.

† Protein Source: Milk protein isolate

†† Fat Source: Palm olein, soy, coconut, high-oleic sunflower oils, and M. alpina[1] and C. codinium[2] oils.

[1] A source of arachidonic acid (ARA) ARA- 0.64% of fatty acids (w/w).

[2] A source of docosahexaenoic acid (DHA) DHA- 0.32% of fatty acids (w/w).

§ Carbohydrate Source: Corn syrup solids

Enfamil® ProSobee® 20

20 Cal/fl oz

Nutrient	per 100 Cal	per Liter
Energy, Cal	100	676
Volume, mL	148	1000
Protein, g	2.50	17.30
% of total calories †	10	10
Fat, g	5.30	37
% of total calories ††	48	48
Linoleic acid, mg	860	5760
Carbohydrate, g	10.60	73
% of total calories §	42	42
Water, g	134	910
Minerals		
Calcium, mg (mEq)	105 (5.3)	710 (36)
Phosphorus, mg	83	560
Magnesium, mg	11	74
Iron, mg	1.8*	12.2*
Zinc, mg	1.2	8.1
Manganese, mcg	25	169
Copper, mcg	75	510
Molybdenum, mcg	0	0
Iodine, mcg	15	101
Selenium, mcg	2.8	18.9
Sodium, mg (mEq)	36 (1.6)	240 (10.4)
Potassium, mg (mEq)	120 (3.1)	810 (21)
Chloride, mg (mEq)	80 (2.3)	540 (15.2)
Vitamins		
Vitamin A, IU	300	2000
Vitamin D, IU	60	410
Vitamin E, IU	2	13.5
Vitamin K, mcg	8	54
Thiamine (B_1), mcg	80	540
Riboflavin (B_2), mcg	90	610
Vitamin B_6, mcg	60	410
Vitamin B_{12}, mcg	0.3	2
Niacin, mcg	1000	6800
Folic acid (Folacin), mcg	16	108
Pantothenic acid, mcg	500	3400
Biotin, mcg	3	20
Vitamin C (Ascorbic acid), mg	12	81
Choline, mg	12	81
Inositol, mg	6	41
L-Carnitine, mg	2	13.5
Taurine, mg	6	41
Nucleotide fortification, mg	0	0
Renal Solute Load, mOsm	24	164
Osmolality, mOsm/kg water	200	200
Osmolarity, mOsm/L	182	182

* The addition of iron to this formula conforms to the recommendation of the Committee on Nutrition of the American Academy of Pediatrics.

† Protein Source: Soy protein isolate

†† Fat Source: Palm olein, soy, coconut, high-oleic sunflower oils

§ Carbohydrate Source: Corn syrup solids

NUTRITIONALS

Enfamil® ProSobee® LIPIL® 20

20 Cal/fl oz

Nutrient	per 100 Cal	per Liter
Energy, Cal	100	676
Volume, mL	148	1000
Protein, g	205	16.9
% of total calories [†]	10	10
Fat, g	5.3	36
% of total calories [††]	48	48
Linoleic acid, mg	860	5800
Carbohydrate, g	10.6	72
% of total calories [§]	42	42
Water, g	133	900
Minerals		
Calcium, mg (mEq)	105 (5.3)	710 (36)
Phosphorus, mg	83	560
Magnesium, mg	11	74
Iron, mg	1.8	12.2
Zinc, mg	1.2	8.1
Manganese, mcg	25	169
Copper, mcg	75	510
Molybdenum, mcg		
Iodine, mcg	15	101
Selenium, mcg	2.8	18.9
Sodium, mg (mEq)	36 (1.6)	240 (10.4)
Potassium, mg (mEq)	120 (3.1)	810 (21)
Chloride, mg (mEq)	80 (2.3)	540 (15.2)
Vitamins		
Vitamin A, IU	300	2000
Vitamin D, IU	60	410
Vitamin E, IU	2	13.5
Vitamin K, mcg	8	54
Thiamine (B_1), mcg	80	540
Riboflavin (B_2), mcg	90	610
Vitamin B_6, mcg	60	410
Vitamin B_{12}, mcg	0.3	2
Niacin, mcg	1000	6800
Folic acid (Folacin), mcg	16	108
Pantothenic acid, mcg	500	3400
Biotin, mcg	3	20
Vitamin C (Ascorbic acid), mg	12	81
Choline, mg	12	81
Inositol, mg	6	81
L-Carnitine, mg	2	13.5
Taurine, mg	6	41
Nucleotide fortification, mg	0	0
Renal Solute Load, mOsm	24	161
Osmolality, mOsm/kg water	200	200
Osmolarity, mOsm/L	180	180

[†] Protein Source: Soy protein isolate

[††] Fat Source: Palm olein, soy, coconut, high-oleic sunflower, and M. alpina[1] and C. codinium[2] oils
[1] A source of arachidonic acid (ARA) ARA- 0.64% of fatty acids (w/w).
[2] A source of docosahexaenoic acid (DHA) DHA- 0.32% of fatty acids (w/w).

[§] Carbohydrate Source: Corn syrup solids

Enfamil® Nutramigen® 20

20 Cal/fl oz

Nutrient	per 100 Cal	per Liter
Energy, Cal	100	676
Volume, mL	148	1000
Protein, g	2.80	19
% of total calories [†]	11	11
Fat, g	5	34
% of total calories [††]	45	45
Linoleic acid, mg	820	5490
Carbohydrate, g	11	74
% of total calories [§]	44	44
Water, g	134	910
Minerals		
Calcium, mg (mEq)	94 (4.7)	640 (32)
Phosphorus, mg	63	430
Magnesium, mg	11	74
Iron, mg	1.8*	12.2*
Zinc, mg	1	6.8
Manganese, mcg	25	169
Copper, mcg	75	510
Molybdenum, mcg	0	0
Iodine, mcg	15	101
Selenium, mcg	2.8	18.9
Sodium, mg (mEq)	47 (2.0)	320 (13.8)
Potassium, mg (mEq)	110 (2.8)	740 (18.9)
Chloride, mg (mEq)	86 (2.4)	580 (16.3)
Vitamins		
Vitamin A, IU	300	2000
Vitamin D, IU	50	340
Vitamin E, IU	2	13.5
Vitamin K, mcg	8	54
Thiamine (B_1), mcg	80	540
Riboflavin (B_2), mcg	90	610
Vitamin B_6, mcg	60	410
Vitamin B_{12}, mcg	0.3	2
Niacin, mcg	1000	6800
Folic acid (Folacin), mcg	16	108
Pantothenic acid, mcg	500	3400
Biotin, mcg	3	20
Vitamin C (Ascorbic acid), mg	12	81
Choline, mg	12	81
Inositol, mg	17	115
L-Carnitine, mg	2	13.5
Taurine, mg	6	41
Nucleotide fortification, mg	0	0
Renal Solute Load, mOsm	25	173
Osmolality, mOsm/kg water	320	320
Osmolarity, mOsm/L	290	290

* The addition of iron to this formula conforms to the recommendation of the Committee on Nutrition of the American Academy of Pediatrics.

† Protein Source: Casein hydrolysate

†† Fat Source: Palm olein, soy, coconut, high-oleic sunflower oils

§ Carbohydrate Source: Corn syrup solids, modified corn starch

NUTRITIONALS

Enfamil® Pregestimil® 20

20 Cal/fl oz

Nutrient	per 100 Cal	per Liter
Energy, Cal	100	676
Volume, mL	148	1000
Protein, g	2.80	19
% of total calories [†]	11	11
Fat, g	5.60	38
% of total calories [††]	48	48
Linoleic acid, mg	940	6300
Carbohydrate, g	10.20	69
% of total calories [§]	41	41
Water, g	133	900
Minerals		
Calcium, mg (mEq)	115 (5.8)	780 (39.3)
Phosphorus, mg	75	510
Magnesium, mg	12	81
Iron, mg	1.88*	12.7*
Zinc, mg	1.1	7.4
Manganese, mcg	30	200
Copper, mcg	110	740
Molybdenum, mcg	0	0
Iodine, mcg	11	74
Selenium, mcg	2.8	18.9
Sodium, mg (mEq)	47 (2.0)	320 (13.9)
Potassium, mg (mEq)	110 (2.8)	740 (18.9)
Chloride, mg (mEq)	86 (2.4)	580 (16.3)
Vitamins		
Vitamin A, IU	380	2600
Vitamin D, IU	50	340
Vitamin E, IU	3.8	26
Vitamin K, mcg	18.8	127
Thiamine (B_1), mcg	80	540
Riboflavin (B_2), mcg	90	610
Vitamin B_6, mcg	60	410
Vitamin B_{12}, mcg	0.3	2
Niacin, mcg	1000	6800
Folic acid (Folacin), mcg	16	108
Pantothenic acid, mcg	500	3400
Biotin, mcg	3	20
Vitamin C (Ascorbic acid), mg	12	81
Choline, mg	12	81
Inositol, mg	17	115
L-Carnitine, mg	2	13.5
Taurine, mg	6	41
Nucleotide fortification, mg	0	0
Renal Solute Load, mOsm	26	174
Osmolality, mOsm/kg water	280	280
Osmolarity, mOsm/L	250	250

* The addition of iron to this formula conforms to the recommendation of the Committee on Nutrition of the American Academy of Pediatrics.

† Protein Source: Casein hydrolysate

†† Fat Source: Medium-chain triglycerides, soy oil, and high-oleic safflower oils

§ Carbohydrate Source: Corn syrup solids and modified cornstarch

24 Cal/fl oz

Nutrient	per 100 Cal	per Liter
Energy, Cal	100	812
Volume, mL	123	1000
Protein, g	2.80	23
% of total calories †	11	11
Fat, g	5.60	45
% of total calories ††	48	48
Linoleic acid, mg	940	7600
Carbohydrate, g	10.20	83
% of total calories §	41	41
Water, g	108	880
Minerals		
Calcium, mg (mEq)	115 (5.8)	930 (47)
Phosphorus, mg	75	610
Magnesium, mg	12	97
Iron, mg	1.88*	15.3*
Zinc, mg	1.1	8.9
Manganese, mcg	30	240
Copper, mcg	110	890
Molybdenum, mcg	0	0
Iodine, mcg	11	89
Selenium, mcg	2.8	23
Sodium, mg (mEq)	47 (2.0)	380 (16.5)
Potassium, mg (mEq)	110 (2.8)	890 (23)
Chloride, mg (mEq)	86 (2.4)	700 (20)
Vitamins		
Vitamin A, IU	380	3100
Vitamin D, IU	50	410
Vitamin E, IU	3.8	31
Vitamin K, mcg	18.8	153
Thiamine (B_1), mcg	80	650
Riboflavin (B_2), mcg	90	730
Vitamin B_6, mcg	60	490
Vitamin B_{12}, mcg	0.3	2.4
Niacin, mcg	1000	8100
Folic acid (Folacin), mcg	16	130
Pantothenic acid, mcg	500	4100
Biotin, mcg	3	24
Vitamin C (Ascorbic acid), mg	12	97
Choline, mg	12	97
Inositol, mg	17	138
L-Carnitine, mg	2	16.2
Taurine, mg	6	49
Nucleotide fortification, mg	0	0
Renal Solute Load, mOsm	26	210
Osmolality, mOsm/kg water	320	320
Osmolarity, mOsm/L	280	280

 * The addition of iron to this formula conforms to the recommendation of the Committee on Nutrition of the American Academy of Pediatrics.

 † Protein Source: Casein hydrolysate

 †† Fat Source: Medium-chain triglycerides, soy oil, and high-oleic safflower oils

 § Carbohydrate Source: Corn syrup solids and modified cornstarch

NUTRITIONALS

Enfamil® Pregestimil® Powder

When mixed as normal dilution, 20 Cal/fl oz

Nutrient	per 100 Cal	per Liter
Energy, Cal	100	676
Volume, mL	148	1000
Protein, g	2.80	19
% of total calories [†]	11	11
Fat, g	5.60	38
% of total calories [††]	48	48
Linoleic acid, mg	1040	7000
Carbohydrate, g	10.2	69
% of total calories [§]	41	41
Water, g	134	910
Minerals		
Calcium, mg (mEq)	115	740
Phosphorus, mg	75	510
Magnesium, mg	11	74
Iron, mg	1.8*	12.2*
Zinc, mg	1	6.8
Manganese, mcg	25	169
Copper, mcg	75	510
Molybdenum, mcg	0	0
Iodine, mcg	15	101
Selenium, mcg	2.8	18.9
Sodium, mg (mEq)	47	320
Potassium, mg (mEq)	110	740
Chloride, mg (mEq)	86	580
Vitamins		
Vitamin A, IU	380	2600
Vitamin D, IU	50	340
Vitamin E, IU	4	27
Vitamin K, mcg	12	81
Thiamine (B_1), mcg	80	540
Riboflavin (B_2), mcg	90	610
Vitamin B_6, mcg	60	410
Vitamin B_{12}, mcg	0.3	2
Niacin, mcg	1000	680
Folic acid (Folacin), mcg	16	108
Pantothenic acid, mcg	500	3400
Biotin, mcg	3	20
Vitamin C (Ascorbic acid), mg	12	81
Choline, mg	12	81
Inositol, mg	17	115
L-Carnitine, mg	2	13.5
Taurine, mg	6	41
Nucleotide fortification, mg	0	0
Renal Solute Load, mOsm	26	176
Osmolality, mOsm/kg water	340	340
Osmolarity, mOsm/L	310	310

* The addition of iron to this formula conforms to the recommendation of the Committee on Nutrition of the American Academy of Pediatrics.

† Protein Source: Casein hydrolysate

†† Fat Source: Medium-chain triglycerides, soy oil, and high-oleic safflower oils

§ Carbohydrate Source: Corn syrup solids, starch, and dextrose

SMA® 20* and SMA Lo-Iron 20**
20 Cal/fl oz

Nutrient	per 100 Cal	per Liter
Energy, Cal	100	676
Volume, mL	148	1000
Protein, g	2.20	15
% of total calories †	8.90	8.90
Fat, g	5.30	36
% of total calories ††	48.20	48.20
Linoleic acid, mg	500	3300
Carbohydrate, g	10.60	72
% of total calories §	42.90	42.90
Water, g	134	904
Minerals		
Calcium, mg (mEq)	63 (3.1)	420 (20.9)
Phosphorus, mg	42	280
Magnesium, mg	7	45
Iron, mg	1.8* (0.2)**	12* (1.5)**
Zinc, mg	0.8	5
Manganese, mcg	15	100
Copper, mcg	70	470
Molybdenum, mcg	0	0
Iodine, mcg	9	60
Selenium, mcg	0	0
Sodium, mg (mEq)	22 (1.0)	150 (6.5)
Potassium, mg (mEq)	83 (2.1)	560 (14.3)
Chloride, mg (mEq)	55.5 (1.6)	375 (10.6)
Vitamins		
Vitamin A, IU	300	2000
Vitamin D, IU	60	400
Vitamin E, IU	1.5	10
Vitamin K, mcg	8	55
Thiamine (B_1), mcg	100	670
Riboflavin (B_2), mcg	150	1000
Vitamin B_6, mcg	62.5	420
Vitamin B_{12}, mcg	0.15	1.0
Niacin, mcg	750	5000
Folic acid (Folacin), mcg	7.5	50
Pantothenic acid, mcg	315	2100
Biotin, mcg	2.2	15
Vitamin C (Ascorbic acid), mg	8.5	55
Choline, mg	15	100
Inositol, mg	4.1	27
L-Carnitine, mg	0	0
Taurine, mg	0	0
Nucleotide fortification, mg	0	0
Renal Solute Load, mOsm	13.5	91.4
Osmolality, mOsm/kg water	321	321
Osmolarity, mOsm/L	290	290

* With iron: The addition of iron to this formula conforms to the recommendation of the Committee on Nutrition of the American Academy of Pediatrics.

** Low-Iron: Additional iron should be supplied from other sources.

† Protein Source: Casein

†† Fat Source: Palm, high oleic safflower or sunflower, coconut and soybean oils

§ Carbohydrate Source: Corn syrup solids and lactose

Nursoy® 20

20 Cal/fl oz

Nutrient	per 100 Cal	per Liter
Energy, Cal	100	672
Volume, mL	148	1000
Protein, g	2.70	18
% of total calories [†]	11	11
Fat, g	5.30	36
% of total calories [††]	48	48
Linoleic acid, mg	500	3300
Carbohydrate, g	10.20	69
% of total calories [§]	41	41
Water, g	134	904
Minerals		
Calcium, mg (mEq)	90 (4.5)	600 (29.9)
Phosphorus, mg	63	420
Magnesium, mg	10	67
Iron, mg	1.8*	12*
Zinc, mg	0.80	5
Manganese, mcg	30	200
Copper, mcg	70	470
Iodine, mcg	9	60
Selenium, mcg	N/A	N/A
Sodium, mg (mEq)	30 (1.3)	200 (8.7)
Potassium, mg (mEq)	105 (2.7)	700 (17.9)
Chloride, mg (mEq)	56 (1.6)	375 (10.6)
Vitamins		
Vitamin A, IU	300	2000
Vitamin D, IU	60	400
Vitamin E, IU	1.5	10
Vitamin K, mcg	8.25	55
Thiamine (B_1), mcg	100	670
Riboflavin (B_2), mcg	150	1000
Vitamin B_6, mcg	62.50	420
Vitamin B_{12}, mcg	0.30	2
Niacin, mcg	750	5000
Folic acid (Folacin), mcg	7.50	50
Pantothenic acid, mcg	450	3000
Biotin, mcg	5.50	35
Vitamin C (Ascorbic acid), mg	8.30	55
Choline, mg	13	85
Inositol, mg	4.10	27
Renal Solute Load, mOsm	18	109.20
Osmolality, mOsm/kg water	245	245
Osmolarity, mOsm/L	220	220

* The addition of iron to this formula conforms to the recommendation of the Committee on Nutrition of the American Academy of Pediatrics.

† Protein Source: Soy protein isolate and L-methionine

†† Fat Source: Palm, high oleic safflower or sunflower, coconut and soybean oils

§ Carbohydrate Source: Corn syrup solids and sucrose

Neocate® With Iron 20 Infant Formula *
20 Cal/fl oz

Nutrient	per 100 Cal	per Liter
Energy, Cal	100	676
Volume, mL	148	1000
Protein, g	3.1	20.9
% of total calories [†]	12	11
Fat, g	4.5	30
% of total calories [††]	41	48
Linoleic acid, mg	677	4574
Carbohydrate, g	11.7	79
% of total calories [§]	47	41
Water, g	131	904
Minerals		
Calcium, mg (mEq)	124 (6.2)	838 (41.9)
Phosphorus, mg	93.1	629
Magnesium, mg	12.4	84
Iron, mg	1.85*	12.5*
Zinc, mg	1.66	11
Manganese, mcg	90	608
Copper, mcg	124	838
Iodine, mcg	15.4	104
Molybdenum, mcg	4.75	32
Selenium, mcg	3.73	25
Sodium, mg (mEq)	37.3 (1.6)	252 (11)
Potassium, mg (mEq)	155.1 (4)	1048 (27)
Chloride, mg (mEq)	77.2 (2.2)	522 (14.9)
Vitamins		
Vitamin A, IU	409	2764
Vitamin D, IU	87	588
Vitamin E, IU	1.14	7.7
Vitamin K, mcg	8.79	59.4
Thiamine (B_1), mcg	92.6	626
Riboflavin (B_2), mcg	137.8	931
Vitamin B_6, mcg	123.5	834
Vitamin B_{12}, mcg	0.17	1.15
Niacin, mcg	1544	10432
Folic acid (Folacin), mcg	10.2	68.9
Pantothenic acid, mcg	620	4189
Biotin, mcg	3.1	20.9
Vitamin C (Ascorbic acid), mg	9.26	62.6
Choline, mg	13.1	89
Inositol, mg	23.3	157
Renal Solute Load, mOsm	18	122
Osmolality, mOsm/kg water	342	342
Osmolarity, mOsm/L	296	296

* The addition of iron to this formula conforms to the recommendation of the Committee on Nutrition of the American Academy of Pediatrics.

† Protein Source: L-amino acids

†† Fat Source: Soy oil, coconut oil, and medium-chain triglycerides

§ Carbohydrate Source: Corn syrup solids

NUTRITIONALS

Medium Chain Triglyceride Oil

Medium chain triglycerides (MCT) are lipid fractions of coconut oil consisting of triglycerides with chain lengths of 6 to 10 carbons. Used to supplement orally, or added to tube feeding formulas. Mixes easily with enteral formulas.

Nutrient	per mL	per 15 mL (1 Tbsp)	per 89 mL (3 fl oz)
Calories	7.7	115	685.3
Protein, g	0	0	0
Fat, g	0.94	14	44.5
Carbohydrate, g	0	0	0
Water	0	0	0
Linoleic Acid, g	0.367	5.50	32.63

Fatty Acid Distribution

Shorter than carbon 8	<6%
Caprylic C8:0	67%
Capric C10:0	23%
Longer than C10:0	<4%

Osmolality (mOsm/kg water): Not Available

Supplied: 1 quart glass bottles.

Ingredients: Medium chain tryglycerides.

For oral use only. Do not give parenterally (IV). Use within 60 to 90 days after a bottle is opened. Do not store in plastic container. MCT may break or soften plastic containers.

Microlipid is a 50% safflower oil fat emulsion with 4.5 Cal/mL. Used to supplement orally, or added to tube feeding formulas. Mixes easily with enteral formulas.

Nutrient	per mL	per 15 mL (1 Tbsp)	per 89 mL (3 fl oz)
Energy, Cal	4.5	67.5	400
Protein, g	0	0	0
Fat, g	0.5	7.5	44
Carbohydrate, g	0	0.04	0
Water	0.45	6.7	40
Linoleic Acid, g	0.4	5.9	35

Fatty Acid Distribution

Polyunsaturated	78%
Monounsaturated	12%
Saturated	10%
PUFA:SFA	8:1

Osmolality (mOsm/kg water): Not available

Supplied: 48 three ounce bottles per case.

Ingredients: Safflower oil, water, polyglycerol esters of fatty acids, soy lecithin, xanthan gum, ascorbic acid.

For oral use only. Do not give parenterally (IV). Shake well before opening. Opened product should be recapped, refrigerated, and discarded after 5 days. Store unopened bottles at room temperature. Protect from freezing.

Fat Emulsion

Dose and Administration

Begin at 0.5 g/kg per day IV increasing by 0.5 g/kg per day to a maximum of 3 g/kg per day. Infusion rate should not exceed 0.15 g/kg per hour. 24 hour infusion times are preferred. Essential fatty acid deficiency maybe prevented with 0.5 to 1 g/kg per day.

	Intralipid® 20%	Products Liposyn II® 20%	Liposyn III® 20%
Oils (%)			
Safflower	0	10	0
Soybean	20	10	20
Fatty Acid Content (%)			
Linoleic	50	65.8	54.5
Oleic	26	17.7	22.4
Palmitic	10	8.8	10.5
Linolenic	9	4.2	8.3
Stearic	3.5	3.4	4.2
Egg yolk			
phospholipid (%)	1.2	1.2	1.2
Glycerine (%)	2.25	2.5	2.5
Calories per mL	2	2	2
Osmolarity (mOsm/L)	260	258	292

Uses

Parenteral nutrition source of calories and essential fatty acids.

Monitoring

Monitor serum triglycerides (<200 mg/dL), liver function test, platelet count, albumin, glucose, and bilirubin.

Adverse Effects/Precautions

Hypertriglyceridemia and hyperglycemia. The minimum dose should be used in infants with severe hyperbilirubinemia, sepsis, or severe pulmonary dysfunction. Extravasation may cause tissue inflammation and necrosis.

Pharmacology

Intravenous fat emulsions are high caloric (2 Cal/mL) isotonic emulsions of either soybean or safflower oil. Fat particle size is between 0.4 and 0.5 microns in diameter, similar to endogenous chylomicrons. Clearance is via endogenous lipoprotein lipase activity, which is limited in very premature (<28 weeks gestation) and infected infants. Twenty percent emulsions are preferred due to lower total phospholipid and liposome content per gram of triglyceride. Ten percent emulsions have been associated with hypercholesterolemia and hyperphospholipidemia. Destabilization of lipid emulsions (flocculation and separation) may occur when they are co-infused with Dex/AA solutions containing calcium and high concentrations (> 1 U/mL) of heparin. This risk may be decreased by 1) minimizing the contact time; 2) using low (≤ 1 U/mL) concentrations of heparin; and 3) adding a multivitamin preparation to the Dex/AA solution.

Special Considerations/Preparation

Liposyn® and Intralipid® are available in 50, 100, 250, and 500 mL bottles. Store at room temperature.

Do not freeze.

Use within 24 hours when dispensed in syringes.

Solution compatibility: D_5W, $D_{10}W$, and NS.

Terminal injection site compatibility: Dex/AA. Aminophylline, ampicillin, aztreonam, bumetanide, caffeine citrate, calcium chloride, calcium gluconate, cefazolin, cefotaxime, cefoxitin, ceftazidime, ceftriaxone, chloramphenicol, cimetidine, clindamycin, dexamethasone, digoxin, dobutamine, dopamine, enalaprilat, erythromycin lactobionate, famotidine, fentanyl, fluconazole, furosemide, gentamicin, heparin (≤ 1 U/mL), hydrocortisone, imipenem/cilastatin, insulin, isoproterenol, lidocaine, meropenem, metoclopramide, metronidazole, morphine, nafcillin, netilmicin, norepinephrine, oxacillin, penicillin G, piperacillin, piperacillin/tazobactam, potassium chloride, pyridoxine, ranitidine, sodium bicarbonate, sodium nitroprusside, ticarcillin, ticarcillin/clavulanate, tobramycin, trimethoprim/sulfamethoxazole, vancomycin, and zidovudine.

Incompatibility: Acyclovir, amikacin, amphotericin B, lorazepam, magnesium chloride, midazolam, pentobarbital, phenobarbital, and phenytoin.

Selected References

♦ Silvers KM, Darlow BA, Winterbourn CC: Pharmacologic levels of heparin do not destabilize neonatal parenteral nutrition. *J Parenter Enteral Nutr* 1998;22:311-314.

♦ Lipsky CL, Spear ML: Recent advances in parenteral nutrition. *Clin Perinatol* 1995;22:141-155.

♦ Haumont D, Deckelbaum RJ, Richelle M, Dahlan W, et al: Plasma lipid and plasma lipoprotein concentration in low birth weight infants given parenteral nutrition with twenty or ten percent lipid emulsion. *J Pediatr* 1989;115:787-93.

♦ Brans YW, Andrews DS, Carrillo DW, Dutton EP, et al: Tolerance of fat emulsions in very-low-birth-weight neonates. *Am J Dis Child* 1988;142:145-152.

♦ Kao LC, Cheng MH, Warburton D: Triglycerides, free fatty acids, free fatty acids/albumin molar ratio, and cholesterol levels in serum of neonates receiving long-term lipid infusions: Controlled trial of continuous and intermittent regimens. *J Pediatr* 1984;104:429-435.

Added 3/99
Compatibilities updated 3/2001

NUTRITIONALS

RECOMMENDED CONCENTRATIONS FOR ADMINISTRATION

Generic Name	Route	Units	Available	Low	Default	High
				Concentration		
Acyclovir	IV	mg/mL	50*	5	7	10
Amikacin	IV	mg/mL	50*	5	10	10
Amikacin	IM	mg/mL	50	50	50	50
Amphotericin B	IV	mg/mL	5*	0.05	0.1	0.1
Amphotericin B Lipid Complex	IV	mg/mL	5*	0.5	1	2
Amphotericin B Liposome	IV	mg/mL	4*	0.5	1	2
Ampicillin	IV	mg/mL	125 or 250*	50	100	100
Ampicillin	IM	mg/mL	250	125	250	250
Aztreonam	IV	mg/mL	50	25	50	50
Aztreonam	IM	mg/mL	125 or 250	125	250	250
Cefepime	IV	mg/mL	100	100	100	100
Cefepime	IM	mg/mL	280	160	280	280
Cefazolin	IV	mg/mL	225*	75	100	125
Cefazolin	IM	mg/mL	225	225	225	225
Cefotaxime	IV	mg/mL	50 or 100	50	100	100
Cefotaxime	IM	mg/mL	230 or 300	230	300	300
Cefoxitin	IV	mg/mL	100*	40	100	100
Cefoxitin	IM	mg/mL	400*	100	200	400
Ceftazidime	IV	mg/mL	100 or 200	50	100	200
Ceftazidime	IM	mg/mL	280	100	280	280
Ceftriaxone	IV	mg/mL	40 or 100*	10	40	40
Ceftriaxone	IM	mg/mL	250	250	250	250
Chloramphenicol	IV	mg/mL	100 *	20	50	100
Clindamycin	IV	mg/mL	150*	6	6	18
Erythromycin Lactobionate	IV	mg/mL	50*	2.5	5	5
Fluconazole	IV	mg/mL	2	2	2	2
Gentamicin	IV	mg/mL	10	10	10	10
Gentamicin	IM	mg/mL	40	20	40	40
Imipenem - Cilastatin	IV	mg/mL	2.5 or 5	2.5	5	5
Linezolid	IV	mg/mL	2	2	2	2
Meropenem	IV	mg/mL	50	25	50	50
Metronidazole	IV	mg/mL	5	5	5	5
Nafcillin	IV	mg/mL	250*	25	40	40
Netilmicin	IV	mg/mL	100*	5	10	10
Netilmicin	IM	mg/mL	100*	20	40	40

* See Neofax Special Consideration/Preparation section for dilution details

Generic Name	Route	Units	Concentration			
			Available	Low	Default	High
Oxacillin	IV	mg/mL	167*	25	40	40
Penicillin G	IV	U/mL	500,000	100,000	500,000	500,000
Piperacillin	IV	mg/mL	200*	50	100	200
Piperacillin	IM	mg/mL	400	400	400	400
Piperacillin - Tazobactam	IV	mg/mL	200*	50	100	200
Rifampin	IV	mg/mL	60*	3	6	6
Ticarcillin - Clavulanate	IV	mg/mL	200	100	100	100
Tobramycin	IV	mg/mL	10	5	10	10
Tobramycin	IM	mg/mL	40	20	40	40
Vancomycin	IV	mg/mL	50*	5	5	5
Zidovudine (ZDV, AZT)	IV	mg/mL	10*	2	4	4

Biologicals

Generic Name	Route	Units	Concentration			
			Available	Low	Default	High
Epoetin alfa	IV	U/mL	2,000	2,000	2,000	2,000
Epoetin alfa	SC	U/mL	2,000	2,000	2,000	2,000

Cardiovascular

Generic Name	Route	Units	Concentration			
			Available	Low	Default	High
Adenosine	IV	mcg/mL	3,000*	200	300	3,000
Alteplase	IV	mg/mL	1	1	1	1
Amiodarone	IV	mg/mL	50*	2	2	2
Atropine	IV	mg/mL	0.4*	0.05	0.08	0.4
Digoxin	IV	mcg/mL	100*	10	20	100
Enalaprilat	IV	mcg/mL	1250*	25	25	50
Enoxaparin	IV	mg/mL	100	100	100	100
Hydralazine	IV	mg/mL	20*	0.5	1	2
Indomethacin	IV	mg/mL	0.5 to 1	0.5	0.5	1
Propranolol	IV	mg/mL	1*	0.1	1	1
Prostaglandin E1	IV	mcg/mL	500*	5	10	20
Sodium nitroprusside	IV	mg/mL	10*	0.2	0.2	0.2

* See Neofax Special Consideration/Preparation section for dilution details

Generic Name	Route	Units	Concentration			
			Available	Low	Default	High
Fentanyl	IV	mcg/mL	50	5	5	50
Fosphenytoin	IV	mg PE/mL	50	1.5	25	25
Fosphenytoin	IM	mg PE/mL	50	50	50	50
Lorazepam	IV	mg/mL	2 or 4*	0.2	0.4	2
Methadone	IV	mg/mL	10*	0.1	0.5	0.5
Midazolam	IV	mg/mL	1 or 5*	0.1	0.5	1
Morphine	IV	mg/mL	0.5 to 50*	0.1	0.5	1
Pancuronium	IV	mg/mL	1 or 2	0.5	1	2
Pentobarbital	IV	mg/mL	50*	5	5	50
Vecuronium	IV	mg/mL	1*	0.1	0.1	1

Diuretics

Generic Name	Route	Units	Concentration			
			Available	Low	Default	High
Bumetanide	IV	mg/mL	0.25*	0.1	0.125	0.25
Furosemide	IV	mg/mL	10*	2	5	10

* See Neofax Special Consideration/Preparation section for dilution details

Generic Name	Route	Units	Concentration Available	Low	Default	High
Cimetidine	IV	mg/mL	150*	6	15	15
Famotidine	IV	mg/mL	10*	1	1	2
Metoclopramide	IV	mg/mL	5*	0.1	0.1	1
Ranitidine	IV	mg/mL	1 and 25*	0.5	1	5

Respiratory

Generic Name	Route	Units	Concentration Available	Low	Default	High
Aminophylline	IV	mg/mL	25*	5	5	25
Dexamethasone	IV	mg/mL	4 to 24	0.1	0.2	1

Miscellaneous

Generic Name	Route	Units	Concentration Available	Low	Default	High
Hydrocortisone succinate	IV	mg/mL	125*	1	1	5
Insulin	IV	U/mL	100*	1	1	1
Levothyroxine (T4)	IV	mcg/mL	20 or 50*	20	20	50

* See Neofax Special Consideration/Preparation section for dilution details

NEWBORN METRIC CONVERSION TABLES

Newborn Metric Conversion Tables

Temperature in Fahrenheit (F) to Celsius (C)

°F	°C	°F	°C	°F	°C	°F	°C
95.0 · · · 35.0		98.0 · · · 36.7		101.0 · · · 38.3		104.0 · · · 40.0	
95.2 · · · 35.1		98.2 · · · 36.8		101.2 · · · 38.4		104.2 · · · 40.1	
95.4 · · · 35.2		98.4 · · · 36.9		101.4 · · · 38.6		104.4 · · · 40.2	
95.6 · · · 35.3		98.6 · · · 37.0		101.6 · · · 38.7		104.6 · · · 40.3	
95.8 · · · 35.4		98.8 · · · 37.1		101.8 · · · 38.8		104.8 · · · 40.4	
96.0 · · · 35.6		99.0 · · · 37.2		102.0 · · · 38.9		105.0 · · · 40.6	
96.2 · · · 35.7		99.2 · · · 37.3		102.2 · · · 39.0		105.2 · · · 40.7	
96.4 · · · 35.8		99.4 · · · 37.4		102.4 · · · 39.1		105.4 · · · 40.8	
96.6 · · · 35.9		99.6 · · · 37.6		102.6 · · · 39.2		105.6 · · · 40.9	
96.8 · · · 36.0		99.8 · · · 37.7		102.8 · · · 39.3		105.8 · · · 41.0	
97.0 · · · 36.1		100.0 · · · 37.8		103.0 · · · 39.4		106.0 · · · 41.1	
97.2 · · · 36.2		100.2 · · · 37.9		103.2 · · · 39.6		106.2 · · · 41.2	
97.4 · · · 36.3		100.4 · · · 38.0		103.4 · · · 39.7		106.4 · · · 41.3	
97.6 · · · 36.4		100.6 · · · 38.1		103.6 · · · 39.8		106.6 · · · 41.4	
97.8 · · · 36.6		100.8 · · · 38.2		103.8 · · · 39.9		106.8 · · · 41.6	

Note: $°C = (°F - 32) \times {}^5/_9$. Celsius temperature equivalents rounded to one decimal place by adding 0.1 when second decimal place is 5 or greater. The metric system replaces the term *Centigrade* with *Celsius* (name of the inventor of the scale).

$$BSA (m^2) = (0.05 \times kg) + 0.05$$

Weight (kg)	Approximate Surface Area (m^2)	Weight (kg)	Approximate Surface Area (m^2)
0.5 . . . . 0.075		4.25 . . . . . . 0.2625	
0.75 . . . . 0.0875		4.5 . . . . 0.275	
1 . . . . 0.1		4.75 . . . . . . 0.2875	
1.25 . . . . 0.1125		5 . . . . 0.3	
1.5 . . . . 0.125		5.25 . . . . . . 0.3125	
1.75 . . . . 0.1375		5.5 . . . . 0.325	
2 . . . . 0.15		5.75 . . . . . . 0.3375	
2.25 . . . . 0.1625		6 . . . . 0.35	
2.5 . . . . 0.175		6.25 . . . . . . 0.3625	
2.75 . . . . 0.1875		6.5 . . . . 0.375	
3 . . . . 0.2		6.75 . . . . . . 0.3875	
3.25 . . . . 0.2125		7 . . . . 0.4	
3.5 . . . . 0.225		7.25 . . . . . . 0.4125	
3.75 . . . . 0.2375		7.5 . . . . 0.425	
4 . . . . 0.25		7.75 . . . . . . 0.4375	

Newborn Metric
Conversion Tables

Length in inches (in.) to centimeters (cm)

1-in. increments. Example: To obtain centimeters equivalent to 22 in., read "20" on top scale, "2" on side scale; equivalent is 55.9 cm.

Inches	0	10	20	30	40
0	0	25.4	50.8	76.2	101.6
1	2.5	27.9	53.3	78.7	104.1
2	5.1	30.5	55.9	81.3	106.7
3	7.6	33.0	58.4	83.8	109.2
4	10.2	35.6	61.0	86.4	111.8
5	12.7	38.1	63.5	88.9	114.3
6	15.2	40.6	66.0	91.4	116.8
7	17.8	43.2	68.6	94.0	119.4
8	20.3	45.7	71.1	96.5	121.9
9	22.9	48.3	73.7	99.1	124.5

$1/4$-in. increments. Example: To obtain centimeters equivalent to $14\,3/4$ in., read "14" on top scale, "$3/4$" on side scale; equivalent is 37.5 cm.

Inches	10	11	12	13	14	15
0	25.4	27.9	30.5	33.0	35.6	38.1
1/4	26.0	28.6	31.1	33.7	36.2	38.7
1/2	26.7	29.2	31.8	34.3	36.8	39.4
3/4	27.3	29.8	32.4	34.9	37.5	40.0

Inches	16	17	18	19	20	21
0	40.6	43.2	45.7	48.3	50.8	53.3
1/4	41.3	43.8	46.4	48.9	51.4	54.0
1/2	41.9	44.5	47.0	49.5	52.1	54.6
3/4	42.5	45.1	47.6	50.2	52.7	55.2

Note: 1 in. = 2.540 cm. Centimeter equivalents are rounded one decimal place by adding 0.1 when second decimal place is 5 or greater; for example, 33.48 becomes 33.5.

Newborn Metric
Conversion Tables

Weight (mass) pounds (lb) and ounces (oz) to grams (g). Example: To obtain grams equivalent to 6 lb, 8 oz read "6" on top scale, "8" on side scale; equivalent is 2948 g.

	Pounds						
Oz	0	1	2	3	4	5	6
0	0	454	907	1361	1814	2268	2722
1	28	482	936	1389	1843	2296	2750
2	57	510	964	1417	1871	2325	2778
3	85	539	992	1446	1899	2353	2807
4	113	567	1021	1474	1928	2381	2835
5	142	595	1049	1503	1956	2410	2863
6	170	624	1077	1531	1984	2438	2892
7	198	652	1106	1559	2013	2466	2920
8	227	680	1134	1588	2041	2495	2948
9	255	709	1162	1616	2070	2523	2977
10	283	737	1191	1644	2098	2551	3005
11	312	765	1219	1673	2126	2580	3033
12	340	794	1247	1701	2155	2608	3062
13	369	822	1276	1729	2183	2637	3090
14	397	850	1304	1758	2211	2665	3118
15	425	879	1332	1786	2240	2693	3147

	Pounds						
Oz	7	8	9	10	11	12	13
0	3175	3629	4082	4536	4990	5443	5897
1	3203	3657	4111	4564	5018	5471	5925
2	3232	3685	4139	4593	5046	5500	5953
3	3260	3714	4167	4621	5075	5528	5982
4	3289	3742	4196	4649	5103	5557	6010
5	3317	3770	4224	4678	5131	5585	6038
6	3345	3799	4252	4706	5160	5613	6067
7	3374	3827	4281	4734	5188	5642	6095
8	3402	3856	4309	4763	5216	5670	6123
9	3430	3884	4337	4791	5245	5698	6152
10	3459	3912	4366	4819	5273	5727	6180
11	3487	3941	4394	4848	5301	5755	6209
12	3515	3969	4423	4876	5330	5783	6237
13	3544	3997	4451	4904	5358	5812	6265
14	3572	4026	4479	4933	5386	5840	6294
15	3600	4054	4508	4961	5415	5868	6322

Note: 1 lb = 453.59237 g; 1 oz = 28.349523 g; 1000 g = 1 kg. Gram equivalents have been rounded to whole numbers by adding 1 when the first decimal place is 5 or greater.

Index

Index

Index

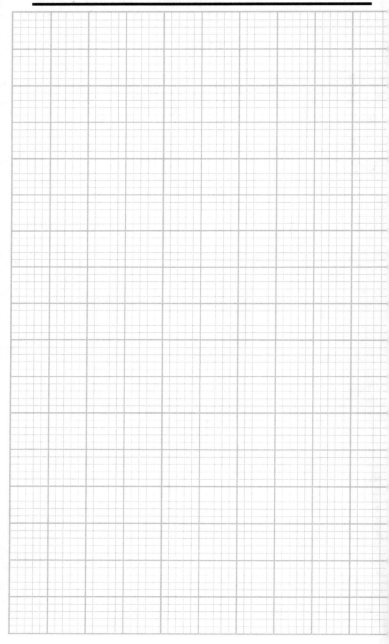

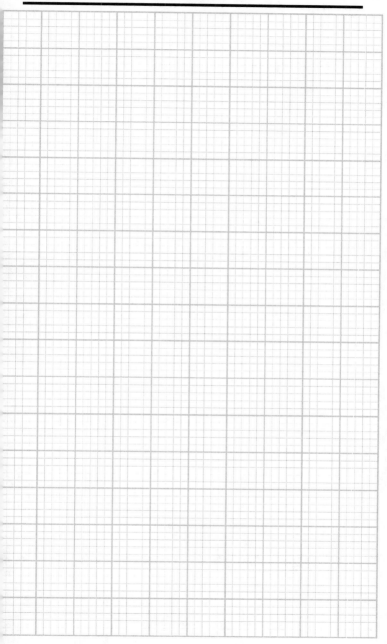

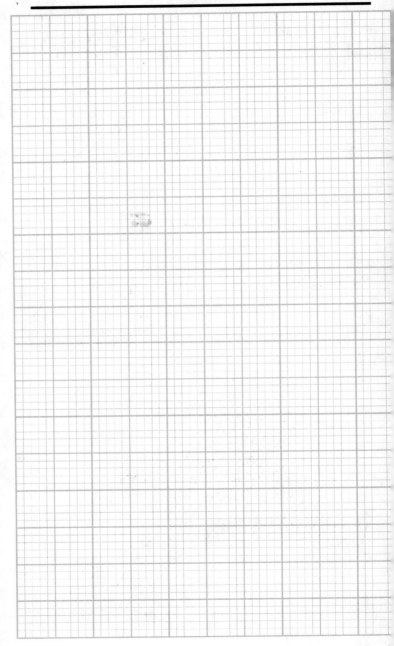